Lyme Borreliosis

Klaus-Peter Hunfeld • Jeremy Gray
Editors

Lyme Borreliosis

Springer

Editors
Klaus-Peter Hunfeld
Institute for Laboratory Medicine
Microbiology, and Infection Control
Northwest Medical Centre, Medical
Faculty, Goethe University
Frankfurt/Main, Hessen, Germany

Jeremy Gray
UCD School of Biology &
Environmental Science
University College Dublin
Belfield, Dublin, Ireland

ISBN 978-3-030-93679-2 ISBN 978-3-030-93680-8 (eBook)
https://doi.org/10.1007/978-3-030-93680-8

This Springer imprint is published by the registered company Springer Nature Switzerland AG
The registered company address is: Gewerbestrasse 11, 6330 Cham, Switzerland

Contents

Introduction

26.03.2022

Historically, tick-associated pathogens can be tracked back to the book of Exodus in the Hebrew Bible. The plague ("murrain") visited upon the cattle of Pharaoh Ramses II is probably the first historical reference to a disease transmitted by ticks [1]. It took until the late eighteenth century, however, to gather scientific evidence for the existence of tick-borne microorganisms and to attain a better understanding of the circumstances of transmission and the life cycles of such pathogens. In 1893, Smith and Kilbourne discovered that the causative agent of Texas cattle fever, now known as the protozoan *Babesia bigemina*, is transmitted by ticks and were the first to determine these arthropods as important vectors of pathogens [2]. McCalla and Brereton further substantiated the importance of ticks in the transmission of disease in 1908 in the USA. A tick from a patient with Rocky Mountain spotted fever was at that time used to transmit the infection to two healthy volunteers [3]. In 1909, Ricketts discovered the eponymous genus of bacteria responsible for Rocky Mountain spotted fever—*Rickettsia* [4]. Up to now, more than 50 tick-borne pathogens—parasites, bacteria and viruses—have been found to be of considerable concern to humans exposed to tick bites in Europe [5].

Today, Lyme borreliosis (LB)—an infectious disease caused by tick-borne spirochetes of the *Borrelia burgdorferi* sensu lato (s.l.) complex—is the most commonly reported vector-borne infection in the northern hemisphere [6, 7]. The geographical presence of the disease thereby follows a belt-like distribution and mirrors the distribution of ixodid ticks in this part of the world [6]. In central Europe, *Ixodes ricinus* is primarily known as the main vector of *B. burgdorferi* s.l. and tick-borne encephalitis (TBE) virus, which taken together are estimated to infect some 100,000 individuals per year. Moreover, studies based on polymerase chain reaction (PCR) and DNA sequence analyses have shown that tick-borne pathogens other than *B. burgdorferi* s.l., such as *Borrelia miyamotoi, Anaplasma phagocytophilum, Neoehrlichia mikurensis, Rickettsia* spp. and *Babesia* spp., are also widely prevalent in the three-host tick *I. ricinus*, whose larvae, nymphs, and adults feed on different hosts, including virtually any warm-blooded animal and humans [5, 8].

According to the Centers for Disease Control and Prevention (CDC), the incidence in the USA was 7.9/100,000 in 2014, with the majority of cases reported in the Northeastern and upper Midwestern States [9]. In the USA, 30,000–40,000 cases are reported annually through surveillance each year with an estimated

476,000 patients treated during 2010–2018 [7]. In Europe, incidence ranges of 0.001/100,000 in Italy (2001–2005) up to 188.7/100,000 in Slovenia (2014) have been published [8]. "Lyme disease", as it was called, emerged when Steere et al. [10] investigated an arthritis epidemic among young children in the community of Old Lyme, Connecticut, USA, in the late 1970s [10], but the infection was known to medicine in Europe much earlier.

Typical cutaneous manifestations are the most frequent signs of the disease and was described at the end of the nineteenth century and the beginning of the twentieth century by physicians such as Buchwald, Pick, Herxheimer, Hartman, Afzelius and Lipschütz [11]. Additionally, two French physicians, Garin and Bujadoux, in a landmark paper published in 1922, reported a patient who developed erythema chronicum migrans followed by painful meningoradiculitis [12]. This patient was reportedly bitten by a tick and had a positive Bordet-Wasserman test, which was used at that time to diagnose syphilis. Although the test was positive, the patient obviously did not have syphilis, and the authors concluded he had a tick-borne disease caused by a spirochete that induced cutaneous and neurological manifestations and was different from the causative agent of syphilis, *Treponema pallidum* [12]. The causative agent of LB, however, remained a mystery until the discovery of spirochetal bacteria in the midgut of ticks collected from Long Island, New York, in 1982 by the Swiss-borne entomologist Willy Burgdorfer [13]. The subsequent epidemiological and laboratory establishment of LB as a new multi-system infectious disease entity is one of the most important biomedical discoveries of the twentieth century [14]. In the years after the isolation of the causative bacterium, it was quickly shown that there were significant differences in disease expression between North America and Europe. Furthermore, it was established that in North America there was just one predominant pathogenic species of borrelia (*B. burgdorferi* sensu stricto) and one recently discovered minor one (*B. mayonii*), while there were at least four different pathogenic species in Europe [6]. The infection may occur without signs and symptoms, but in clinically apparent cases, typical symptoms associated with infection include erythema migrans (EM), neurological manifestations (e.g. polymeningoradiculoneuritis, also known as Bannwarth's syndrome), Lyme arthritis (LA) and acrodermatitis chronica atrophicans (ACA). Such manifestations, together with some other rare ones, had been well recognized in Europe years before the final discovery of the causative pathogen *B. burgdorferi* s.l. [11]. Over the last few decades, tremendous progress has been achieved in well-recognized treatment options [6]. Nevertheless, LB, like syphilis, can behave as a chameleon of clinical medicine for inexperienced clinicians, resulting in a cornucopia of problems, especially when it comes to direct and indirect laboratory diagnosis of the pathogen and consideration of the many potential differential diagnoses [15].

This is why we see an urgent need for a practical medical textbook for doctors and students devoted to all the different facets of the diagnosis and clinical management of Lyme borreliosis. In addition, special chapters cover differences in disease manifestations between Europe and North America, the pathogenicity of the pathogens, the life cycle and biology of the vectors, and also important tick-borne pathogens other than *B. burgdorferi* s.l. that are important for the differential diagnosis of tick-borne diseases in Europe. The contributors to this book are all internationally well-known specialists in the field of infectious diseases and tick-borne pathogens. We aim to provide a well-structured and practice-oriented presentation of clinical management, and laboratory diagnosis of LB, and other important tick-borne diseases in Europe. We also discuss the current pitfalls and limitations, as well as future prospects in this challenging and rapidly moving area of medicine.

Frankfurt/Main, Hessen, Germany Klaus-Peter Hunfeld
Belfield, Dublin, Ireland Jeremy Gray

References

1. Gelfand JA. Babesia. In: Mandell GL, Douglas RG, Bennett JE, Dolin R. editors. Mandell, Douglas, and Bennett's principles and practice of infectious diseases, 5th ed. Churchill Livingstone, New York; 2000, pp. 2899–2902.
2. Smith T, Kilbourne EL. Investigation into the nature, causation, and prevention of southern cattle fever. US Dept Agr Bur Anim Indust Bull 1893; 1.
3. Weiss E. History of rickettsiology. In Walker DH, editor. Biology of rickettsial diseases. CRC Press, Boca Raton; 1988, pp. 15–32.
4. Ricketts HT. Some aspects of Rocky Mountain spotted fever as shown by recent investigations. 1909. Rev Infect Dis 1991;13(6):1227-40. doi: 10.1093/clinids/13.6.1227. PMID: 1775857.
5. Kernif T, Leulmi H, Raoult D, Parola P. Emerging tick-borne bacterial pathogens. Microbiol Spectr 2016;4(3). doi: 10.1128/microbiolspec. EI10-0012-2016. PMID: 27337487.
6. Lohr B, Fingerle V, Norris DE, Hunfeld KP. Laboratory diagnosis of Lyme borreliosis: current state of the art and future perspectives. Crit Rev Clin Lab Sci 2018;55(4):219-245. doi: 10.1080/10408363.2018.1450353. Epub 2018 Apr 2. PMID: 29606016.
7. Kugeler KJ, Schwartz AM, Delorey MJ, Mead PS, Hinckley AF. Estimating the frequency of Lyme disease diagnoses, United States, 2010–2018. Emerg Infect Dis 2021;27(2):616-9. doi: 10.3201/eid2702.202731.
8. Azagi T, Hoornstra D, Kremer K, Hovius JWR, Sprong H. Evaluation of disease causality of rare *Ixodes ricinus*-borne infections in Europe. Pathogens 2020; 24;9(2):150. doi: 10.3390/pathogens9020150.
9. Nelson CA, Saha S, Kugeler KJ, et al. Incidence of clinician-diagnosed Lyme disease, United States, 2005–2010. Emerg Infect Dis. 2015;21:1625–1631.
10. Steere AC, Hardin JA, Malawista SE. Lyme arthritis: a new clinical entity. Hosp Pract. 1978;13(4):143-58. doi: 10.1080/21548331.1978.11707320. PMID: 658948.
11. Lipsker D and Jaulhac B. Preface. Curr Probl Dermatol 2009;37:167–177. doi: 10.1159/000213074. Epub 2009 Apr 8. PMID: 19367101.
12. Garin C, Bujadoux A. Paralysis by ticks. 1922. Clin Infect Dis. 1993;16(1):168–9. doi: 10.1093/clinids/16.1.168. PMID: 8448296.
13. Burgdorfer W, Barbour AG, Hayes SF, Péter O, Aeschlimann A. Erythema chronicum migrans--a tickborne spirochetosis. Acta Trop. 1983;40(1):79-83. PMID: 6134457.
14. Gern L, Aeschlimann A, Schwan T, et al. A tribute to Dr. Willy Burgdorfer, medical entomologist extraordinaire. Ticks Tick Borne Dis. 2016;7:66–7.
15. Santino I, Comite P, Gandolfo GM. Borrelia burgdorferi, a great chameleon: know it to recognize it! Neurol Sci. 2010;31:193–6.

Characteristics of *Borrelia burgdorferi* sensu lato

1

Gabriele Margos, Sabrina Hepner, and Volker Fingerle

1.1 Introduction

The microorganisms that can cause Lyme borreliosis in humans are spirochetal bacteria (Fig. 1.1) that comprise the *Borrelia burgdorferi* sensu lato (s.l.; Latin: in the broad sense) species complex. The bacteria live a parasitic lifestyle and are maintained in natural transmission cycles between tick vectors of the *Ixodes ricinus–persulcatus* species complex and small- to medium-sized vertebrate reservoir hosts [1–3].

It had been suspected since the beginning of the last century that tick-borne pathogens may cause symptoms that are now known as Lyme borreliosis (reviewed by [4]). However, it was not until the early 1980s that the causative agent was shown to be a spirochetal bacterium that utilizes ticks as vectors [5]. The bacterium was named *Borrelia burgdorferi* Johnson et al. 1984 [6]. Subsequent studies unraveled the genetic and ecological heterogeneity of borreliae in Europe, Asia, and North America and several new genospecies were named, e.g., *Borrelia garinii* Baranton et al. 1992 and *Borrelia afzelii* Baranton et al. 1992; (Table 1.1) [7–25]. Since then, the name *B. burgdorferi* s.l. has been used to refer to the species complex, while *B. burgdorferi* sensu stricto (s.s.; Latin: in the strict sense) refers to the species first discovered by W. Burgdorfer and colleagues [5, 6]. Today the species complex contains 23 named and proposed genospecies (Table 1.1). The species are non-uniformly distributed mainly between the northern 40° and 60° latitude (Fig. 1.3). This distribution reflects the presence of competent tick vector and reservoir host species [26].

G. Margos (✉) · S. Hepner · V. Fingerle
Bavarian Health and Food Safety Authority, German National Reference Centre for Borrelia, Oberschleissheim, Germany
e-mail: Gabriele.margos@lgl.bayern.de; Sabrina.hepner@lgl.bayern.de; volker.fingerle@lgl.bayern.de

K.-P. Hunfeld, J. Gray (eds.), *Lyme Borreliosis*,
https://doi.org/10.1007/978-3-030-93680-8_1

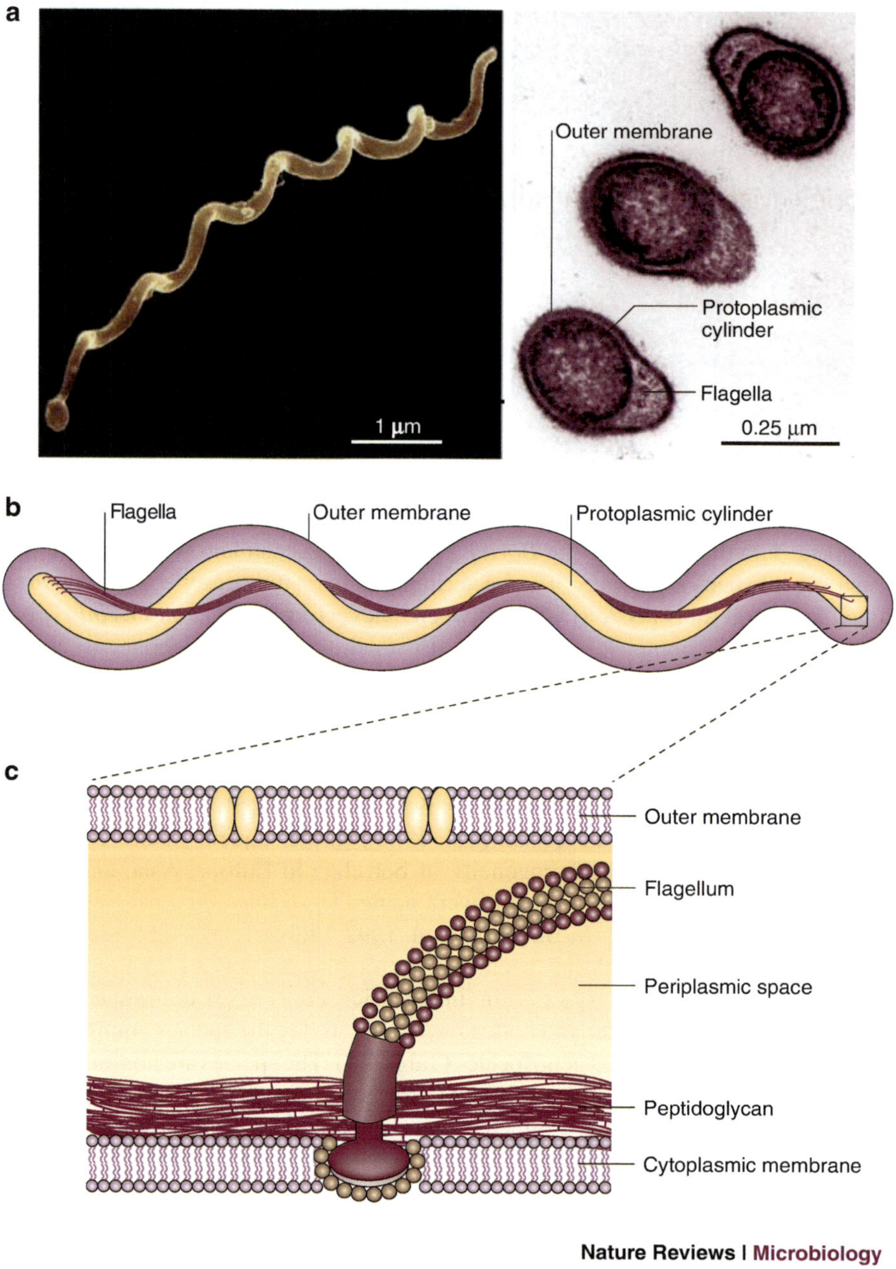

Fig. 1.1 Morphology of *Borrelia* (adapted from [54] with permission from Nature Reviews Microbiology). (**a**) light microscopy of *Borrelia* and schematic drawing of transection of a spirochete; (**b**) schematic representation of a spirochete showing the protoplasmic space with inserted flagella; (**c**) magnification from (**b**) of the insertion site of a flagellum into the cytoplasmic membrane

Table 1.1 The *Borrelia burgdorferi* sensu lato species complex

Borrelia species	Type strain	Reservoir hosts	Vector species	Distribution	Human pathogenicity
B. afzelii	VS461	Rodents, insectivores	*Ixodes ricinus, Ixodes persulcatus, Ixodes hexagonus*	Asia, Europe	Yes
B. americana	SCW-41	Birds, rodents	*Ixodes minor, Ixodes pacificus*	North America	Unknown
B. andersonii (p)	21,038	Birds, rabbits	*Ixodes dentatus*	North America	Unknown
B. bavariensis	PBi	Rodents	*Ixodes ricinus, Ixodes persulcatus*	Asia, Europe	Yes
B. bissettiae [a]	DN-127	Rodents	*Ixodes spinipalpis, Ixodes pacificus, Ixodes ricinus*	Europe, North America	Potentially
B. burgdorferi sensu stricto	B31	Birds, rodents, insectivores, carnivores	*Ixodes ricinus, Ixodes scapularis, Ixodes affinis, Ixodes pacificus, Ixodes minor, Ixodes hexagonus*	Europe, North America	Yes
B. californiensis	CA446	Rodents	*Ixodes pacificus, Ixodes spinipalpis, Ixodes jellisoni*	North America	Unknown
B. carolinensis	SCW-22	Rodents	*Ixodes minor*	North America	Unknown
B. chilensis (p)	VA1 (p)	Rodents	*Ixodes stilesi*	South America	Unknown
B. garinii	20047	Birds	*Ixodes ricinus, Ixodes persulcatus, Ixodes uriae* [b]	Asia, Europe	Yes
B. japonica	HO14	Rodents	*Ixodes ovatus*	Asia	Unknown
B. kurtenbachii	25015	Rodents	?	North America	Potentially
B. lanei	CA28–91	Lagomorphs?	*Ixodes spinipalpis, Ixodes pacificus*	North America	Unknown
B. lusitaniae	PoTiB2	Lizards	*Ixodes ricinus*	Europe	Potentially
B. maritima	CA690	?	?	North America	Unknown
B. mayonii	M14–1420	Rodents?	*Ixodes scapularis*	North America	Yes

(continued)

Table 1.1 (continued)

Borrelia species	Type strain	Reservoir hosts	Vector species	Distribution	Human pathogenicity
B. sinica	CMN3	Rodents	*Ixodes ovatus*	Asia	Unknown
B. spielmanii	PC-Eq17	Rodents	*Ixodes ricinus, Ixodes hexagonus*	Europe	Yes
B. tanukii	Hk501	Rodents	*Ixodes tanuki*	Asia	Unknown
B. turdi	Ya501	Birds	*Ixodes turdus, Ixodes frontalis, Ixodes ricinus*	Asia, Europe	Unknown
B. valaisiana	VS116	Birds	*Ixodes ricinus*	Europe	No
B. yangtzensis	Okinawa CW62	Rodents	*Ixodes granulatus*	Asia	Potentially
Candidatus B. aligera	NA	Birds?	?	Europe	Unknown

(p) proposed, *a* formerly *B. bissettii, b* also in sea bird colonies in Canada, *NA* not applicable

1.2 *Borrelia* Genomics and Cell Biology

Genomics. The first genome of Lyme borreliosis group spirochete to be completely sequenced was that of *B. burgdorferi* s.s. isolate B31 [27]. The genome turned out to be unusual for bacteria: it consisted of a large linear chromosome of about 910 kbp and of 12 linear and 9 circular plasmids which make up another 600 kbp of DNA sequence, a substantial contribution to the total genome of *B. burgdorferi* s.s. [27–29]. The genomic structure, i.e., consisting of a linear chromosome and circular as well as linear plasmids, was found to be maintained in all species investigated so far [19, 24, 30–33]. In B31, the main chromosome contains 820 open reading frames (803 protein-coding sequences, 17 pseudogenes; 5 rRNA, 32 tRNA, 3 ncRNA), 10% of which match hypothetical proteins and 29% have no match in a database. The G + C content of the chromosome is around 28% [27, 34]. The plasmids in B31 range in size from 5 to 60 kbp, contain additional 700 coding sequences of which >90% have no convincing database match outside the genus *Borrelia* [27, 28]. Main chromosome and linear plasmids are terminated by covalently closed hairpin structures [35–37] which are created involving a telomere resolvase, ResT, an enzyme encoded on plasmid cp26 [38, 39]. Plasmids may be lost under *in vitro* culture conditions [40–43], but they are essential for completion of the complex *B. burgdorferi* s.l. life cycle in nature [44, 45].

Initially, plasmids have been named according to whether they are linear or circular and according to size, e.g., lp54 for a 54 kbp linear plasmids, cp26 for a 26 kbp circular plasmid [28]. However, since several plasmids of similar size have been found in a single isolate, and size differences of the same plasmid have been noticed in different isolates, recently plasmids are typed according to their PFam32 locus, which supposedly is homologous to plasmid partitioning protein (ParA) encoding sequences in other bacteria [29]. Apart from PFam32, related loci (PFam49, PFam52, PFam57/60) may be involved in autonomous plasmid replication and maintenance but their function is yet to be confirmed [39, 46].

Perhaps as a result of the parasitic lifestyle, *B. burgdorferi* s.l. has very few genes for biosynthesis of cell constituents [27]. The majority of chromosomal genes encode proteins for housekeeping and metabolic functions, while many of the genes encoding outer surface proteins required for interaction with host or vector are located on plasmids. Analyses of plasmid sequences showed that there have been extensive rearrangements, and plasmid numbers and structures vary not only between genospecies but also between strains of a single species [29, 30, 46, 47]. Plasmids of the cp32 family have been shown to contain prophages, perhaps facilitating rearrangements and/or exchange of genetic material [46, 48, 49]. Information on *B. burgdorferi* s.l. genome content and structure has been largely gained from strains of the genospecies *B. burgdorferi* s.s. [29, 47, 50]. Although for other *Borrelia* genospecies genomes have been sequenced, the whole complement of plasmids has not been completed for all of them [30, 32, 33, 46, 51], (http://BorreliaBase.org).

Cell biology. Borreliae are helical bacteria. Their size is 0.2–0.3 μm wide and 10–30 μm long. *Borrelia* are not gram-negative, they lack the lipopolysaccharide (LPS) and the protein richness that are typical for the cell surface membrane of gram-negative bacteria [52, 53]. Instead, they have a diderm cell envelope consisting of an outer surface membrane separated by a periplasmic space from the cytoplasmic membrane, which is covered by a peptidoglycan layer. Usually 7–11 flagella are inserted near the end of the protoplasmic cylinder of the cell extending into the periplasmic space (Fig. 1.1) [54]. These endoflagella give the bacteria a unique form of motility permitting them to move in viscous media. They can flex and bend, propel themselves forwards and backwards and rotate (non-translational mode of motility) [55, 56] and this motility is crucial for host/vector infection [57].

Inserted in the outer surface membrane via lipid moieties are outer surface membrane proteins (Osps); >150 potential Osps have been identified [27]. They have been named alphabetically in order of their identification, e.g., OspA, OspB, OspC, etc. Many of these proteins have functions in the interaction of the bacteria with their environment (host or vector). Table 1.2 provides a non-exhaustive list.

Apart from these Osps, there are outer membrane proteins (OMPs) that are integral membrane proteins and may serve as transporters for nutrients or other essential molecules that borreliae take up from the host environment. Freeze fracture electron microscopy has shown that the outer membrane contains relatively few transmembrane proteins [53]. These studies also provided evidence that blebs, surrounded by a membrane(s) resembling the outer membrane and/or the cytoplasmic membrane, are shed from *Borrelia* cells suggesting that blebs are pinched off sections of the cells.

Many other outer membrane and internal proteins are important for the life cycle of *B. burgdorferi* s.l. and intensive research efforts are being made to understand their function and role in the life cycle of these bacteria (e.g., [44, 58–60]).

Table 1.2 A non-exhaustive list of outer surface proteins and transmembrane proteins of *B. burgdorferi* s.l.

Protein name		Gene designation B31	Proposed biological role	Size
Outer surface proteins (Osp)				
OspA/ OspB	Outer surface protein A/B	BB_A15/ BB_A16	Interaction with tick receptor TROSPA	31 kDa/34 kDa
OspC	Outer surface protein C	BB_B19	Early infection of vertebrate host	22 kDa
OspD	Outer surface protein D		Unknown, potentially adherence to the tick midgut	28 kDa
BptA	Borrelial persistence in ticks A	BBE16		
P35		BBA64	Unknown, tick-to-host transmission or vertebrate infection	35 kDa
DbpA/ DbpB	Decorin-binding protein A/B	BBA24/BBA25	Interaction with collagen fibers; decorin binding	18 kDa/17 kDa
BBK32		BBK32	Binding to fibronectin	47 kDa
OspF	Outer surface protein F protein family	BBM38/ BBO39/ BBR42	Unknown, potential adhesin	29 kDa/26 kDa /25 kDa
VLsE	Variable major protein-like sequence expressed	BB_F0041	Immune evasion	35 kDa
OspE	Outer surface protein E protein family	BBL39/ BBN38, (BBP38 identical to BBL39)	Evasion of complement lysis (CRASP)	
ErpG, ErpL, ErpX, ErpY	OspE-related proteins		Complement evasion?	
CspA	CRASP-1	BBA68	Evasion of complement lysis	27 kDa
CspZ	CRASP-2	BBH06	Evasion of complement lysis	27 kDa
BBA36		BBA36	Unknown	
BBA65		BBA65	Unknown	
BBA66		BBA66	Unknown	
BBA69		BBA69	Unknown	
BBA71		BBA71	Unknown	
BBA73		BBA73	Unknown	

Table 1.2 (continued)

Protein name		Gene designation B31	Proposed biological role	Size
BBI42		BBI42	Unknown	
Integral outer membrane proteins (OMP)				
P66		BB0603	Putative porin	66 kDa
P13		BB0034	Putative porin	13 kDa
Lmp1	Surface-located membrane protein 1	BB0210	Protection from host adaptive immunity	128 kDa
BesA/ BesB/ BesC	*Borrelia* efflux system proteins A, B, C	Bb0141/ Bb0140/ Bb0142	Putative bacterial resistance-nodulation-division (RND)-type multidrug-efflux system	
BamA	β-Barrel assembly machine protein	bb0795	β-Barrel assembly machine	94 kDa
BB0405		BB0405	Unknown	22 kDa
Bgp	*Borrelia* glycosaminoglycan-binding protein	bb0588	Glycosaminoglycan (GAG)-binding protein; cell adhesion	

1.3 The *Borrelia burgdorferi* Sensu Lato Species Complex

The phylum Spirochaetes Cavalier-Smith 2002 comprises a group of helically shaped bacteria, several of which cause human diseases such as *Leptospira, Treponema, Brachyspira,* and *Borrelia*. The genus *Borrelia* contains the relapsing fever group of spirochetes (e.g., *Borrelia recurrentis* causing louse-borne human relapsing fever and several species causing tick-borne relapsing fever), the Lyme borreliosis group of spirochetes (*B. burgdorferi* s.l. complex), and a group of reptile- and echidna-associated spirochetes [61–64]. In 2014, based on investigations on conserved signature proteins (CSP), conserved signature insertions/deletions (indels) (CSI), and average nucleotide identity (ANI), the genus was divided into two genera: *Borrelia* containing the relapsing fever species and *Borreliella* for the Lyme borreliosis species [65]. The third clade, reptile- and echidna-associated species were not considered. Using different methodology of genus delimitation, namely the percentage of conserved proteins (PCOP) [66], recently all groups were reunited in the genus *Borrelia* [62]. This work also showed that reptile- and echidna-associated species do not genetically resemble relapsing fever species but take a somewhat intermediate position between relapsing fever and Lyme borreliosis spirochetes [64].

The *B. burgdorferi* s.l. species complex currently consists of 23 named species (Table 1.1), six of which are assured human pathogens. Five of the species pathogenic to humans occur in Europe including *B. afzelii*, *Borrelia bavariensis* Margos et al. 2013, *B. burgdorferi* s.s., *B. garinii*, and *Borrelia spielmanii* Richter et al. 2006 [67, 68]. *Borrelia afzelii*, *B. bavariensis,* and *B. garinii* also occur in Eastern Europe and Asia [69–71].

In North America, two species are the cause of human Lyme disease, these are *B. burgdorferi* s.s. and *Borrelia mayonii* Pritt et al. 2016 [72–75]. The latter species was only discovered in 2016 in patients visiting the Mayo Clinic in Wisconsin [73]. Since then more symptomatic patients have been found to be infected with *B. mayonii* [72].

Two additional species have been discussed as putative human pathogens; these are *Borrelia lusitaniae* Le Fleche et al. 1997 and *Borrelia bissettiae* Margos et al. 2016. *Borrelia lusitaniae* can be commonly found in questing ticks in countries neighboring the Mediterranean Sea [76–81], and so far two cases have been described in the literature incriminating *B. lusitaniae* as a suspected human pathogen [82, 83]. On the other hand, *B. bissettiae* has rarely been found in questing ticks in Europe [84–86]. So far one human case (where an isolate was obtained) of *B. bissettiae* causing symptoms resembling mild neuroborreliosis has been described [11, 67]. In North America where *B. bissettiae* can be commonly found at a regional scale and in certain habitat types [87–91], no patient isolates have been obtained from humans although *B. bissettiae* DNA was recovered from serum [92]. *Borrelia valaisiana* Wang et al. 1997, has been asserted to be nonpathogenic for humans [93]. This *Borrelia* species is transmitted by *Ixodes ricinus* Linnaeus 1758, the main vector of human pathogenic *Borrelia* species in Europe (reviewed by [94, 95], see chapter "Pathogenesis and Immune Defense"), it utilizes avian reservoir hosts and is being found as frequently as *B. garinii* in certain regions [96]. Although it is found commonly in ticks, to date not a single human isolate of *B. valaisiana* has been acquired [93]. For the remaining species shown in Table 1.1, the human pathogenic potential is unknown. Many of these species are transmitted by ticks that do not bite humans, which may explain why these spirochetes have not emerged as pathogens, although their lack of human pathogenicity may be because of their genetic makeup.

1.4 Ecology and Transmission Cycles

As the geographical distribution of the different *Borrelia* species depends on vector and host associations (putatively also their pathogenic potential), it may be worth to briefly consider the biology of ticks and hosts, both of which will be discussed in more detail in chapter "Tick ecology and the eco-epidemiology of *Borrelia burgdorferi* sensu lato" in this book.

Only hard ticks of the genus *Ixodes* serve as vectors for *B. burgdorferi* s.l. (reviewed by [71, 94, 95, 97, 98]. *Ixodes* ticks have three life stages that require a blood meal from a host: larvae, nymphs, and adult females. In between blood meals, the ticks drop off the host, digest the blood meal, and molt into the next developmental stage in the undergrowth or leaf litter of their habitats. Ticks with a generalist feeding behavior serve as bridge vectors for agents of human Lyme borreliosis. The most important vectors for *B. burgdorferi* s.l. include *I. pacificus* (west of the Rocky Mountains) and *I. scapularis* (east of Rocky Mountains, Northeast, Midwest and Southeast USA, and Canada) in North America, *I. ricinus* in Europe, and *I. persulcatus* in Eastern Europe and Asia [99]. Host-specific or nidicolous ticks such as *I. uriae* [100], *I. hexagonus* [101], *I. frontalis* [102, 103], or *I. spinipalpis* [104], have more or less strong host preferences and are thus less prone to bite (and therefore only rarely transmit *Borrelia* to) humans. However, these specialist ticks in many cases use identical hosts to more generalist vectors (such as *I. ricinus*, *I. scapularis*, *I. pacificus*, and *I. persulcatus*); in this way, a potential connection arises between *Borrelia* transmission cycles of nonhuman-biting and human-biting ticks [105].

Ticks are armed with a cocktail of components that deflect adverse reactions by the host to the attached tick [106–110]. Microorganisms that utilize ticks as vectors can use tick salivary molecules to their own advantage during transmission, e.g., not being recognized by the host's immune system (reviewed by [110–113]). This phenomenon has been termed saliva-assisted transmission or SAT [114]. Nevertheless, some natural hosts are able to develop immune responses toward ticks leading to premature detachment of the feeding tick [115] and that can have an effect on pathogen transmission (see section *Reservoir hosts*).

Tick immunity to pathogens. In recent years, progress has been made in recognizing the complexity of the tick's immune system (reviewed in [113, 116–118]). *Ixodes* possess a number of immune effectors and modulators such as recognition molecules that serve as lectins labeling foreign cells for immune attack, phagocytotic hemocytes, antimicrobial peptides, lysozymes, defensins, and a dityrosine network (DTN) [119]. Signaling pathways such as Toll, an atypical IMD (Immunodeficiency), and JAK-STAT (Janus Kinase/Signal Transducers and Activators of Transcription) regulate the immune system and, interestingly, ticks also possess an indirect, cross-species signaling pathway that recognizes the cytokine interferon gamma in the blood of the host [113, 116, 120–122]. The tick's immune system may even be exploited by *Borrelia* as RNA interference studies of genes involved in the tick's immune response have shown that depletion of expression may lead to suppression of *Borrelia* colonization in ticks [123]. Furthermore, induction of a protein of *I. scapularis* with a Reeler domain (PIXR) by *Borrelia* limits bacterial biofilm formation in the tick's gut, thereby preventing alterations in the microbiome and promoting colonization by *Borrelia* [123]. Thus, it is likely that immune effectors play an important role in determining the competence of *Ixodes* species for *Borrelia* species and/or *vice versa*.

The microbiome of ticks. In the past decade, efforts have been devoted to study the tick's microbiome in detail. Using high-throughput sequencing methods, initial studies on different *Ixodes* species (e.g., *I. scapularis, I. ricinus, I. pacificus,* and *I. persulcatus*) discovered a whole range of bacterial taxa associated with ticks. It showed that the microbiome of ticks consists of microorganisms associated with the outer surface of ticks, the gut, and endosymbiotic bacteria (reviewed by [124]). Bacterial genera that were found constituted known tick symbionts like *Arsenophonus*, *Cardinium*, *Coxiella*, *Francisella*, *Lariskella*, *Midichloria*,

Rickettsia, *Rickettsiella*, *Spiroplasma*, and *Wolbachia* [125–131]. A more recent study used dissected tick tissues of questing *I. scapularis* to determine the "internal" microbiome and the "surface" microbiome. The authors found that in the majority of adults the gut microbiome of *I. scapularis* was limited in diversity [132]. The dominating bacteria were *Rickettsia* and *B. burgdorferi*. Only a minority of samples showed a high microbiome diversity with bacteria of the genera *Bacillus* and *Pseudomonas*, and the family Enterobacteriaceae in their midguts [132]. It remains to be investigated what impact the different "layers" of the microbiome have on the tick itself and the microorganisms it transmits.

Reservoir hosts (see also chapter "Pathogenesis and Immune Defense"). More than 100 vertebrate species can serve as host for generalist *Ixodes* ticks such as *I. ricinus*. Most of these species belong to the orders Rodentia, Eulipotyphla (formerly part of the Insectivores), Carnivores, Lagomorphs, as well as the classes Aves (here mostly Passeriformes and sea birds) and Reptiles. A fraction of these tick hosts can serve as hosts for *Borrelia*, among them various species of mice (genera *Apodemus*, *Peromyscus*, *Neotoma*), voles (genus *Myodes*, *Microtus*), shrews (genera *Sorex*, *Blarina*), squirrels (*Tamias, Sciurus*), lizards, and ground-feeding passerine birds (genera *Turdus*, *Parus*) (e.g., [25, 71, 78, 88, 133–147]).

However, experimental studies have shown that not all hosts that become infected with *Borrelia* species also serve as reservoirs (e.g., [147–149]. Complement sensitivity or resistance matches the reservoir host association of *Borrelia* species well, with *B. garinii* surviving bird complement but lysed by rodent complement, while rodent-associated species such as *B. afzelii* survive rodent complement but are lysed by bird complement. Complement-active deer serum lysed all tested *Borrelia* species suggesting that deer are nonpermissive as hosts for *Borrelia* [150–152]. The expression "host association" has been used to refer to "true" reservoir hosts of *Borrelia* as defined by Kahl and co-authors and Martin and co-authors [153, 154], i.e., only those hosts are considered reservoir competent that are able to acquire the bacteria from a competent vector tick and (critically) also to transmit it back to new vector ticks [1, 155]. The term "host association" was used instead of "host specialization" because *Borrelia* spirochetes are not "specialized" to infect *only* their reservoir hosts, as may be the case for other directly transmitted or vector-borne infectious agents, e.g., [148].

The development of resistance to tick bites by a host may reduce the ability to transmit tick-borne pathogens to vector ticks [109, 156, 157]. One such example is the bank vole, *Myodes glareolus*. In comparison to the wood mouse, *Apodemus sylvaticus*, repeated exposure of *M. glareolus* to tick bites reduced the engorgement time and weight of ticks making them drop-off the host prematurely (i.e., before complete engorgement) [115]. Reduction of engorgement time limits the transmission of tick-borne pathogens [158–161].

Some studies have suggested that hosts, once infected with *Borrelia*, carry the infection lifelong [162]. However, experimental transmission studies using different isolates of *B. burgdorferi* s.s. have shown that the duration of infection may differ between strains of *Borrelia* [163, 164].

1.4.1 Infection of Ticks by *Borrelia burgdorferi* s.l.

Infection of ticks by Borrelia burgdorferi s.l. Borreliae are taken up by the tick during the blood meal although the transmission efficiency may be variable depending on tick species, *Borrelia* species, or concomitant infections [161, 165–172]. The tick may feed for 16–48 h before the bacterium enters the tick gut [160, 173]. In the tick gut, the bacteria adhere to midgut cells via outer surface proteins. It has been suggested that OspA interacts with a tick midgut protein that was named tick receptor for OspA (TROSPA) [118, 174]. Upon entering the tick midgut, during blood meal digestion, molting, and questing periods, the bacteria remain adhered to the midgut. When the tick takes the next blood meal, changes in environmental conditions and the provided nutrients prompt the bacteria to divide and migrate through the midgut into the hemocoel and the salivary glands [175]. This is accompanied by changes in patterns of protein expression [45] due to regulatory factors responding to environmental cues, e.g., temperature and other physiological changes (reviewed by [3, 176]) (Fig. 1.2).

Although some studies have suggested that *B. burgdorferi* s.l. may create a biofilm in vitro and in vivo [189, 190], biofilm production seems not to be required in the ticks' midgut for spirochete colonization [123]. The spirochetes induce the expression of a tick protein of *I. scapularis* with a Reeler domain (PIXR), which prevents biofilm formation and appears to inhibit changes in the gut microbiome, supposedly giving *Borrelia* an advantage during the tick phase of their development [123].

When characterization of the first genome of *Borrelia* isolate B31 was completed, it was quite astonishing to find that many of the genes encoded hypothetical proteins with unknown functions and no match in databases [27, 28]. In spite of intensive research efforts, the genetic basis for the host- or vector association is still not clear [3, 26, 98, 130, 187]. In contrast to other human pathogenic bacteria, *B. burgdorferi* s.l. lack pathogenicity islands or virulence factors and although several proteins have been identified as virulence determinants, which factor exactly trigger human pathogenicity is currently still unknown (reviewed by [191, 192]).

1.5 Geographic Ranges of the Lyme Borreliosis Spirochetes

The interplay between competent vector ticks and reservoir hosts, their ecology, and migration pattern determines the geographic distribution of LB species (Fig. 1.3). The geographic ranges of the various *B. burgdorferi* s. l. species [193] are in each case limited to those locations in which both reservoir hosts and vector ticks are able to maintain natural transmission cycles [1, 2, 155, 194] (Fig. 1.3). Thus, one should be able to define the fundamental niche of each *Borrelia* species simply by taking account of where its vectors and hosts occur. However, many *B. burgdorferi* s.l. species can utilize multiple vertebrate host species and a number can utilize more than one vector. In addition, ecological associations between borreliae, ticks, and

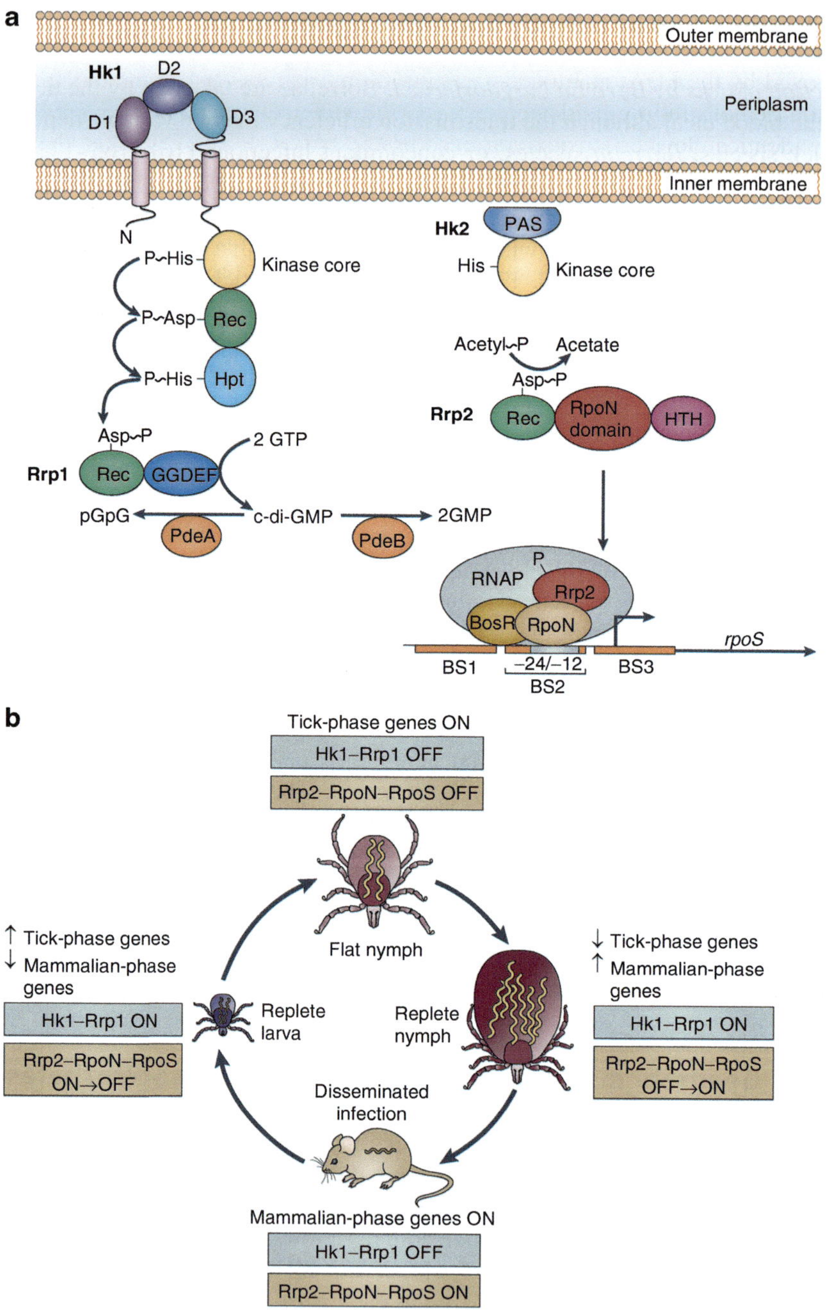

Nature Reviews | Microbiology

reservoir hosts are not all equivalent in strength, thus, the realized niche actually occupied by each *B. burgdorferi* s.l. species is likely to be less than its fundamental niche [26, 155]. The actual spatial limitation for each spirochete species (i.e., its realized niche) will be roughly equivalent to the sum of all those areas in which both at least one vector species and one host species occur at sufficiently high density to maintain its transmission cycle. The basic reproduction number R_0 presents a quantification of the biological framework and efficiency of the transmission cycle and its value can serve as a measure for population fitness [195]. For every local population of the bacterium, the value of R_0, summed over all its hosts and vectors, must be >1 for transmission cycles to be sustained [155, 196, 197]. As the presence of less efficient vectors and hosts will impact negatively on the value of R_0 achieved by the "best" vectors and hosts, one cannot simply add up values of R_0 that have been determined for each vector and each host under laboratory conditions [195, 198]. The effects caused by nonpermissive vectors and/or hosts are very important to consider as they can influence the success of the bacterium in entirely opposite ways

Fig. 1.2 Regulation of gene expression in *Borrelia burgdorferi* sensu lato (modified from [3] with permission from Nature Reviews Microbiology, and with special thanks to Melissa Caimano). (**a**) The histidine kinase 1 (Hk1)–response regulatory protein 1 (Rrp1) and alternative RNA polymerase σ-factor RpoS global regulatory systems. Binding of ligands to the periplasmic sensor domains (D1, D2, and D3) of the hybrid histidine kinase Hk1 initiates the activation of the diguanylyl cyclase activity of Rrp1, resulting in the production of cyclic di-GMP (c-di-GMP) [177–179]. Phosphodiesterase A (PdeA) and PdeB degrade c-di-GMP to 5′-phosphoguanylyl-(3′–5′)-guanosine (pGpG) and GMP, respectively [180, 181]. Activation of Rrp2 *in vitro* and *in vivo* occurs via the high-energy phosphoryl donor acetyl-phosphate rather than by its presumptive cognate histidine kinase, Hk2 [182]. The function of Hk2 is currently unknown. Phosphorylated Rrp2, *Borrelia* oxidative stress regulator (BosR), and RpoN initiate transcription of *rpoS* ([183, 184] and references therein). This is depicted as a trimeric complex, but the precise interactions between these proteins have yet to be determined. Putative BosR-binding sites (BSs) containing the direct repeat sequence TAAATTAAAT are shown; −24/−12 is the RpoN-binding site in the *rpoS* promoter [185]. RpoS in turn induces the expression of genes that are required during the mammalian-host phase of the spirochaete life cycle and represses the expression of tick-phase genes. (**b**) Expression of the Hk1–Rrp1 and RpoS global regulatory systems during the *B. burgdorferi* life cycle [177–179, 183, 184, 186]. In the flat nymph, both the Hk1–Rrp1 and the Rrp2–RpoN–RpoS systems are inactive and only tick-phase genes are expressed. The nymphal blood meal activates both the Hk1-Rrp1 and Rrp2–RpoN–RpoS pathways. Expression of mammalian phase genes begins in concert with downregulation of tick-phase genes. Following inoculation into a mammalian host, the spirochaetes complete the process of adaptation; the Hk1–Rrp1 pathway is inactive, the Rrp2–RpoN–RpoS pathway is active, mammalian phase genes are expressed, and tick-phase genes are repressed. During larval acquisition of spirochaetes, Hk1–Rrp1 is activated, probably at the feeding site, whereas the Rrp2–RpoN–RpoS system is inactivated. Mammalian-phase genes are repressed, expression of tick-phase genes begins, and ingested spirochaetes bind to the larval midgut epithelium via OspA and possibly other receptors [186–188]. GGDEF, a conserved motif present in diguanylyl cyclases; Hpt, histidine-containing phosphotransfer domain; HTH, helix–turn–helix domain; N, amino; PAS, putative sensor domain for Hk2; Rec, receiver domain

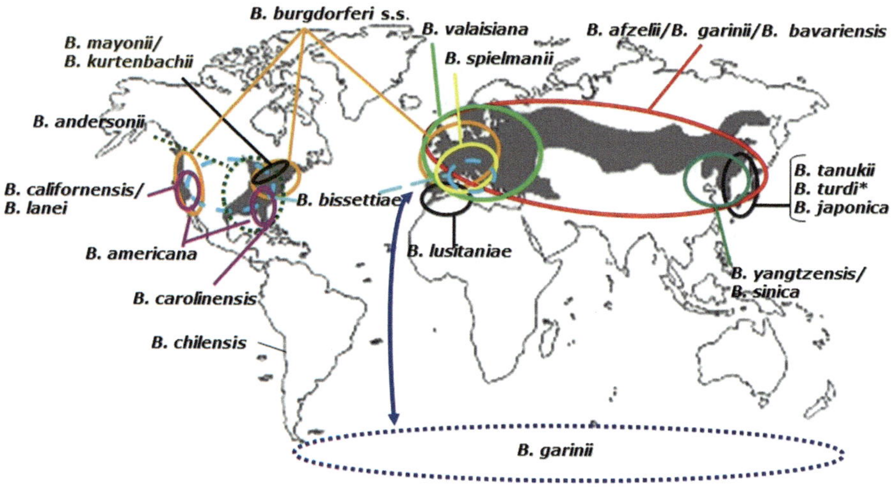

Fig. 1.3 Global distribution of *B. burgdorferi* sensu lato (from [26]). *In recent years, *B. turdi* has also been found in Europe in enzootic cycles driven by *I. frontalis* and passerine bird species [145]. For sake of clarity this is not indicated in the figure

[194]. For example, some potential mammalian hosts (e.g., large animals such as deer) may be colonized by *B. burgdorferi* s.l. spirochetes when bitten by an infected tick vector. They are, however, nonpermissive when it comes to transmission of the bacteria to a new tick and feeding on a deer may actually clear a *B. burgdorferi* s.l. infection in a tick [150, 199]. Following this, the presence of large numbers of deer may actually suppress the spirochete infection rate of true reservoir hosts in that location because ticks are more likely to feed on deer than on small mammals. On the other hand, the presence of deer in a particular geographic region may permit the population density of vector ticks to rise, which would increase the likelihood of successful transmission of spirochetes from infected reservoir hosts to ticks and thus increase R_0 [200–203].

The nonuniform distribution pattern of *Borrelia* genospecies observed in field studies suggests that apart from host associations, vector associations do indeed play an important role in limiting their geographic distribution ranges [193]. Some *Borrelia* species are able to utilize a wide range of vectors [71, 204], for example, *B. burgdorferi* s.s. are able to utilize *I. scapularis, I. pacificus, I. spinipalpis,* and *I. affinis* as vector in North America, as well as *I. ricinus* in Europe but they have not been found in *I. persulcatus* [69, 138]. *Borrelia garinii* can be vectored by *I. persulcatus, I. pavlovskyi, I. ricinus*, and *I. uriae*. Consequently, *B. garinii*'s geographic distribution ranges from France to Japan and it can be found in sea bird colonies in the Northern and Southern Hemisphere. *Borrelia garinii* has been found in sea bird colonies in Newfoundland [205] but it has not been discovered in North America in *I. scapularis* dominated regions or in *I. pacificus* [90, 206–209]. *Borrelia valaisiana*, also a bird-adapted *Borrelia* species, is frequently found in Europe associated with *I. ricinus* but only a single occurrence in Russia has been recorded [210] suggesting that *I. persulcatus* is not a competent vector. Accordingly, in the overlapping zone of *I. ricinus* and *I. persulcatus* in Eastern Europe, the prevalence of *B. valaisiana* is higher in *I. ricinus* than in *I. persulcatus* [211].

A particular interesting case showing that differential vector adaptation plays an essential role in the geographic distribution of *Borrelia* species is that of *B. bavariensis* [13]. The *B. bavariensis* population in Western Europe differs genetically from that in Eastern Europe and Asia and they form sister clades in phylogenies not only based on MLST housekeeping genes but also based on >100 single-copy genes [212]. In addition, the Eastern population of *B. bavariensis* appears to be present only in regions where *I. persulcatus* serves as vector and it shows much higher genetic diversity than the populations in Western Europe. The population that is adapted to *I. ricinus* (Western Europe) shows very little genetic heterogeneity and appears almost clonal suggesting that this population arose recently via a vector switch [13, 26, 32].

1.6 Molecular Typing of *B. burgdorferi* s.l.

Because species of the genus *Borrelia* are difficult to distinguish by morphological criteria, approaches that can accurately identify species and strains within species are critical for epidemiological, clinical, and evolutionary studies. Early tools to discriminate between different *Borrelia* species included DNA-DNA hybridization, ribotyping, DNA sequencing of 16S rRNA or other conserved genes, PCR-based restriction fragment length polymorphism (RFLP) analysis, random amplified polymorphic DNA (RAPD) fingerprinting, or pulsed-field gel electrophoresis (RFLP) [213]. Single loci such as the outer surface proteins A (OspA), outer surface protein C (OspC), the intergenic spacer (IGS) region between the duplicated 5S and 23S rRNA [214], the 23S rRNA locus or flagellin (*flaB*) have been used for species and strain discrimination and are still popular targets for diagnostic purposes, e.g., [7, 23, 89, 215–223]. These targets have been used either individually or in combination for molecular characterization of *B. burgdorferi* s.l. from cultured isolates or directly on clinical samples, samples from mammalian hosts or ticks.

Since 2006/2007 multilocus sequence analysis (MLSA) has replaced DNA–DNA hybridization for species delimitation, epidemiological studies, or strain identification in *B. burgdorferi* s.l. and various multilocus sequence typing (MLST) schemes have been proposed (e.g., [14, 16, 224–227]). Not all of them use exclusively housekeeping genes as originally proposed for bacterial epidemiology and population-level studies [228, 229]. The system currently maintained at the Pubmlst database (http://pubmlst.org/borrelia/) at the University of Oxford [230] uses eight housekeeping loci that are encoded on the main chromosome; these are *clpA, clpX, nifS, pepX, pyrG, recG, rplB,* and *uvrA* [224, 225]. This MLST scheme has been shown to have great potential not only for *Borrelia* species discrimination [10–13, 15, 19, 24, 73, 90] but also for dissecting relationships of bacterial populations [25, 69, 70, 81, 205, 208, 209, 231–237].

In recent years, next-generation sequencing methods giving additional power for species and isolate determination have been explored for *Borrelia* typing and draft genome assembly, population genetics studies, improvement of MLST sequencing, or investigation of pathogenicity [31–33, 72, 238–240]. Currently various technologies for next-generation sequencing are available, the most popular are Illumina Sequencing, Pacific Biosciences single-molecule real-time (SMRT), and Oxford Nanopore technologie (ONT). While Illumina provides highly accurate consensus contigs, long read methods (SMRT, ONT) vastly improve genome assemblies, and hybrid assemblies of both, accurate short and long reads, have been shown to give best results for assembly of *Borrelia* genomes [24, 46, 61, 240, 241]. In future, such methods will undoubtedly help to unveil the genetic basis of host and vector adaptation and factors involved in human pathogenicity via comparative genomics.

1.7 Outlook

In this chapter, we have briefly summarized characteristics of the pathogen(s) that can cause Lyme disease and related bacterial genospecies. Much progress has been made in recent years to understand the diversity of the bacteria, their complex ecology and evolution. Host- and vector associations have been identified as the main drivers of diversification. However, more research needs to be conducted to understand the genetic basis for such associations and to understand what confers human pathogenicity on *B. burgdorferi* s.l.

References

1. Kurtenbach K, Hanincova K, Tsao JI, Margos G, Fish D, Ogden NH. Fundamental processes in the evolutionary ecology of Lyme borreliosis. Nat Rev Microbiol. 2006;4:660–9.
2. Kurtenbach K, Hoen AG, Bent SJ, Vollmer SA, Ogden NH, Margos G. Population biology of Lyme Borreliosis spirochetes. In: Robinson DA, Falush D, Feil EJ, editors. Bacterial population genetics in infectious disease. 1st ed. Hoboken: John Wiley & Sons, Inc; 2010.
3. Radolf JD, Caimano MJ, Stevenson B, Hu LT. Of ticks, mice and men: understanding the dual-host lifestyle of Lyme disease spirochaetes. Nat Rev Microbiol. 2012;10:87–99.
4. Stanek G, Strle F, Gray J, Wormser GP. History and characteristics of Lyme Borreliosis. In: Gray J, Kahl O, Lane RS, Stanek G, editors. Lyme Borreliosis: biology, epidemiology and control. Oxford: CABI Publishing; 2002. p. 1–28.
5. Burgdorfer W, Barbour AG, Hayes SF, Benach JL, Grunwaldt E, Davis JP. Lyme disease-a tick-borne spirochetosis? Science. 1982;216:1317–9.
6. Johnson RC, Schmidt GP, Hyde FW, Steigerwalt AG, Brenner DJ. *Borrelia burgdorferi* sp. nov.: etiological agent of Lyme disease. Int J Syst Bacteriol. 1984;34:496–7.
7. Baranton G, Postic D, Saint Girons I, Boerlin P, Piffaretti JC, Assous M, Grimont PA. Delineation of *Borrelia burgdorferi* sensu stricto, *Borrelia garinii* sp. nov., and group VS461 associated with Lyme borreliosis. Int J Syst Bacteriol. 1992;42:378–83.
8. Fukunaga M, Hamase A, Okada K, Nakao M. *Borrelia tanukii* sp. nov. and *Borrelia turdae* sp. nov. found from ixodid ticks in Japan: rapid species identification by 16S rRNA gene-targeted PCR analysis. Microbiol Immunol. 1996;40:877–81.

9. Le Fleche A, Postic D, Girardet K, Peter O, Baranton G. Characterization of *Borrelia lusitaniae* sp. nov. by 16S ribosomal DNA sequence analysis. Int J Syst Bacteriol. 1997;47:921–5.
10. Margos G, Chu CY, Takano A, Jiang BG, Liu W, Kurtenbach K, Masuzawa T, Fingerle V, Cao WC, Kawabata H. 2015. *Borrelia yangtzensis* sp. nov. a rodent associated species in Asia is related to *B. valaisiana*. Int J Syst Evol Microbiol. 2015
11. Margos G, Lane RS, Fedorova N, Koloczek J, Piesman J, Hojgaard A, Sing A, Fingerle V. *Borrelia bissettiae* sp. nov. and *Borrelia californiensis* sp. nov. prevail in diverse enzootic transmission cycles. Int J Syst Evol Microbiol. 2016.
12. Margos G, Piesman J, Lane RS, Ogden NH, Sing A, Straubinger RK, Fingerle V. *Borrelia kurtenbachii* sp. nov., a widely distributed member of the *Borrelia burgdorferi* sensu lato species complex in North America. Int J Syst Evol Microbiol. 2014;64:128–30.
13. Margos G, Wilske B, Sing A, Hizo-Teufel C, Cao WC, Chu C, Scholz H, Straubinger RK, Fingerle V. *Borrelia bavariensis* sp. nov. is widely distributed in Europe and Asia. Int J Syst Evol Microbiol. 2013;63:4284–8.
14. Postic D, Garnier M, Baranton G. Multilocus sequence analysis of atypical *Borrelia burgdorferi* sensu lato isolates - description of *Borrelia californiensis* sp. nov., and genomospecies 1 and 2. Int J Med Microbiol. 2007;297:263–71.
15. Ivanova LB, Tomova A, Gonzalez-Acuna D, Murua R, Moreno CX, Hernandez C, Cabello J, Cabello C, Daniels TJ, Godfrey HP, Cabello FC. *Borrelia chilensis*, a new member of the *Borrelia burgdorferi* sensu lato complex that extends the range of this genospecies in the southern hemisphere. Environ Microbiol. 2014;16:1069–80.
16. Richter D, Postic D, Sertour N, Livey I, Matuschka FR, Baranton G. Delineation of *Borrelia burgdorferi* sensu lato species by multilocus sequence analysis and confirmation of the delineation of *Borrelia spielmanii* sp. nov. Int J Syst Evol Microbiol. 2006;56:873–81.
17. Rudenko N, Golovchenko M, Grubhoffer L, Oliver JH Jr. *Borrelia carolinensis* sp. nov., a novel species of the *Borrelia burgdorferi* sensu lato complex isolated from rodents and a tick from the South-Eastern USA. Int J Syst Evol Microbiol. 2011;61:381–3.
18. Rudenko N, Golovchenko M, Lin T, Gao L, Grubhoffer L, Oliver JH Jr. Delineation of a new species of the *Borrelia burgdorferi* sensu lato complex, *Borrelia Americana* sp.nov. J Clin Microbiol. 2009;47:3875–80.
19. Margos G, Fedorova N, Kleinjan JE, Hartberger C, Schwan TG, Sing A, Fingerle V. *Borrelia lanei* sp. nov. extends the diversity of *Borrelia* species in California. Int J Syst Evol Microbiol. 2017;67:3872–6.
20. Pritt BS, Respicio-Kingry LB, Sloan LM, Schriefer ME, Replogle AJ, Bjork J, Liu G, Kingry LC, Mead PS, Neitzel DF, Schiffman E, Hoang Johnson DK, Davis JP, Paskewitz SM, Boxrud D, Deedon A, Lee X, Miller TK, Feist MA, Steward CR, Theel ES, Patel R, Irish CL, Petersen JM. *Borrelia mayonii* sp. nov., a member of the *Borrelia burgdorferi* sensu lato complex, detected in patients and ticks in the upper midwestern United States. Int J Syst Evol Microbiol. 2016;66:4878–80.
21. Kawabata H, Masuzawa T, Yanagihara Y. Genomic analysis of *Borrelia japonica* sp. nov. isolated from *Ixodes ovatus* in Japan. Microbiol Immunol. 1993;37:843–8.
22. Anderson JF, Magnarelli LA, LeFebvre RB, Andreadis TG, McAninch JB, Perng GC, Johnson RC. Antigenically variable *Borrelia burgdorferi* isolated from cottontail rabbits and Ixodes dentatus in rural and urban areas. J Clin Microbiol. 1989;27:13–20.
23. Postic D, Belfaiza J, Isogai E, Saint Girons I, Grimont PA, Baranton G. A new genomic species in *Borrelia burgdorferi* sensu lato isolated from Japanese ticks. Res Microbiol. 1993;144:467–73.
24. Margos G, Fedorova N, Becker NS, Kleinjan JE, Marosevic D, Krebs S, Hui L, Fingerle V, Lane RS. *Borrelia maritima* sp. nov., a novel species of the *Borrelia burgdorferi* sensu lato complex, occupying a basal position to North American species. Int J Syst Evol Microbiol. 2020;70:849–56.
25. Norte AC, Margos G, Becker NS, Albino Ramos J, Nuncio MS, Fingerle V, Araujo PM, Adamik P, Alivizatos H, Barba E, Barrientos R, Cauchard L, Csorgo T, Diakou A, Dingemanse

NJ, Doligez B, Dubiec A, Eeva T, Flaisz B, Grim T, Hau M, Heylen D, Hornok S, Kazantzidis S, Kovats D, Krause F, Literak I, Mand R, Mentesana L, Morinay J, Mutanen M, Neto JM, Novakova M, Sanz JJ, Pascoal da Silva L, Sprong H, Tirri IS, Torok J, Trilar T, Tyller Z, Visser ME, Lopes de Carvalho I. Host dispersal shapes the population structure of a tick-borne bacterial pathogen. Mol Ecol. 2020;29:485–501.
26. Margos G, Fingerle V, Reynolds SE. *Borrelia bavariensis*: vector switch, niche invasion, and geographical spread of a tick-borne bacterial parasite. Front Ecol Evolut. 2019;7:401.
27. Fraser CM, Casjens S, Huang WM, Sutton GG, Clayton R, Lathigra R, White O, Ketchum KA, Dodson R, Hickey EK, Gwinn M, Dougherty B, Tomb JF, Fleischmann RD, Richardson D, Peterson J, Kerlavage AR, Quackenbush J, Salzberg S, Hanson M, van Vugt R, Palmer N, Adams MD, Gocayne J, Weidman J, Utterback T, Watthey L, McDonald L, Artiach P, Bowman C, Garland S, Fuji C, Cotton MD, Horst K, Roberts K, Hatch B, Smith HO, Venter JC. Genomic sequence of a Lyme disease spirochaete, *Borrelia burgdorferi*. Nature. 1997;390:580–6.
28. Casjens S, Palmer N, van Vugt R, Huang WM, Stevenson B, Rosa P, Lathigra R, Sutton G, Peterson J, Dodson RJ, Haft D, Hickey E, Gwinn M, White O, Fraser CM. A bacterial genome in flux: the twelve linear and nine circular extrachromosomal DNAs in an infectious isolate of the Lyme disease spirochete *Borrelia burgdorferi*. Mol Microbiol. 2000;35:490–516.
29. Casjens SR, Mongodin EF, Qiu WG, Luft BJ, Schutzer SE, Gilcrease EB, Huang WM, Vujadinovic M, Aron JK, Vargas LC, Freeman S, Radune D, Weidman JF, Dimitrov GI, Khouri HM, Sosa JE, Halpin RA, Dunn JJ, Fraser CM. Genome stability of Lyme disease spirochetes: comparative genomics of *Borrelia burgdorferi* plasmids. PLoS One. 2012;7:e33280.
30. Casjens SR, Di L, Akther S, Mongodin EF, Luft BJ, Schutzer SE, Fraser CM, Qiu WG. Primordial origin and diversification of plasmids in Lyme disease agent bacteria. BMC Genomics. 2018;19:218.
31. Margos G, Becker NS, Fingerle V, Sing A, Ramos JA, Carvalho IL, Norte AC. Core genome phylogenetic analysis of the avian associated *Borrelia turdi* indicates a close relationship to *Borrelia garinii*. Mol Phylogenet Evol. 2019;131:93–8.
32. Becker NS, Margos G, Blum H, Krebs S, Graf A, Lane RS, Castillo-Ramirez S, Sing A, Fingerle V. Recurrent evolution of host and vector association in bacteria of the *Borrelia burgdorferi* sensu lato species complex. BMC Genomics. 2016;17:734.
33. Becker NS, Rollins RE, Nosenko K, Paulus A, Martin S, Krebs S, Takano A, Sato K, Kovalev SY, Kawabata H, Fingerle V, Margos G. High conservation combined with high plasticity: genomics and evolution of *Borrelia bavariensis*. BMC Genomics. 2020;21:702.
34. Mongodin EF, Casjens SR, Bruno JF, Xu Y, Drabek EF, Riley DR, Cantarel BL, Pagan PE, Hernandez YA, Vargas LC, Dunn JJ, Schutzer SE, Fraser CM, Qiu WG, Luft BJ. Inter- and intra-specific pan-genomes of *Borrelia burgdorferi* sensu lato: genome stability and adaptive radiation. BMC Genomics. 2013;14:693.
35. Casjens S, Murphy M, DeLange M, Sampson L, van Vugt R, Huang WM. Telomeres of the linear chromosomes of Lyme disease spirochaetes: nucleotide sequence and possible exchange with linear plasmid telomeres. Mol Microbiol. 1997;26:581–96.
36. Barbour AG, Garon CF. Linear plasmids of the bacterium *Borrelia burgdorferi* have covalently closed ends. Science. 1987;237:409–11.
37. Hinnebusch J, Bergstrom S, Barbour AG. Cloning and sequence analysis of linear plasmid telomeres of the bacterium *Borrelia burgdorferi*. Mol Microbiol. 1990;4:811–20.
38. Kobryn K, Chaconas G. Hairpin telomere resolvases. Microbiol Spectr. 2014;2(6)
39. Chaconas G, Kobryn K. Structure, function, and evolution of linear replicons in *Borrelia*. Annu Rev Microbiol. 2010;64:185–202.
40. Biskup UG, Strle F, Ruzic-Sabljic E. Loss of plasmids of *Borrelia burgdorferi* sensu lato during prolonged *in vitro* cultivation. Plasmid. 2011;66:1–6.
41. Labandeira-Rey M, Skare JT. Decreased infectivity in *Borrelia burgdorferi* strain B31 is associated with loss of linear plasmid 25 or 28-1. Infect Immun. 2001;69:446–55.

42. Norris SJ, Howell JK, Garza SA, Ferdows MS, Barbour AG. High- and low-infectivity phenotypes of clonal populations of in vitro-cultured *Borrelia burgdorferi*. Infect Immun. 1995;63:2206–12.
43. Schwan TG, Burgdorfer W, Garon CF. Changes in infectivity and plasmid profile of the Lyme disease spirochete, *Borrelia burgdorferi*, as a result of *in vitro* cultivation. Infect Immun. 1988;56:1831–6.
44. Lin T, Troy EB, Hu LT, Gao L, Norris SJ. Transposon mutagenesis as an approach to improved understanding of *Borrelia* pathogenesis and biology. Front Cell Infect Microbiol. 2014;4:63.
45. Iyer R, Caimano MJ, Luthra A, Axline D Jr, Corona A, Iacobas DA, Radolf JD, Schwartz I. Stage-specific global alterations in the transcriptomes of Lyme disease spirochetes during tick feeding and following mammalian host adaptation. Mol Microbiol. 2015;95:509–38.
46. Schwartz I, Margos G, Casjens SR, Qiu WG, Eggers CH. Multipartite genome of Lyme disease *Borrelia*: structure, variation and prophages. Curr Issues Mol Biol. 2021;42:409–54.
47. Casjens SR, Gilcrease EB, Vujadinovic M, Mongodin EF, Luft BJ, Schutzer SE, Fraser CM, Qiu WG. Plasmid diversity and phylogenetic consistency in the Lyme disease agent *Borrelia burgdorferi*. BMC Genomics. 2017;18:165.
48. Eggers CH, Samuels DS. Molecular evidence for a new bacteriophage of *Borrelia burgdorferi*. J Bacteriol. 1999;181:7308–13.
49. Eggers CH, Kimmel BJ, Bono JL, Elias AF, Rosa P, Samuels DS. Transduction by phiBB-1, a bacteriophage of *Borrelia burgdorferi*. J Bacteriol. 2001;183:4771–8.
50. Casjens S, Eggers CH, Schwartz I. *Borrelia* genomics: chromosome, plasmids, Bacteriohpages and genetic variation. In: Samuels DS, Radolf J, editors. Borrelia - molecular biology, host interaction and pathogenesis. Norfolk: Caister Academic Press; 2010. p. 27–53.
51. Tyler S, Tyson S, Dibernardo A, Drebot M, Feil EJ, Graham M, Knox NC, Lindsay LR, Margos G, Mechai S, Van Domselaar G, Thorpe HA, Ogden NH. Whole genome sequencing and phylogenetic analysis of strains of the agent of Lyme disease *Borrelia burgdorferi* from Canadian emergence zones. Sci Rep. 2018;8:10552.
52. Takayama K, Rothenberg RJ, Barbour AG. Absence of lipopolysaccharide in the Lyme disease spirochete, *Borrelia burgdorferi*. Infect Immun. 1987;55:2311–3.
53. Radolf JD, Bourell KW, Akins DR, Brusca JS, Norgard MV. Analysis of *Borrelia burgdorferi* membrane architecture by freeze-fracture electron microscopy. J Bacteriol. 1994;176:21–31.
54. Rosa PA, Tilly K, Stewart PE. The burgeoning molecular genetics of the Lyme disease spirochaete. Nat Rev Microbiol. 2005;3:129–43.
55. Barbour AG, Hayes SF. Biology of *Borrelia* species. Microbiol Rev. 1986;50:381–400.
56. Charon NW, Cockburn A, Li C, Liu J, Miller KA, Miller MR, Motaleb MA, Wolgemuth CW. The unique paradigm of spirochete motility and chemotaxis. Annu Rev Microbiol. 2012;66:349–70.
57. Sultan SZ, Manne A, Stewart PE, Bestor A, Rosa PA, Charon NW, Motaleb MA. Motility is crucial for the infectious life cycle of *Borrelia burgdorferi*. Infect Immun. 2013;81:2012–21.
58. Lin T, Gao L, Zhang C, Odeh E, Jacobs MB, Coutte L, Chaconas G, Philipp MT, Norris SJ. Analysis of an ordered, comprehensive STM mutant library in infectious *Borrelia burgdorferi*: insights into the genes required for mouse infectivity. PLoS One. 2012;7:e47532.
59. Petzke M, Schwartz I. *Borrelia burgdorferi* pathogenesis and the immune response. Clin Lab Med. 2015;35:745–64.
60. Rosa PA, Jewett MW. Genetic manipulation of *Borrelia*. Curr Issues Mol Biol. 2021;42:307–32.
61. Gofton AW, Margos G, Fingerle V, Hepner S, Loh SM, Ryan U, Irwin P, Oskam CL. Genome-wide analysis of *Borrelia turcica* and '*Candidatus* Borrelia tachyglossi' shows relapsing fever-like genomes with unique genomic links to Lyme disease *Borrelia*. Infect Genet Evol. 2018;66:72–81.
62. Margos G, Gofton A, Wibberg D, Dangel A, Marosevic D, Loh SM, Oskam C, Fingerle V. The genus *Borrelia* reloaded. PLoS One. 2018;13:e0208432.

63. Takano A, Fujita H, Kadosaka T, Konnai S, Tajima T, Watanabe H, Ohnishi M, Kawabata H. Characterization of reptile-associated *Borrelia* sp. in the vector tick, *Amblyomma geoemydae*, and its association with Lyme disease and relapsing fever *Borrelia* spp. Environ Microbiol Rep. 2011;3:632–7.
64. Margos G, Fingerle V, Cutler S, Gofton A, Stevenson B, Estrada-Pena A. Controversies in bacterial taxonomy: the example of the genus *Borrelia*. Ticks Tick Borne Dis. 2020;11:101335.
65. Adeolu M, Gupta RS. A phylogenomic and molecular marker based proposal for the division of the genus *Borrelia* into two genera: the emended genus *Borrelia* containing only the members of the relapsing fever *Borrelia*, and the genus *Borreliella* gen. Nov. containing the members of the Lyme disease *Borrelia* (*Borrelia burgdorferi* sensu lato complex). Antonie Van Leeuwenhoek. 2014;105:1049–72.
66. Qin Q-L, Xie B-B, Zhang X-Y, Chen X-L, Zhou B-C, Zhou J, Oren A, Zhang Y-Z. A proposed genus boundary for the prokaryotes based on genomic insights. J Bacteriol. 2014;196:2210–5.
67. Fingerle V, Schulte-Spechtel UC, Ruzic-Sabljic E, Leonhard S, Hofmann H, Weber K, Pfister K, Strle F, Wilske B. Epidemiological aspects and molecular characterization of *Borrelia burgdorferi* s.l. from southern Germany with special respect to the new species *Borrelia spielmanii* sp. nov. Int J Med Microbiol. 2008;298:279–90.
68. Stanek G, Fingerle V, Hunfeld KP, Jaulhac B, Kaiser R, Krause A, Kristoferitsch W, O'Connell S, Ornstein K, Strle F, Gray J. Lyme borreliosis: clinical case definitions for diagnosis and management in Europe. Clin Microbiol Infect. 2010;17:69–79.
69. Mukhacheva TA, Kovalev SY. Multilocus sequence analysis of *Borrelia burgdorferi* s.l. in Russia. Ticks Tick Borne Dis. 2013;4:275–9.
70. Takano A, Nakao M, Masuzawa T, Takada N, Yano Y, Ishiguro F, Fujita H, Ito T, Ma X, Oikawa Y, Kawamori F, Kumagai K, Mikami T, Hanaoka N, Ando S, Honda N, Taylor K, Tsubota T, Konnai S, Watanabe H, Ohnishi M, Kawabata H. Multilocus sequence typing implicates rodents as the main reservoir host of human-pathogenic *Borrelia garinii* in Japan. J Clin Microbiol. 2011;49:2035–9.
71. Masuzawa T. Terrestrial distribution of the Lyme borreliosis agent *Borrelia burgdorferi* sensu lato in East Asia. Jpn J Infect Dis. 2004;57:229–35.
72. Kingry LC, Anacker M, Pritt B, Bjork J, Respicio-Kingry L, Liu G, Sheldon S, Boxrud D, Strain A, Oatman S, Berry J, Sloan L, Mead P, Neitzel D, Kugeler KJ, Petersen JM. Surveillance for and discovery of *Borrelia* species in US patients suspected of tickborne illness. Clin Infect Dis. 2018;66:1864–71.
73. Pritt BS, Mead PS, Johnson DK, Neitzel DF, Respicio-Kingry LB, Davis JP, Schiffman E, Sloan LM, Schriefer ME, Replogle AJ, Paskewitz SM, Ray JA, Bjork J, Steward CR, Deedon A, Lee X, Kingry LC, Miller TK, Feist MA, Theel ES, Patel R, Irish CL, Petersen JM. Identification of a novel pathogenic *Borrelia* species causing Lyme borreliosis with unusually high spirochaetaemia: a descriptive study. Lancet Infect Dis. 2016.
74. Spielman A. The emergence of Lyme disease and human babesiosis in a changing environment. Ann N Y Acad Sci. 1994;740:146–56.
75. Steere AC, Coburn J, Glickstein L. The emergence of Lyme disease. J Clin Invest. 2004;113:1093–101.
76. Amore G, Tomassone L, Grego E, Ragagli C, Bertolotti L, Nebbia P, Rosati S, Mannelli A. *Borrelia lusitaniae* in immature *Ixodes ricinus* (Acari: Ixodidae) feeding on common wall lizards in Tuscany, Central Italy. J Med Entomol. 2007;44:303–7.
77. De Michelis S, Sewell HS, Collares-Pereira M, Santos-Reis M, Schouls LM, Benes V, Holmes EC, Kurtenbach K. Genetic diversity of *Borrelia burgdorferi* sensu lato in ticks from mainland Portugal. J Clin Microbiol. 2000;38:2128–33.
78. Dsouli N, Younsi-Kabachii H, Postic D, Nouira S, Gern L, Bouattour A. Reservoir role of lizard *Psammodromus algirus* in transmission cycle of *Borrelia burgdorferi* sensu lato (Spirochaetaceae) in Tunisia. J Med Entomol. 2006;43:737–42.
79. Younsi H, Sarih M, Jouda F, Godfroid E, Gern L, Bouattour A, Baranton G, Postic D. Characterization of *Borrelia lusitaniae* isolates collected in Tunisia and Morocco. J Clin Microbiol. 2005;43:1587–93.

80. Zhioua E, Bouattour A, Hu CM, Gharbi M, Aeschliman A, Ginsberg HS, Gern L. Infection of *Ixodes ricinus* (Acari: Ixodidae) by *Borrelia burgdorferi* sensu lato in North Africa. J Med Entomol. 1999;36:216–8.
81. Norte AC, Boyer PH, Castillo-Ramirez S, Chvostac M, Brahami MO, Rollins RE, Woudenberg T, Didyk YM, Derdakova M, Nuncio MS, Carvalho IL, Margos G, Fingerle V. The population structure of *Borrelia lusitaniae* is reflected by a population division of its *Ixodes* vector. Microorganisms. 2021;9.
82. Collares-Pereira M, Couceiro S, Franca I, Kurtenbach K, Schafer SM, Vitorino L, Goncalves L, Baptista S, Vieira ML, Cunha C. First isolation of *Borrelia lusitaniae* from a human patient. J Clin Microbiol. 2004;42:1316–8.
83. de Carvalho IL, Fonseca JE, Marques JG, Ullmann A, Hojgaard A, Zeidner N, Nuncio MS. Vasculitis-like syndrome associated with *Borrelia lusitaniae* infection. Clin Rheumatol. 2008;27:1587–91.
84. Coipan EC, Jahfari S, Fonville M, Oei GA, Spanjaard L, Takumi K, Hovius JW, Sprong H. Imbalanced presence of *Borrelia burgdorferi* s.l. multilocus sequence types in clinical manifestations of Lyme borreliosis. Infect Genet Evol. 2016;42:66–76.
85. Hanincova K, Taragelova V, Koci J, Schafer SM, Hails R, Ullmann AJ, Piesman J, Labuda M, Kurtenbach K. Association of *Borrelia garinii* and *B. valaisiana* with songbirds in Slovakia. Appl Environ Microbiol. 2003;69:2825–30.
86. Blazejak K, Raulf MK, Janecek E, Jordan D, Fingerle V, Strube C. Shifts in *Borrelia burgdorferi* (s.l.) geno-species infections in *Ixodes ricinus* over a 10-year surveillance period in the city of Hanover (Germany) and *Borrelia miyamotoi*-specific reverse line blot detection. Parasit Vectors. 2018;11:304.
87. Picken RN, Picken MM. Molecular characterization of *Borrelia* spp. isolates from greater metropolitan Chicago reveals the presence of *Borrelia bissettii*. Preliminary report. J Mol Microbiol Biotechnol. 2000;2:505–7.
88. Brown RN, Peot MA, Lane RS. Sylvatic maintenance of *Borrelia burgdorferi* (Spirochaetales) in northern California: untangling the web of transmission. J Med Entomol. 2006;43:743–51.
89. Postic D, Ras NM, Lane RS, Hendson M, Baranton G. Expanded diversity among Californian borrelia isolates and description of *Borrelia bissettii* sp. nov. (formerly *Borrelia* group DN127). J Clin Microbiol. 1998;36:3497–504.
90. Fedorova N, Kleinjan JE, James D, Hui LT, Peeters H, Lane RS. Remarkable diversity of tick or mammalian-associated borreliae in the metropolitan San Francisco Bay Area, California. Ticks Tick Borne Dis. 2014;5:951–61.
91. Eisen L, Eisen RJ, Mun J, Salkeld DJ, Lane RS. Transmission cycles of *Borrelia burgdorferi* and *B. bissettii* in relation to habitat type in northwestern California. J Vector Ecol. 2009;34:81–91.
92. Girard YA, Fedorova N, Lane RS. Genetic diversity of *Borrelia burgdorferi* and detection of *B. bissettii*-like DNA in serum of North-Coastal California residents. J Clin Microbiol. 2011;49:945–54.
93. Margos G, Sing A, Fingerle V. Published data do not support the notion that *Borrelia valaisiana* is human pathogenic. Infection. 2017;45:567–9.
94. Eisen L, Lane RS. Vectors of *Borrelia burgdorferi* sensu lato. In: Gray J, Kahl O, Lane RS, Stanek G, editors. Lyme Borreliosis: biology, epidemiology and control. Wallingford: CABI Publishing; 2002. p. 91–115.
95. Eisen L. Vector competence studies with hard ticks and *Borrelia burgdorferi* sensu lato spirochetes: a review. Ticks Tick Borne Dis. 2020;11:101359.
96. Rauter C, Hartung T. Prevalence of *Borrelia burgdorferi* sensu lato genospecies in *Ixodes ricinus* ticks in Europe: a metaanalysis. Appl Environ Microbiol. 2005;71:7203–16.
97. Padgett KA, Lane RS. Life cycle of *Ixodes pacificus* (Acari: Ixodidae): timing of developmental processes under field and laboratory conditions. J Med Entomol. 2001;38:684–93.
98. Piesman J, Schwan TG. Ecology of borreliae and their arthropod vectors. In: Samuels DS, Radolf JD, editors. *Borrelia*: molecular biology, host Interaction and Pathogenesis. Norfolk: Caister Academic Press; 2010. p. 251–78.

99. Swanson SJ, Neitzel D, Reed KD, Belongia EA. Coinfections acquired from *Ixodes* ticks. Clin Microbiol Rev. 2006;19:708–27.
100. McCoy KD, Chapuis E, Tirard C, Boulinier T, Michalakis Y, Bohec CL, Maho YL, Gauthier-Clerc M. Recurrent evolution of host-specialized races in a globally distributed parasite. Proc Biol Sci. 2005;272:2389–95.
101. Gern L, Humair P. Ecology of *Borrelia burgdorferi* sensu lato in Europe. In: Gray JS, Kahl O, Lane RS, Stanek G, editors. Lyme borreliosis: biology, epidemiology and control. Wallingford: CABI Publishing; 2002. p. 149–74.
102. Norte AC, da Silva LP, Tenreiro PJ, Felgueiras MS, Araujo PM, Lopes PB, Matos C, Rosa A, Ferreira PJ, Encarnacao P, Rocha A, Escudero R, Anda P, Nuncio MS, Lopes de Carvalho I. Patterns of tick infestation and their *Borrelia burgdorferi* s.l. infection in wild birds in Portugal. Ticks Tick Borne Dis. 2015;6:743–50.
103. Heylen D, Sprong H, van Oers K, Fonville M, Leirs H, Matthysen E. Are the specialized bird ticks, *Ixodes arboricola* and *I. frontalis*, competent vectors for *Borrelia burgdorferi* sensu lato? Environ Microbiol. 2014;16:1081–9.
104. Burkot TR, Maupin GO, Schneider BS, Denatale C, Happ CM, Rutherford JS, Zeidner NS. Use of a sentinel host system to study the questing behavior of *Ixodes spinipalpis* and its role in the transmission of *Borrelia bissettii*, human granulocytic ehrlichiosis, and *Babesia microti*. Am J Trop Med Hyg. 2001;65:293–9.
105. Heylen D, Krawczyk A, Lopes de Carvalho I, Nuncio MS, Sprong H, Norte AC. Bridging of cryptic *Borrelia* cycles in European songbirds. Environ Microbiol. 2017;19:1857–67.
106. Wikel SK. Tick-host-pathogen systems immunobiology: an interactive trio. Front Biosci (Landmark Ed). 2018;23:265–83.
107. Chmelar J, Kotal J, Kopecky J, Pedra JHF, Kotsyfakis M. All for one and one for all on the tick-host battlefield. Trends Parasitol. 2016;32:368–77.
108. Shaw DK, Kotsyfakis M, Pedra JH. For whom the bell tolls (and nods): spit-acular saliva. Curr Trop Med Rep. 2016;3:40–50.
109. Brossard M, Wikel SK. Tick immunobiology. In: Bowman AS, Nuttall PA, editors. Ticks. Biology, diasease and control. Cambridge: Cambridge University Press; 2008. p. 186–204.
110. Martins LA, Bensaoud C, Kotal J, Chmelar J, Kotsyfakis M. Tick salivary gland transcriptomics and proteomics. Parasite Immunol. 2021;43:e12807.
111. Simo L, Kazimirova M, Richardson J, Bonnet SI. The essential role of tick salivary glands and saliva in tick feeding and pathogen transmission. Front Cell Infect Microbiol. 2017;7:281.
112. Mason LM, Veerman CC, Geijtenbeek TB, Hovius JW. Menage a trois: *Borrelia*, dendritic cells, and tick saliva interactions. Trends Parasitol. 2014;30:95–103.
113. Kurokawa C, Lynn GE, Pedra JHF, Pal U, Narasimhan S, Fikrig E. Interactions between *Borrelia burgdorferi* and ticks. Nat Rev Microbiol. 2020;18:587–600.
114. Nuttall PA, Labuda M. Saliva-assisted transmission of tick-borne pathogens. In: Bowman AS, Nuttall PA, editors. Ticks. Cambridge: Cambridge University Press; 2008. p. 205–19.
115. Dizij A, Kurtenbach K. *Clethrionomys glareolus*, but not *Apodemus flavicollis*, acquires resistance to *Ixodes ricinus* L., the main European vector of *Borrelia burgdorferi*. Parasite Immunol. 1995;17:177–83.
116. Hajdusek O, Sima R, Ayllon N, Jalovecka M, Perner J, de la Fuente J, Kopacek P. Interaction of the tick immune system with transmitted pathogens. Front Cell Infect Microbiol. 2013;3:26.
117. Kitsou C, Pal U. *Ixodes* immune responses against Lyme disease pathogens. Front Cell Infect Microbiol. 2018;8:176.
118. Pal U, Kitsou C, Drecktrah D, Yas OB, Fikrig E. Interactions between ticks and Lyme disease spirochetes. Curr Issues Mol Biol. 2021;42:113–44.
119. Yang X, Smith AA, Williams MS, Pal U. A dityrosine network mediated by dual oxidase and peroxidase influences the persistence of Lyme disease pathogens within the vector. J Biol Chem. 2014;289:12813–22.
120. Urbanova V, Hajdusek O, Honig Mondekova H, Sima R, Kopacek P. Tick thioester-containing proteins and phagocytosis do not affect transmission of *Borrelia afzelii* from the competent vector *Ixodes ricinus*. Front Cell Infect Microbiol. 2017;7:73.

121. Sonenshine DE, Macaluso KR. Microbial invasion vs. tick immune regulation. Front Cell Infect Microbiol. 2017;7:390.
122. Johns R, Ohnishi J, Broadwater A, Sonenshine DE, De Silva AM, Hynes WL. Contrasts in tick innate immune responses to *Borrelia burgdorferi* challenge: immunotolerance in *Ixodes scapularis* versus immunocompetence in *Dermacentor variabilis* (Acari: Ixodidae). J Med Entomol. 2001;38:99–107.
123. Narasimhan S, Schuijt TJ, Abraham NM, Rajeevan N, Coumou J, Graham M, Robson A, Wu MJ, Daffre S, Hovius JW, Fikrig E. Modulation of the tick gut milieu by a secreted tick protein favors *Borrelia burgdorferi* colonization. Nat Commun. 2017;8:184.
124. Narasimhan S, Fikrig E. Tick microbiome: the force within. Trends Parasitol. 2015;31:315–23.
125. Abraham NM, Liu L, Jutras BL, Yadav AK, Narasimhan S, Gopalakrishnan V, Ansari JM, Jefferson KK, Cava F, Jacobs-Wagner C, Fikrig E. Pathogen-mediated manipulation of arthropod microbiota to promote infection. Proc Natl Acad Sci U S A. 2017;114:E781–90.
126. Carpi G, Cagnacci F, Wittekindt NE, Zhao F, Qi J, Tomsho LP, Drautz DI, Rizzoli A, Schuster SC. Metagenomic profile of the bacterial communities associated with *Ixodes ricinus* ticks. PLoS One. 2011;6:e25604.
127. Mukhacheva TA, Kovalev SY. Bacteria of the family '*Candidatus* Midichloriaceae' in sympatric zones of *Ixodes* ticks: genetic evidence for vertical transmission. Microb Ecol. 2017;74:185–93.
128. Benson MJ, Gawronski JD, Eveleigh DE, Benson DR. Intracellular symbionts and other bacteria associated with deer ticks (*Ixodes scapularis*) from Nantucket and Wellfleet, Cape Cod, Massachusetts. Appl Environ Microbiol. 2004;70:616–20.
129. Swei A, Kwan JY. Tick microbiome and pathogen acquisition altered by host blood meal. ISME J. 2017;11:813–6.
130. de la Fuente J, Antunes S, Bonnet S, Cabezas-Cruz A, Domingos AG, Estrada-Pena A, Johnson N, Kocan KM, Mansfield KL, Nijhof AM, Papa A, Rudenko N, Villar M, Alberdi P, Torina A, Ayllon N, Vancova M, Golovchenko M, Grubhoffer L, Caracappa S, Fooks AR, Gortazar C, ROM R. Tick-pathogen interactions and vector competence: identification of molecular drivers for tick-borne diseases. Front Cell Infect Microbiol. 2017;7:114.
131. Bonnet SI, Paul RE, Bischoff E, Cote M, Le Naour E. First identification of *Rickettsia helvetica* in questing ticks from a French northern Brittany Forest. PLoS Negl Trop Dis. 2017;11:e0005416.
132. Ross BD, Hayes B, Radey MC, Lee X, Josek T, Bjork J, Neitzel D, Paskewitz S, Chou S, Mougous JD. *Ixodes scapularis* does not harbor a stable midgut microbiome. ISME J. 2018;12:2596–607.
133. Brisson D, Dykhuizen DE. A modest model explains the distribution and abundance of *Borrelia burgdorferi* strains. Am J Trop Med Hyg. 2006;74:615–22.
134. Brisson D, Dykhuizen DE, Ostfeld RS. Conspicuous impacts of inconspicuous hosts on the Lyme disease epidemic. Proc Biol Sci. 2008;275:227–35.
135. Gern L, Estrada-Pena A, Frandsen F, Gray JS, Jaenson TG, Jongejan F, Kahl O, Korenberg E, Mehl R, Nuttall PA. European reservoir hosts of *Borrelia burgdorferi* sensu lato. Zentralbl Bakteriol. 1998;287:196–204.
136. Gern L, Humair PF. Natural history of *Borrelia burgdorferi* sensu lato. Wien Klin Wochenschr. 1998;110:856–8.
137. Hanincova K, Kurtenbach K, Diuk-Wasser M, Brei B, Fish D. Epidemic spread of Lyme borreliosis, northeastern United States. Emerg Infect Dis. 2006;12:604–11.
138. Korenberg EI, Gorelova NB, Kovalevskii YV. Ecology of *Borrelia burgdorferi* sensu lato in Russia. In: Gray J, Kahl O, Lane RS, Stanek G, editors. Lyme borreliosis: biology, epidemiology and control. Wallingford: CABI Publishing; 2002.
139. Piesman J, Gern L. Lyme borreliosis in Europe and North America. Parasitology. 2004;129(Suppl):S191–220.
140. Lane RS, Brown RN. Wood rats and kangaroo rats: potential reservoirs of the Lyme disease spirochete in California. J Med Entomol. 1991;28:299–302.

141. Lane RS, Loye JE. Lyme disease in California: interrelationship of ixodid ticks (Acari), rodents, and *Borrelia burgdorferi*. J Med Entomol. 1991;28:719–25.
142. Miyamoto K, Masuzawa T. Ecology of *Borrelia burgdorferi* sensu lato in Japan and East Asia. In: Gray J, Kahl O, Lane RS, Stanek G, editors. Lyme Borreliosis: biology, epidemiology and control. Wallingford: CABI Publishing; 2002. p. 201–22.
143. Taragel'ova V, Koci J, Hanincova K, Kurtenbach K, Derdakova M, Ogden NH, Literak I, Kocianova E, Labuda M. Blackbirds and song thrushes constitute a key reservoir of *Borrelia garinii*, the causative agent of borreliosis in Central Europe. Appl Environ Microbiol. 2008;74:1289–93.
144. Dubska L, Literak I, Kocianova E, Taragelova V, Sychra O. Differential role of passerine birds in distribution of *Borrelia* spirochetes, based on data from ticks collected from birds during the postbreeding migration period in Central Europe. Appl Environ Microbiol. 2009;75:596–602.
145. Norte AC, Lopes de Carvalho I, Nuncio MS, Ramos JA, Gern L. Blackbirds *Turdus merula* as competent reservoirs for *Borrelia turdi* and *Borrelia valaisiana* in Portugal: evidence from a xenodiagnostic experiment. Environ Microbiol Rep. 2013;5:604–7.
146. Norte AC, Ramos JA, Gern L, Nuncio MS, Lopes de Carvalho I. Birds as reservoirs for *Borrelia burgdorferi* s.l. in Western Europe: circulation of *B. turdi* and other genospecies in bird-tick cycles in Portugal. Environ Microbiol. 2013;15:386–97.
147. Heylen D, Matthysen E, Fonville M, Sprong H. Songbirds as general transmitters but selective amplifiers of *Borrelia burgdorferi* sensu lato genotypes in *Ixodes rinicus* ticks. Environ Microbiol. 2014;16:2859–68.
148. Kurtenbach K, Peacey M, Rijpkema SG, Hoodless AN, Nuttall PA, Randolph SE. Differential transmission of the genospecies of *Borrelia burgdorferi* sensu lato by game birds and small rodents in England. Appl Environ Microbiol. 1998;64:1169–74.
149. Lane RS, Quistad GB. Borreliacidal factor in the blood of the western fence lizard (*Sceloporus occidentalis*). J Parasitol. 1998;84:29–34.
150. Kurtenbach K, De Michelis S, Etti S, Schafer SM, Sewell HS, Brade V, Kraiczy P. Host association of *Borrelia burgdorferi* sensu lato-the key role of host complement. Trends Microbiol. 2002;10:74–9.
151. Kurtenbach K, Sewell HS, Ogden NH, Randolph SE, Nuttall PA. Serum complement sensitivity as a key factor in Lyme disease ecology. Infect Immun. 1998;66:1248–51.
152. Kurtenbach K, De Michelis S, Sewell HS, Etti S, Schafer SM, Holmes E, Hails R, Collares-Pereira M, Santos-Reis M, Hanincova K, Labuda M, Bormane A, Donaghy M. The key roles of selection and migration in the ecology of Lyme borreliosis. Int J Med Microbiol. 2002;291(Suppl 33):152–4.
153. Martin LB, Burgan SC, Adelman JS, Gervasi SS. Host competence: an organismal trait to integrate immunology and epidemiology. Integr Comp Biol. 2016;56:1225–37.
154. Kahl O, Gern L, Eisen L, Lane RS. Ecological research on *Borrelia burgdorferi* sensu lato: terminology and some methodological pitfalls. In: Gray JS, Kahl O, Lane RS, Stanek G, editors. Lyme borreliosis: biology, epidemiology and control. Wallingford: CABI Publishing; 2002.
155. Tsao JI. Reviewing molecular adaptations of Lyme borreliosis spirochetes in the context of reproductive fitness in natural transmission cycles. Vet Res. 2009;40:36.
156. Wikel SK. Host immunity to ticks. Annu Rev Entomol. 1996;41:1–22.
157. Wikel SK. The induction of host resistance to tick infestation with a salivary gland antigen. Am J Trop Med Hyg. 1981;30:284–8.
158. Nazario S, Das S, de Silva AM, Deponte K, Marcantonio N, Anderson JF, Fish D, Fikrig E, Kantor FS. Prevention of *Borrelia burgdorferi* transmission in guinea pigs by tick immunity. Am J Trop Med Hyg. 1998;58:780–5.
159. Wikel SK, Ramachandra RN, Bergman DK, Burkot TR, Piesman J. Infestation with pathogen-free nymphs of the tick *Ixodes scapularis* induces host resistance to transmission of *Borrelia burgdorferi* by ticks. Infect Immun. 1997;65:335–8.

160. Kahl O, Janetzki-Mittmann C, Gray JS, Jonas R, Stein J, de Boer R. Risk of infection with *Borrelia burgdorferi* sensu lato for a host in relation to the duration of nymphal *Ixodes ricinus* feeding and the method of tick removal. Zentralbl Bakteriol. 1998;287:41–52.
161. Kurtenbach K, Dizij A, Seitz HM, Margos G, Moter SE, Kramer MD, Wallich R, Schaible UE, Simon MM. Differential immune responses to *Borrelia burgdorferi* in European wild rodent species influence spirochete transmission to Ixodes ricinus L. (Acari: Ixodidae). Infect Immun. 1994;62:5344–52.
162. Gern L, Siegenthaler M, Hu CM, Leuba-Garcia S, Humair PF, Moret J. *Borrelia burgdorferi* in rodents (*Apodemus flavicollis* and *A. sylvaticus*): duration and enhancement of infectivity for *Ixodes ricinus* ticks. Eur J Epidemiol. 1994;10:75–80.
163. Hanincova K, Ogden NH, Diuk-Wasser M, Pappas CJ, Iyer R, Fish D, Schwartz I, Kurtenbach K. Fitness variation of *Borrelia burgdorferi* sensu stricto strains in mice. Appl Environ Microbiol. 2008;74:153–7.
164. Derdakova M, Dudioak V, Brei B, Brownstein JS, Schwartz I, Fish D. Interaction and transmission of two *Borrelia burgdorferi* sensu stricto strains in a tick-rodent maintenance system. Appl Environ Microbiol. 2004;70:6783–8.
165. Dolan MC, Lacombe EH, Piesman J. Vector competence of *Ixodes muris* (Acari: Ixodidae) for *Borrelia burgdorferi*. J Med Entomol. 2000;37:766–8.
166. Dolan MC, Maupin GO, Panella NA, Golde WT, Piesman J. Vector competence of *Ixodes scapularis*, *I. spinipalpis*, and *Dermacentor andersoni* (Acari:Ixodidae) in transmitting *Borrelia burgdorferi*, the etiologic agent of Lyme disease. J Med Entomol. 1997;34:128–35.
167. Dolan MC, Piesman J, Mbow ML, Maupin GO, Peter O, Brossard M, Golde WT. Vector competence of *Ixodes scapularis* and *Ixodes ricinus* (Acari: Ixodidae) for three genospecies of *Borrelia burgdorferi*. J Med Entomol. 1998;35:465–70.
168. Donahue JG, Piesman J, Spielman A. Reservoir competence of white-footed mice for Lyme disease spirochetes. Am J Trop Med Hyg. 1987;36:92–6.
169. Gern L, Toutoungi LN, Hu CM, Aeschlimann A. *Ixodes* (Pholeoixodes) *hexagonus*, an efficient vector of *Borrelia burgdorferi* in the laboratory. Med Vet Entomol. 1991;5:431–5.
170. Humair PF, Rais O, Gern L. Transmission of *Borrelia afzelii* from *Apodemus* mice and *Clethrionomys* voles to *Ixodes ricinus* ticks: differential transmission pattern and overwintering maintenance. Parasitology. 1999;118(Pt 1):33–42.
171. Nakao M, Miyamoto K. Susceptibility of *Ixodes persulcatus* and *I. ovatus* (Acari: Ixodidae) to Lyme disease spirochetes isolated from humans in Japan. J Med Entomol. 1994;31:467–73.
172. Mather TN, Piesman J, Spielman A. Absence of spirochaetes (*Borrelia burgdorferi*) and piroplasms (*Babesia microti*) in deer ticks (*Ixodes dammini*) parasitized by chalcid wasps (*Hunterellus hookeri*). Med Vet Entomol. 1987;1:3–8.
173. Eisen L. Pathogen transmission in relation to duration of attachment by *Ixodes scapularis* ticks. Ticks Tick Borne Dis. 2018;9:535–42.
174. Pal U, Li X, Wang T, Montgomery RR, Ramamoorthi N, Desilva AM, Bao F, Yang X, Pypaert M, Pradhan D, Kantor FS, Telford S, Anderson JF, Fikrig E. TROSPA, an *Ixodes scapularis* receptor for *Borrelia burgdorferi*. Cell. 2004;119:457–68.
175. Dunham-Ems SM, Caimano MJ, Pal U, Wolgemuth CW, Eggers CH, Balic A, Radolf JD. Live imaging reveals a biphasic mode of dissemination of *Borrelia burgdorferi* within ticks. J Clin Invest. 2009;119:3652–65.
176. Grove AP, Liveris D, Iyer R, Petzke M, Rudman J, Caimano MJ, Radolf JD, Schwartz I. Two distinct mechanisms govern RpoS-mediated repression of tick-phase genes during mammalian host adaptation by *Borrelia burgdorferi*, the Lyme disease spirochete. MBio. 2017;8(4):e01204–17.
177. Medrano MS, Policastro PF, Schwan TG, Coburn J. Interaction of *Borrelia burgdorferi* Hbb with the p66 promoter. Nucleic Acids Res. 2010;38:414–27.
178. Caimano MJ, Kenedy MR, Kairu T, Desrosiers DC, Harman M, Dunham-Ems S, Akins DR, Pal U, Radolf JD. The hybrid histidine kinase Hk1 is part of a two-component system that is essential for survival of *Borrelia burgdorferi* in feeding *Ixodes scapularis* ticks. Infect Immun. 2011;79:3117–30.

179. He M, Ouyang Z, Troxell B, Xu H, Moh A, Piesman J, Norgard MV, Gomelsky M, Yang XF. Cyclic di-GMP is essential for the survival of the Lyme disease spirochete in ticks. PLoS Pathog. 2011;7:e1002133.
180. Kostick JL, Szkotnicki LT, Rogers EA, Bocci P, Raffaelli N, Marconi RT. The diguanylate cyclase, Rrp1, regulates critical steps in the enzootic cycle of the Lyme disease spirochetes. Mol Microbiol. 2011;81:219–31.
181. Pitzer JE, Sultan SZ, Hayakawa Y, Hobbs G, Miller MR, Motaleb MA. Analysis of the *Borrelia burgdorferi* cyclic-di-GMP-binding protein PlzA reveals a role in motility and virulence. Infect Immun. 2011;79:1815–25.
182. Xu H, Caimano MJ, Lin T, He M, Radolf JD, Norris SJ, Gherardini F, Wolfe AJ, Yang XF. Role of acetyl-phosphate in activation of the Rrp2-RpoN-RpoS pathway in *Borrelia burgdorferi*. PLoS Pathog. 2010;6:e1001104.
183. Samuels DS. Gene regulation in *Borrelia burgdorferi*. Annu Rev Microbiol. 2011;65:479–99.
184. Skare JT, Carroll JA, Yang XF, Samuels DS, Akins DR. Gene regulation, transcriptomics and proteomics. In: Samuels DS, Radolf JD, editors. Borrelia - molecular biology, host interaction and pathogenesis. Norfolk: Caister Academic Press; 2010. p. 67–101.
185. Ouyang Z, Deka RK, Norgard MV. BosR (BB0647) controls the RpoN-RpoS regulatory pathway and virulence expression in *Borrelia burgdorferi* by a novel DNA-binding mechanism. PLoS Pathog. 2011;7:e1001272.
186. Battisti JM, Bono JL, Rosa PA, Schrumpf ME, Schwan TG, Policastro PF. Outer surface protein a protects Lyme disease spirochetes from acquired host immunity in the tick vector. Infect Immun. 2008;76:5228–37.
187. Pal U, Fikrig E. Tick interactions. In: Samuels DS, Radolf J, editors. *Borrelia* - molecular biology, host interaction and pathogenesis. Norfolk: Caister Academic Press; 2010. p. 279–98.
188. Yang XF, Pal U, Alani SM, Fikrig E, Norgard MV. Essential role for OspA/B in the life cycle of the Lyme disease spirochete. J Exp Med. 2004;199:641–8.
189. Sapi E, Balasubramanian K, Poruri A, Maghsoudlou JS, Socarras KM, Timmaraju AV, Filush KR, Gupta K, Shaikh S, Theophilus PA, Luecke DF, MacDonald A, Zelger B. Evidence of in vivo existence of borrelial biofilm in Borrelial lymphocytomas. Eur J Microbiol Immunol. 2016;6:9–24.
190. Timmaraju VA, Theophilus PA, Balasubramanian K, Shakih S, Luecke DF, Sapi E. Biofilm formation by *Borrelia burgdorferi* sensu lato. FEMS Microbiol Lett. 2015;362:fnv120.
191. Norris SJ, Coburn J, Leong JM, Hu LT, Höök M. Pathobiology of Lyme disease *Borrelia*. In: Samuels DS, Radolf JD, editors. *Borrelia* - molecular biology, host interaction and pathogenesis. Norfolk: Caister Academic Press; 2010. p. 299–332.
192. Coburn J, Garcia B, Hu LT, Jewett MW, Kraiczy P, Norris SJ, Skare J. Lyme disease pathogenesis. Curr Issues Mol Biol. 2021;42:473–518.
193. Margos G, Vollmer SA, Ogden NH, Fish D. Population genetics, taxonomy, phylogeny and evolution of *Borrelia burgdorferi* sensu lato. Infect Genet Evol. 2011;11:1545–63.
194. Mannelli A, Bertolotti L, Gern L, Gray J. Ecology of *Borrelia burgdorferi* sensu lato in Europe: transmission dynamics in multi-host systems, influence of molecular processes and effects of climate change. FEMS Microbiol Rev. 2012;36:837–61.
195. Randolph SE, Craine NG. General framework for comparative quantitative studies on transmission of tick-borne diseases using Lyme borreliosis in Europe as an example. J Med Entomol. 1995;32:765–77.
196. Randolph SE. Ticks are not insects: consequences of contrasting vector biology for transmission potential. Parasitol Today. 1998;14:186–92.
197. Hartemink NA, Randolph SE, Davis SA, Heesterbeek JA. The basic reproduction number for complex disease systems: defining R(0) for tick-borne infections. Am Nat. 2008;171:743–54.
198. Ostfeld RS, Canham CD, Oggenfuss K, Winchcombe RJ, Keesing F. Climate, deer, rodents, and acorns as determinants of variation in Lyme-disease risk. PLoS Biol. 2006;4:e145.
199. Telford SR 3rd, Mather TN, Moore SI, Wilson ML, Spielman A. Incompetence of deer as reservoirs of the Lyme disease spirochete. Am J Trop Med Hyg. 1988;39:105–9.

200. Kilpatrick AM, Dobson ADM, Levi T, Salkeld DJ, Swei A, Ginsberg HS, Kjemtrup A, Padgett KA, Jensen PM, Fish D, Ogden NH, Diuk-Wasser MA. Lyme disease ecology in a changing world: consensus, uncertainty and critical gaps for improving control. Philos Trans R Soc Lond Ser B Biol Sci. 2017;372
201. Ogden NH, Tsao JI. Biodiversity and Lyme disease: dilution or amplification? Epidemics. 2009;1:196–206.
202. LoGiudice K, Ostfeld RS, Schmidt KA, Keesing F. The ecology of infectious disease: effects of host diversity and community composition on Lyme disease risk. Proc Natl Acad Sci U S A. 2003;100:567–71.
203. Ruyts SC, Ampoorter E, Coipan EC, Baeten L, Heylen D, Sprong H, Matthysen E, Verheyen K. Diversifying forest communities may change Lyme disease risk: extra dimension to the dilution effect in Europe. Parasitology. 2016;143:1310–9.
204. Margos G, Castillo-Ramirez S, Hoen AG. Phylogeography of Lyme borreliosis-group spirochetes and methicillin-resistant *Staphylococcus aureus*. Parasitology. 2012;139:1952–65.
205. Munro HJ, Ogden NH, Lindsay LR, Robertson GJ, Whitney H, Lang AS. Evidence for *Borrelia bavariensis* infections of *Ixodes uriae* within seabird colonies of the North Atlantic Ocean. Appl Environ Microbiol. 2017.
206. Hamer SA, Roy PL, Hickling GJ, Walker ED, Foster ES, Barber CC, Tsao JI. Zoonotic pathogens in *Ixodes scapularis*, Michigan. Emerg Infect Dis. 2007;13:1131–3.
207. Hoen AG, Margos G, Bent SJ, Kurtenbach K, Fish D. Phylogeography of *Borrelia burgdorferi* in the eastern United States reflects multiple independent Lyme disease emergence events. Proc Natl Acad Sci U S A. 2009;106:15013–8.
208. Mechai S, Feil EJ, Gariepy TD, Gregory TR, Lindsay LR, Millien V, Ogden NH. Investigation of the population structure of the tick vector of Lyme disease *Ixodes scapularis* (Acari: Ixodidae) in Canada using mitochondrial cytochrome C oxidase subunit I gene sequences. J Med Entomol. 2013;50:560–70.
209. Ogden NH, Bouchard C, Kurtenbach K, Margos G, Lindsay LR, Trudel L, Nguon S, Milord F. Active and passive surveillance and phylogenetic analysis of *Borrelia burgdorferi* elucidate the process of Lyme disease risk emergence in Canada. Environ Health Perspect. 2010;118:909–14.
210. Kurilshikov AM, Fomenko NV, Stronin OV, Tikunov AY, Kabilov MR, Tupikin AE, Tikunova NV. Complete genome sequencing of *Borrelia valaisiana* and *Borrelia afzelii* Isolated from *Ixodes persulcatus* Ticks in Western Siberia. Genome Announc. 2014;2(6):e01315–4.
211. Bormane A, Lucenko I, Duks A, Mavtchoutko V, Ranka R, Salmina K, Baumanis V. Vectors of tick-borne diseases and epidemiological situation in Latvia in 1993-2002. Int J Med Microbiol. 2004;293(Suppl 37):36–47.
212. Gatzmann F, Metzler D, Krebs S, Blum H, Sing A, Takano A, Kawabata H, Fingerle V, Margos G, Becker NS. NGS population genetics analyses reveal divergent evolution of a Lyme Borreliosis agent in Europe and Asia. Ticks Tick Borne Dis. 2015;6:344–51.
213. Wang G, Liveris D, Mukherjee P, Jungnick S, Margos G, Schwartz I. Molecular typing of *Borrelia burgdorferi*. Curr Protoc Microbiol. 2014;34:12C 15 11–31.
214. Schwartz JJ, Gazumyan A, Schwartz I. rRNA gene organization in the Lyme disease spirochete, *Borrelia burgdorferi*. J Bacteriol. 1992;174:3757–65.
215. Wilske B, Busch U, Eiffert H, Fingerle V, Pfister HW, Rossler D, Preac-Mursic V. Diversity of OspA and OspC among cerebrospinal fluid isolates of *Borrelia burgdorferi* sensu lato from patients with neuroborreliosis in Germany. Med Microbiol Immunol. 1996;184:195–201.
216. Wilske B, Preac-Mursic V, Gobel UB, Graf B, Jauris S, Soutschek E, Schwab E, Zumstein G. An OspA serotyping system for *Borrelia burgdorferi* based on reactivity with monoclonal antibodies and *ospA* sequence analysis. J Clin Microbiol. 1993;31:340–50.
217. Strube C, Montenegro VM, Epe C, Eckelt E, Schnieder T. Establishment of a minor groove binder-probe based quantitative real time PCR to detect *Borrelia burgdorferi* sensu lato and differentiation of *Borrelia spielmanii* by ospA-specific conventional PCR. Parasit Vectors. 2010;3:69.

218. Postic D, Assous MV, Grimont PA, Baranton G. Diversity of *Borrelia burgdorferi* sensu lato evidenced by restriction fragment length polymorphism of rrf (5S)-rrl (23S) intergenic spacer amplicons. Int J Syst Bacteriol. 1994;44:743–52.
219. Fukunaga M, Koreki Y. A phylogenetic analysis of *Borrelia burgdorferi* sensu lato isolates associated with Lyme disease in Japan by flagellin gene sequence determination. Int J Syst Bacteriol. 1996;46:416–21.
220. Venczel R, Knoke L, Pavlovic M, Dzaferovic E, Vaculova T, Silaghi C, Overzier E, Konrad R, Kolencik S, Derdakova M, Sing A, Schaub GA, Margos G, Fingerle V. A novel duplex real-time PCR permits simultaneous detection and differentiation of *Borrelia miyamotoi* and *Borrelia burgdorferi* sensu lato. Infection. 2015.
221. Liveris D, Gazumyan A, Schwartz I. Molecular typing of *Borrelia burgdorferi* sensu lato by PCR-restriction fragment length polymorphism analysis. J Clin Microbiol. 1995;33:589–95.
222. Bunikis J, Garpmo U, Tsao J, Berglund J, Fish D, Barbour AG. Sequence typing reveals extensive strain diversity of the Lyme borreliosis agents *Borrelia burgdorferi* in North America and *Borrelia afzelii* in Europe. Microbiology. 2004;150:1741–55.
223. Qiu WG, Bruno JF, McCaig WD, Xu Y, Livey I, Schriefer ME, Luft BJ. Wide distribution of a high-virulence *Borrelia burgdorferi* clone in Europe and North America. Emerg Infect Dis. 2008;14:1097–104.
224. Margos G, Gatewood AG, Aanensen DM, Hanincova K, Terekhova D, Vollmer SA, Cornet M, Piesman J, Donaghy M, Bormane A, Hurn MA, Feil EJ, Fish D, Casjens S, Wormser GP, Schwartz I, Kurtenbach K. MLST of housekeeping genes captures geographic population structure and suggests a European origin of *Borrelia burgdorferi*. Proc Natl Acad Sci U S A. 2008;105:8730–5.
225. Margos G, Vollmer SA, Cornet M, Garnier M, Fingerle V, Wilske B, Bormane A, Vitorino L, Collares-Pereira M, Drancourt M, Kurtenbach K. A new *Borrelia* species defined by multilocus sequence analysis of housekeeping genes. Appl Environ Microbiol. 2009;75:5410–6.
226. Rudenko N, Golovchenko M, Grubhoffer L, Oliver JH Jr. *Borrelia carolinensis* sp.nov. - a new (14th) member of *Borrelia burgdorferi* sensu lato complex from the southeastern United States. J Clin Microbiol. 2009;47:134–41.
227. Crowder CD, Matthews HE, Schutzer S, Rounds MA, Luft BJ, Nolte O, Campbell SR, Phillipson CA, Li F, Sampath R, Ecker DJ, Eshoo MW. Genotypic variation and mixtures of Lyme *Borrelia* in *Ixodes* ticks from North America and Europe. PLoS One. 2010;5:e10650.
228. Enright MC, Spratt BG. Multilocus sequence typing. Trends Microbiol. 1999;7:482–7.
229. Urwin R, Maiden MC. Multi-locus sequence typing: a tool for global epidemiology. Trends Microbiol. 2003;11:479–87.
230. Margos G, Binder K, Dzaferovic E, Hizo-Teufel C, Sing A, Wildner M, Fingerle V, Jolley KA. PubMLST.org - the new home for the *Borrelia* MLSA database. Ticks Tick Borne Dis. 2015;6:869–71.
231. Vollmer SA, Bormane A, Dinnis RE, Seelig F, Dobson AD, Aanensen DM, James MC, Donaghy M, Randolph SE, Feil EJ, Kurtenbach K, Margos G. Host migration impacts on the phylogeography of Lyme borreliosis spirochaete species in Europe. Environ Microbiol. 2011;13:184–92.
232. Vollmer SA, Feil EJ, Chu CY, Raper SL, Cao WC, Kurtenbach K, Margos G. Spatial spread and demographic expansion of Lyme borreliosis spirochaetes in Eurasia. Infect Genet Evol. 2013;14C:147–55.
233. Mechai S, Margos G, Feil EJ, Barairo N, Lindsay LR, Michel P, Ogden NH. Evidence for host-genotype associations of *Borrelia burgdorferi* sensu stricto. PLoS One. 2016;11:e0149345.
234. Mechai S, Margos G, Feil EJ, Lindsay LR, Michel P, Kotchi SO, Ogden NH. Evidence for an effect of landscape connectivity on *Borrelia burgdorferi* sensu stricto dispersion in a zone of range expansion. Ticks Tick Borne Dis. 2018;9:1407–15.
235. Ogden NH, Margos G, Aanensen DM, Drebot MA, Feil EJ, Hanincová K, Schwartz I, Tyler S, Lindsay LR. Investigation of genotypes of *Borrelia burgdorferi* in *Ixodes scapularis* ticks collected in surveillance in Canada. Appl Environ Microbiol. 2011;77:3244–54.

236. Hanincova K, Mukherjee P, Ogden NH, Margos G, Wormser GP, Reed KD, Meece JK, Vandermause MF, Schwartz I. Multilocus sequence typing of *Borrelia burgdorferi* suggests existence of lineages with differential pathogenic properties in humans. PLoS One. 2013;8:e73066.
237. Okeyo M, Hepner S, Rollins RE, Hartberger C, Straubinger RK, Marosevic D, Bannister SA, Bormane A, Donaghy M, Sing A, Fingerle V, Margos G. Longitudinal study of prevalence and spatio-temporal distribution of *Borrelia burgdorferi* sensu lato in ticks from three defined habitats in Latvia, 1999-2010. Environ Microbiol. 2020;22(12):5033–47.
238. Castillo-Ramirez S, Fingerle V, Jungnick S, Straubinger RK, Krebs S, Blum H, Meinel DM, Hofmann H, Guertler P, Sing A, Margos G. Trans-Atlantic exchanges have shaped the population structure of the Lyme disease agent *Borrelia burgdorferi* sensu stricto. Sci Rep. 2016;6:22794.
239. Kingry LC, Batra D, Replogle A, Rowe LA, Pritt BS, Petersen JM. Whole genome sequence and comparative genomics of the novel Lyme Borreliosis causing pathogen, *Borrelia mayonii*. PLoS One. 2016;11:e0168994.
240. Margos G, Hepner S, Mang C, Marosevic D, Reynolds SE, Krebs S, Sing A, Derdakova M, Reiter MA, Fingerle V. Lost in plasmids: next generation sequencing and the complex genome of the tick-borne pathogen *Borrelia burgdorferi*. BMC Genomics. 2017;18:422.
241. Margos G, Hepner S, Mang C, Sing A, Liebl B, Fingerle V. Completed genome sequences of *Borrelia burgdorferi* sensu stricto B31(NRZ) and closely related patient isolates from Europe. Genome Announc. 2017;5(28):e00637-17.

Tick Ecology and the Eco-Epidemiology of *Borrelia burgdorferi* sensu lato

2

Jeremy Gray and Olaf Kahl

2.1 Introduction

The four ixodid tick species mainly responsible for *Borrelia burgdorferi* sensu lato (s.l.) transmission and the vast majority of resulting Lyme borreliosis (LB) cases are *Ixodes ricinus* and *Ixodes persulcatus* in the Old World, and *Ixodes scapularis* and *Ixodes pacificus* in the New World (Fig. 2.1). In general, the geographical distribution of LB coincides with that of the main vectors except for the southern USA, where the disease is rare despite the presence of *I. scapularis* [1, 2]. In southern Europe and northern Africa, the discovery that *Ixodes inopinatus* is a separate species may mean that the role of *I. ricinus* as a vector in these regions needs to be reassessed and that of *I. inopinatus* to be investigated. Several other ixodid tick species have been reported as possible vectors, but generally the proof provided by transmission studies is lacking. Some known vectors of *Borrelia burgdorferi* s.l., such as *I. hexagonus* parasitizing European hedgehogs (*Erinaceus europaeus* and *E. roumanicus* – proven reservoirs of several *Borrelia burgdorferi* genospecies), mainly occur in burrows and very rarely bite humans, but probably contribute to the circulation of those pathogens in nature. The vectors of both pathogenic and non-pathogenic *Borrelia* genospecies are listed by Ogden and others [3].

Although *I. scapularis, I. pacificus* and *I. persulcatus* are considered in this review on the ecology of *Borrelia burgdorferi* s.l., the main focus is on the European vector, *I. ricinus*.

J. Gray (✉)
UCD School of Biology & Environmental Science, University College Dublin, Belfield, Dublin, Ireland
e-mail: Jeremy.gray@ucd.ie

O. Kahl
tick-radar GmbH, Berlin, Germany

K.-P. Hunfeld, J. Gray (eds.), *Lyme Borreliosis*,
https://doi.org/10.1007/978-3-030-93680-8_2

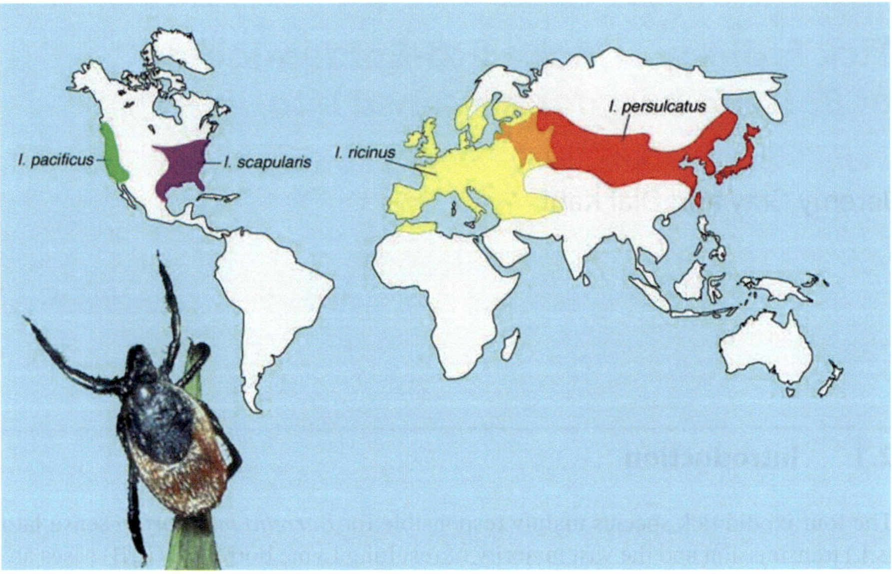

Fig. 2.1 Approximate geographical distribution of *Ixodes pacificus*, *I. persulcatus*, *I. ricinus* and *I. scapularis*. *Ixodes persulcatus* and *I. ricinus* are sympatric over a large area, comprising parts of the Baltic States, Belarus and Russia. © Bernard Kaye and Jeremy Gray

2.2 The Tick Life Cycle

The life cycle of the *Ixodes* spp. vectors of *Borrelia burgdorferi* s.l. consists of four distinct life stages, egg, larva, nymph and adult. The motile stages each take a single large blood meal on a different individual host, drop off and then develop to the next stage or in the case of the adult females, lay eggs. These feeding phases take up less than 1% of their life cycle and for the remaining proportion, the ticks are free-living in the habitat, either in an engorged state after feeding on a host or as unfed (flat) ticks that seek hosts by ambushing them from vegetation as they pass by. All the life stages show some degree of host specificity and although a very wide range of mammals, birds and reptiles can be parasitized, nymphs are less successful on small mammals than larvae, and adults are restricted to large hosts, mainly ungulates, and some medium-sized species, such as hedgehogs, foxes hares and dogs.

2.3 The Feeding Process

The external mouthparts of ixodid ticks consist of two essential components. First, a proboscis (hypostome) enclosing the feeding tube that introduces saliva into the skin and up which blood and inflammatory exudate is sucked during feeding, and second a pair of barbed chelicerae apically, with movable cheliceral digits, blade-like structures that are used for incising the skin (Fig. 2.2). Once the tick has found

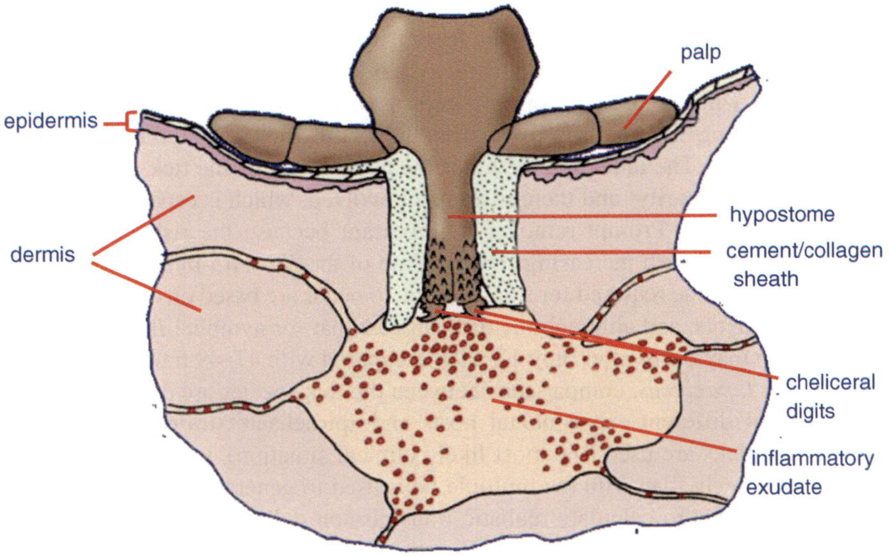

Fig. 2.2 Diagrammatic illustration of tick mouthparts embedded in the skin of a vertebrate host (after Balashov, 1972 [60])

a suitable feeding site on a host it makes an incision with the cheliceral digits and inserts the hypostome into the host skin. Since the tick must feed for several days, firm attachment is essential and is provided by recurved teeth on the hypostome, reflexed chelicerae at the end of the hypostome, and a cement-like salivary secretion. Anchorage is further facilitated by the deposition of collagen around the hypostome (Fig. 2.2). The tick does not neatly pierce blood vessels (as a female mosquito does) but creates a feeding pool by secreting vasoactive mediators and immunomodulators that keep the blood flowing and suppress host attempts to resist the process. Local inflammation may occur around the tick bite, and the tick-bite lesion may persist beneath the epidermis for many days after the tick has fed. During the relatively long initial phase of feeding, the tick grows both gut and cuticle to accommodate a large volume of blood, which is ingested over a relatively short time just before detachment. Detachment is an active process and there is evidence that natural rhythms play a part [4], but little is known about the factors involved. Although a fully engorged tick readily withdraws its mouthparts from the host skin, a partially fed feeding tick resists its removal and considerable force is required, especially for adult females. Much has been written about correct and incorrect ways to remove ticks in order to minimise the risk of pathogen transmission, but Kahl et al. [5] demonstrated experimentally that the method of removal of *Borrelia burgdorferi* s.l.-infected *I. ricinus* nymphs from Mongolian gerbils (*Meriones unguiculatus*), including intensive squeezing of feeding ticks and the use of nail polish to block the tick spiracles, did not affect the likelihood of infection of the host. Thus suggestions that careless and rough removal of a feeding tick, or the application of irritating fluids, might result in the regurgitation of infective spirochaetes into the tick-bite lesion, have proved unfounded. The clear conclusions that emerged from this study were that in every case, it is important that a feeding tick is removed as soon as possible, and that it is much less important how the tick is removed. Although the removal of feeding ticks with the use of proper forceps seems optimal, one may also be successful using long fingernails or by rotating the feeding tick several times around its longitudinal axis. The latter approach has the advantage that the tick withdraws its mouthparts 'voluntarily' and there is no pain involved, which is especially relevant if a child is bitten. Prompt removal is important because the risk of becoming infected increases with increasing feeding time of the *Borrelia*-infected tick. Most estimates of the time required for transmission to occur are based on experiments on laboratory rodents, and although the data suggest that for nymphal *I. ricinus* >50% transmission may occur after only 17–29 h compared with 47–49 h for *I. scapularis* and 72 h for *I. pacificus*, comparisons between the tick species are difficult because of the use of different experimental hosts and spirochaete strains. Additionally, when single ticks are used (the most likely clinical situation), transmission occurs much more slowly than with the multiple ticks used to generate most experimental data [6]. Attempts to calculate realistic transmission delays based on the state of engorgement of ticks removed from LB patients have not been successful, despite the availability of data relating measurements of engorging ticks to the duration of feeding [6].

2.4 Tick Development

Once a feeding tick has fed to repletion, it detaches from the host and locates in the mat of decaying vegetation overlying the soil, where the relative humidity is usually no lower than 80–85%, so that it can avoid desiccation [7]. Although these tick species do not drink, they can actively take in atmospheric water when relative humidity surpasses 80–85% by secreting a hygroscopic fluid from the salivary glands onto the mouthparts, which is then ingested [8–10]. This ability recurs in unfed ticks during the host-seeking phase of the life cycle. Development to the next stage following engorgement takes many weeks and even longer in the case of larvae and nymphs if they feed late in the year, when they show a developmental delay (diapause) that is driven by day length and allows them to overwinter. For females, this diapause tends to manifest as delayed oviposition (*I. scapularis*) or as an egg development (*I. ricinus*) delay [11]. In the absence of ovipositional diapause, egg laying starts a week or two after the fed female drops from its host and has found a suitable microclimate in the leaf litter. In the case of *I. ricinus*, approximately 2,000–3,000 eggs are continuously laid whenever the microclimate temperature exceeds 4–5 °C. In the other three species, some differences are evident. For example, unlike *I. ricinus*, neither engorged females nor eggs of *I. persulcatus* overwinter [12, 13] and oviposition and hatching are completed before the winter. *Ixodes scapularis* females can overwinter in either the engorged or unfed state, with oviposition commencing in the spring [14]. *Ixodes pacificus* shows a similar pattern, but in southern regions, unfed adults do not appear to survive the winter [15].

Following hatching or moulting and after a delay of varying length, the unfed ticks commence questing for a host. This involves climbing to a vantage point in the vegetation, or on the surface of leaf litter, where they wait in ambush, fastening onto a host as it passes by. Questing is punctuated by many visits for water replenishment to the humid microclimate at the base of the vegetation. If the tick fails to acquire a host, it will die once the energy reserves required for this activity have been depleted. The length of time ticks can spend in this questing phase varies and depends on the nature of the habitat and on the weather, but in most cases does not exceed a few weeks.

2.5 Seasonal Activity

The seasonality of human infection with *Borrelia burgdorferi* s.l., indicated by the incidence of erythema migrans, is well established and determined by two basic factors: first, people entering tick habitats most often during the summer and autumn months, and second, to the seasonal activity of the ticks themselves. In *I. ricinus,* most host-seeking by unfed ticks occurs in spring and early summer as air temperatures rise above about 7 °C, and then declines gradually over the summer as a result of accelerating mortality at a rate usually determined by the nature of the habitat [16]. In some regions, a second smaller peak may occur in autumn, which is due to the activity of a part of the population that mostly overwintered in the previous winter as engorged ticks in developmental diapause. Some of these autumn-active ticks may be active in the winter if temperatures are high enough [17]. In the far south of the *I. ricinus* range, the autumn and early winter peaks, especially of adults, are more in evidence and some questing activity may occur throughout the winter [18, 19]. Although seasonal activity patterns can be partly explained by tactical responses to ambient conditions, the main regulating factor is diapause, a physiological response to day length, which in addition to causing delays in development (developmental diapause) referred to above, can also inhibit host-seeking by unfed ticks (behavioural diapause) [11]. These mechanisms ensure that ticks that feed late in the year enter a developmental diapause and overwinter in the engorged state in the case of larvae and nymphs or produce diapausing eggs in the case of females. Ticks that fed earlier in the year and then moulted by late autumn often go into a behavioural diapause, which prevents them becoming active at an inclement time of year. However, many individuals merely become quiescent in response to falling temperatures and can respond to rising temperatures in winter [17–19]. The other main vectors of LB, *I. pacificus, I. persulcatus* and *I. scapularis,* show similar patterns of activity, though with some differences in both timing and behaviour, depending on the region. For example, larval and nymphal *I. persulcatus* tend to remain within the leaf litter and are difficult to collect by flagging, and there is virtually no autumn questing by adults of this species, which seem to undergo a strong behavioural diapause. In the southern part of the *I. scapularis* range, the immature stages also remain in the leaf litter in the United States, but not in the north. In direct contrast to *I. persulcatus*, adult *I. scapularis* quest in the autumn (fall), showing little or no behavioural diapause, though some individuals in the population appear in the spring and early summer. A more detailed comparative account of the seasonal activity of LB vectors can be found in Gray et al. [11].

2.6 Tick Habitats

The requirement of the non-parasitic phases of these tick species for a humid microclimate (>80% RH) at the base of vegetation and in leaf litter is the main factor that determines the suitability of a habitat for colonisation. But host requirements must also be met and since the adults are mostly restricted to large animals, especially deer, the ticks mainly inhabit forests and forest-like habitats and their margins [20]. Deciduous and mixed forests are especially favourable because of the year-round ability of the leaf litter to retain a high humidity, but all these tick species can also be found in some coniferous forests in appreciable densities if there is sufficient precipitation in all seasons. Infection of ticks with pathogenic *Borrelia burgdorferi* s.l. in such habitats depends on the presence of reservoir hosts, which are a range of small mammals and birds. Ticks may also occur in parks and garden areas where hosts for the immature stages can be found, and although the availability of hosts for adult ticks may be more limited, tick numbers may be augmented by roosting birds, hedgehogs and foxes. In the case of *I. scapularis,* the greatest risk of LB probably occurs in periurban habitats, where many deer may be present in woodland close to human dwellings [21]. Deer alone are capable of feeding immature stages as well as adults [22–27] and in habitats where the vast majority of all tick stages feed on large non-reservoir animals, such as deer, the proportion of infected ticks tends to be low. This situation occurs in agricultural settings, especially in the British Isles and Ireland, where sheep and cattle maintain large tick populations in areas of rough grazing with high precipitation [20].

2.7 Factors Affecting Tick Abundance

2.7.1 Weather and Climate

Since all the tick species considered here are susceptible to desiccation, hot dry conditions can be highly detrimental to their survival, and to some extent determine their geographical distribution. However, they can survive limited periods of such weather as long they have access to protected humid microclimates. Very cold winters are also often thought to result in poor survival of these ticks. However, this is simplistic considering that *I. ricinus* is found in regions such as Scandinavia where the winter temperatures can be much lower than in most other parts of Europe. In fact, the main risk to overwintering ticks appears to be very cold weather in the absence of snow cover for prolonged periods [28]. The northern distribution of both *I. ricinus* and *I. scapularis* seems to be primarily limited by spring and summer temperatures that are not high enough for a sufficient period to permit complete development within a season [29–31]. Temperature-limiting effects on questing activity and the availability of appropriate hosts are also relevant factors here.

The factors that limit *I. ricinus* distribution to the east of its range are unknown, but are probably also temperature-based. *Ixodes ricinus* is gradually replaced eastwards by the closely related *I. persulcatus*, and there is a substantial area where the two species are sympatric (Fig. 2.1). It seems likely that *I. persulcatus* is better adapted to continental climates, involving hot summers and prolonged cold winters, than is *I. ricinus*, but this awaits further research.

2.7.2 Hosts

In most LB habitats, deer are the most important tick maintenance hosts, mainly because of their role in feeding the adult females. Not surprisingly, therefore, the density of deer can have a profound effect on local tick abundance [32–35]. However, this relationship is complex and it has been suggested that the mere presence of deer in tick permissive habitats that harbour numerous hosts of the immature stages, may be enough to result in high tick abundance [36]. However, it is commonly found that when deer are absent from a habitat, ticks are relatively scarce, unless there are alternative hosts such as foxes or hedgehogs, for example in city parks, or they are imported from surrounding areas by roosting birds.

While overall host density can affect *I. ricinus* abundance, short-term changes may have a profound effect on year-to-year fluctuations in the size of questing tick populations. For example, masting, the production of tree seeds such as beech nuts and oak acorns, is known to result in major increases in rodent populations after high mast years, which occur every few years [37]. A relationship between high mast years and abundance of *Ixodes* nymphs 2 years later was first explored in the United States for *I. scapularis* [38]. More recently this has been studied in detail in Switzerland for *I. ricinus* by Bregnard and others [39], who found that annual tick abundance over a 15-year period was strongly associated with high mast years 2 and 3 years earlier. Deer are probably also benefited by high mast years, in which case effects on tick abundance are likely to be more prolonged, since deer can feed all active stages of *I. ricinus.* At present, there are no data on this in Europe.

2.8 Transmission and Circulation of *Borrelia burgdorferi* sensu lato

2.8.1 The Transmission Process

During feeding, the blood meal is concentrated by the extraction of water, which is then secreted back into the host by specialised salivary gland cells, an important means by which tick-borne pathogens invade their vertebrate hosts. Furthermore, the immunomodulation, induced by components of tick saliva, that permits successful feeding, has an effect on the establishment of transmitted pathogens, as demonstrated by the increased efficiency of tick-transmitted *Borrelia burgdorferi* s.l. compared with needle injection [40].

When *Borrelia burgdorferi* s.l. spirochaetes are ingested with the blood by a feeding tick, they enter the midgut, a sequestered location for pathogens because of intracellular rather than lumenal enzymatic digestion. The spirochaetes remain in the midgut attached to the gut epithelium through the subsequent tick development and moult, but when the resulting unfed tick acquires a host and starts feeding, the spirochaetes multiply enormously and migrate to the salivary glands. During this migration, crucial changes to the outer surface proteins (Osp) occur and they are upregulated from OspA to OspC, the latter being the form required for migration to the salivary glands and invasion of the vertebrate host [41, 42]. The time taken for these changes and for migration to the salivary glands to occur explains the delay in transmission of the spirochaetes after the commencement of tick feeding.

Several other proteins of vector origin have been shown to have a role in regulating the behaviour of the spirochaetes within the tick and the overall complexity of the transmission process suggests that arthropods other than certain ixodid ticks are unlikely to serve as vectors of *Borrelia burgdorferi* s.l. Therefore circumstantial evidence for transmission by haematophagous arthropods such as mosquitoes and horseflies can most probably be discounted.

Borrelia burgdorferi s.l. is usually transmitted horizontally, a process in which the pathogens are acquired from a vertebrate host by one tick stage, survive the moult and are then transmitted by the next to another host (Fig. 2.3). Most *Borrelia burgdorferi* s.l. infections are acquired by larvae and transmitted by nymphs and in *I. ricinus*, *I. scapularis* and *I. pacificus* it is thought to be the nymphal stage that is mostly responsible for the transmission of Lyme borreliae to humans. However, adult females, infected as nymphs can also transmit the infection to humans, and in *I. persulcatus* the adult female is regarded as the most important vector stage.

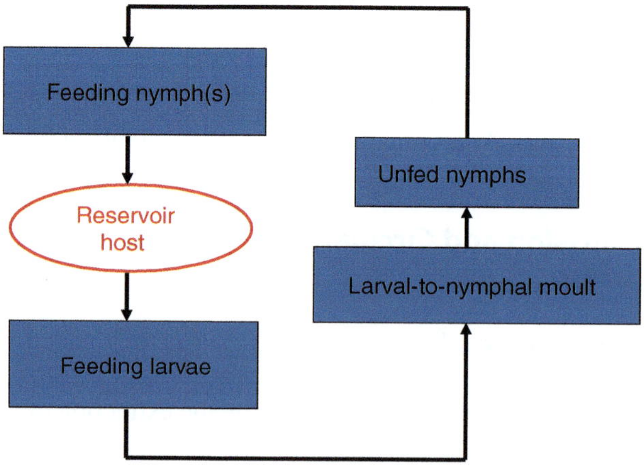

Fig. 2.3 Primary transmission pathway of *Borrelia burgdorferi* s.l. Nymphal ticks can infect hosts from which feeding larvae then acquire the infection. Since reservoir hosts may retain the infection for many months, infections may pass from nymphs to larvae over two seasons

Transovarial transmission of *Borrelia burgdorferi* s.l. is rare [43, 44], and larvae are therefore not considered significant in the epidemiology of human LB, though they may have a role in maintaining circulation of the spirochaetes in nature. Non-systemic transmission (co-feeding transmission), involving transmission of pathogens between ticks feeding close together on the reservoir host, has been demonstrated for *Borrelia burgdorferi* s.l. [45, 46], but has limited epidemiological significance except for the possible promotion of strain variability [47, 48].

Infection prevalences in unfed ticks are highly variable, ranging from 0% to 50% with many variables, including spirochaete genospecies, tick species, nature of habitat (especially in relation to the vertebrate fauna), geographical area, and even the methodology used for detection. In general, higher infection prevalence tends to occur in adults than nymphs, because of the opportunity for adults to acquire infections over two blood meals. Larvae are very rarely infected.

2.8.2 Tick and Spirochaete Reservoir Hosts

The host requirements of zoonotic *Borrelia burgdorferi* genospecies and of their tick vectors that enable them to persist within a habitat differ significantly. Whereas medium-sized to large mammal hosts, usually deer, are essential for successful feeding of adult female ticks, such hosts are usually not reservoir-competent for the spirochaetes, for which various species of small mammals and birds serve as reservoirs [49]. By definition, a reservoir host of *Borrelia burgdorferi* s.l. must be capable of supporting infections, but also serve as hosts to immature stages of the vectors, so that the spirochaetes can then infect a substantial proportion of the tick population. Although the vectors are capable of parasitizing a wide range of hosts, a relatively small proportion of them are significant reservoirs of *Borrelia burgdorferi* s.l. The ecological situation is made more complex by the fact that the pathogenic spirochaete genospecies differ to some extent in their predilections for vertebrate hosts. For example, in Europe, most strains of *B. garinii* utilise certain bird species, notably passerines, *B. afzelii* is found predominantly in rodents, and *B. spielmanii* in two species of dormouse in particular (*Eliomys quercinus* and *Muscardinus avellanarius*) [50]. European strains of *Borrelia burgdorferi* sensu stricto (s.s.) appear to be found only in small mammals, but in North America, these genospecies can infect both birds and rodents [3]. The only other acknowledged pathogenic genospecies in the United States, *B. mayonii,* appears to be associated with small mammals [51]. Additional complexity occurs in Europe in that some species of small mammals such as wood mice (*Apodemus sylvaticus*) are excellent hosts of larval *I. ricinus*, but the spirochaetes are not as infectious for these hosts as they are for bank voles (*Myodes glareolus*), which on the other hand mount a more effective immune response against feeding larval ticks [52]. The circulation in nature of the three main pathogenic *Borrelia burgdorferi* s.l. genospecies in Europe (*B. afzelii, Borrelia burgdorferi* s.s., *B. garinii*), showing their predilections for various reservoir hosts, is illustrated in Fig. 2.4.

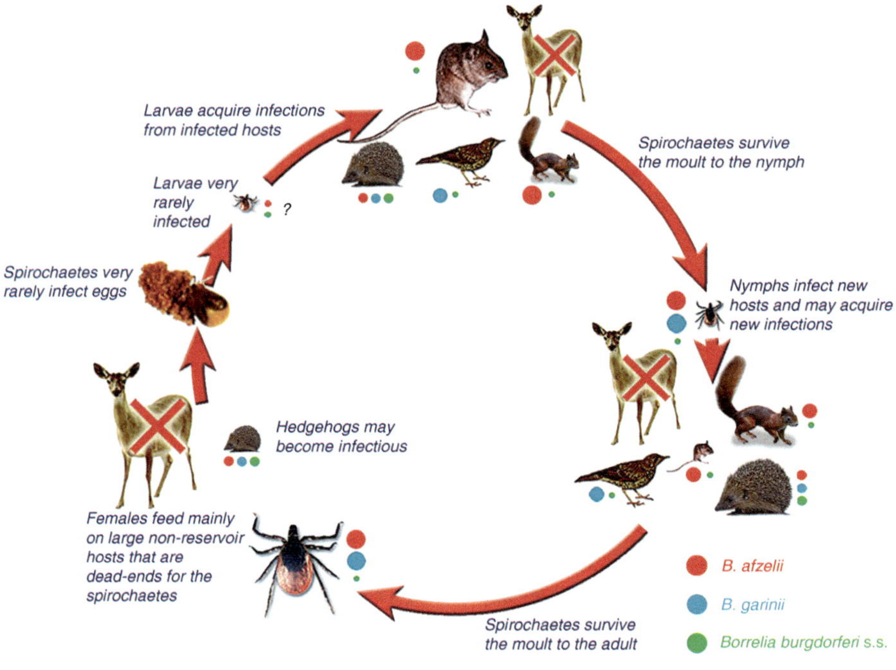

Fig. 2.4 Transmission cycle of the three main pathogenic *Borrelia burgdorferi* sensu lato genospecies in Europe. The size of coloured circles indicates the relative prevalence of the genospecies in the hosts and tick, and the size of the hosts indicates their relative significance in the tick life cycle in a typical woodland habitat. Hedgehogs are known to transmit all three genospecies, but their overall contribution to genospecies circulation is unknown

It is clear that the precise composition of the vertebrate fauna within a habitat can have a profound effect on the abundance of infected ticks, especially in relation to the relative proportions of non-reservoir hosts, such as deer, and the important spirochaete reservoir hosts such as voles, wood mice and ground-feeding passerine birds. In most habitats with high vertebrate diversity, infected tick abundance is likely to be high, but where deer occur at very high densities, tick infection rates may be low [32]. This latter situation is common on tick-infested agricultural land where sheep and cattle, which are of very limited reservoir competence, are the main hosts of all stages [53, 54].

2.9 Environmental Measures for Prevention of Lyme Borreliosis

The overall objective of environmental measures for the prevention and control of LB should be to reduce the contact rate between people and infected ticks. This may be achieved in a variety of ways, preferably in combination. They include the reduction of the abundance of ticks, reduction in the infection rate of ticks, and the management of habitats to reduce exposure of the public to ticks [55].

Since deer are acknowledged to be the most important maintenance host for tick populations in LB habitats, it would seem logical that tick abundance could be reduced by the reduction of deer densities. However, there are ethical and practical problems in such an approach and furthermore, the existence of alternative hosts such as foxes and hedgehogs, and the complexity of the dynamic relationship between deer and tick populations, discussed above, makes it difficult to predict the level of deer control required to obtain worthwhile tick control. Another factor to consider is that reduction of deer density can theoretically divert ticks to other hosts, and if these include reservoir-competent species, such as rodents, the tick infection rate and even the overall abundance of infected ticks may increase, thus increasing risk.

Host-targeted measures in the United States include self-medication systems, involving acaricides for deer and rodents, and these have been deployed commercially in peri-urban habitats [55]. Such measures have not been adopted in Europe, where recreational rather than peri-urban habitats pose the main risk to the public [56] and where ethical and environmental obstacles arise.

Similarly, while area applications of acaricides, particularly in domestic situations, are quite common in the United States, such services are not on offer in Europe [55]. Less environmentally damaging options include dissemination of spores of the fungal entomological pathogen, *Metarhizium anisopliae*, and deployment of parasitic wasps (*Ixodiphagus hookeri*) and entomopathogenic nematodes, but so far, such approaches have been limited by scale and expense. Targeting the spirochaetes within their rodent hosts, with antibiotics or vaccines, has not got beyond experimental stages [55].

Reducing tick habitat by disrupting the humid microhabitat of the non-parasitic tick phases is effective and has long been utilised on agricultural land in Europe, but such habitats are rarely significant for LB transmission, because of the relative scarcity of LB reservoir hosts. However, such an approach has some utility in gardens and peri-urban habitats [55]. Measures designed to reduce contact between ticks and the public include mowing the edges of pathways, removal of leaf litter, and erection of barriers. This last measure is most appropriate for residential properties, small recreational areas and campsites, and usually consists of deer-proof fencing, sometimes combined with borders of materials, such as yellow cedar sawdust that discourage crawling ticks [57].

No single preventive measure has been shown to reduce cases of LB, though several have shown promise. While it is acknowledged that eradication of LB vectors is not possible, suppression of infected-tick abundance and consequently of case incidence could theoretically be achieved by the adoption of an integrated approach. However, an acceptable level of infected-tick density is difficult to determine and depends on risk perceptions by public health authorities and the human population utilizing a particular habitat [58]. Most other LB preventive measures depend on education of the public, particularly concerning personal protection. However, as pointed out by Beaujean et al. [59] in Europe, uptake of recommended measures for implementation by the public is poor, and in the United States, it is variable and of undetermined overall effectiveness [55]. It is clear that more research is required on the technical aspects of integrated pest management as applied to the vectors of LB and also on the promotion of awareness and preventive behaviour among the public, particularly with the continuing absence of a widely acceptable vaccine.

Acknowledgments We are very grateful to Bernard Kaye (UCD School of Agriculture, University College Dublin, Ireland) for creating Figs. 2.1 and 2.4.

Disclosures O. Kahl is an unpaid member of the ESGBOR steering committee, the ESCMID study group for Lyme borreliosis.

References

1. Piesman J. Ecology of *Borrelia burgdorferi* sensu lato in North America. In: Gray JS, Kahl O, Lane RS, Stanek G, editors. Lyme Borreliosis: biology, epidemiology and control. Wallingford/Oxon: CAB international; 2002. p. 347.
2. Arsnoe I, Tsao JI, Hickling GJ. Nymphal *Ixodes scapularis* questing behavior explains geographic variation in Lyme borreliosis risk in the eastern United States. Ticks Tick Borne Dis. 2019;10:553–63.
3. Ogden NH, Artsob H, Margos G, Tsao J. Non-rickettsial tick-borne bacteria and the diseases they cause. In: Sonenshine DE, Roe RM, editors. Biology of ticks, vol. 2. 2nd ed. New York: Oxford University Press; 2014. p. 278–312.
4. Kheisin BN, Lawrenenko LE. Duration of bloodsucking and diurnal rhythm of nutrition and dropping of females of *Ixodes ricinus* L. Zool Zh. 1956;35:379–83. engl. translation by NAMRU-3
5. Kahl O, Janetzki-Mittmann C, Gray JS, Jonas R, Stein J, de Boer R. Risk of infection with *Borrelia burgdorferi* sensu lato for a host in relation to the duration of nymphal *Ixodes ricinus* feeding and the method of tick removal. Zentralbl Bakteriol. 1998;287:41–52.
6. Eisen L. Pathogen transmission in relation to duration of attachment by *Ixodes scapularis* ticks. Ticks Tick Borne Dis. 2018;9:535–42.
7. Kahl O. Investigations on the water balance of ticks (Acari, Ixodoidea) in the course of their postembryonic development with special reference to active water vapour uptake in the engorged phases. PhD Thesis. Germany: Free University of Berlin; 1989. pp. 356, in German.
8. Lees AD. The water balance in *Ixodes ricinus* L. and certain other species of ticks. Parasitology. 1946;37:1–20.
9. Kahl O, Knülle W. Water vapour uptake from subsaturated atmospheres by engorged immature ixodid ticks. Exp Appl Acarol. 1988;4:73–83.
10. Gaede K, Knülle W. On the mechanism of water vapour sorption from unsaturated atmospheres by ticks. J Exp Biol. 1997;200:1491–8.
11. Gray JS, Kahl O, Lane RS, Levin ML, Tsao JI. Diapause in ticks of the medically important *Ixodes ricinus* species complex. Ticks Tick Borne Dis. 2016;7:992–1003.
12. Babenko LV, Rubina MA. Patterns of development of the taiga tick in the vicinity of Kremenchug station. In: Pospelova-Shtrom MV, Rashina MG, editors. Problems of epidemiology of tick-borne encephalitis and biological patterns in its natural focus. Moscow: Meditsina; 1968. p. 138–68. (in Russian).
13. Kachanko NI. Development of ixodid ticks in the northern limits of their geographic range in Amur Province. Parazitologiia. 1978;20:218–25. (in Russian)

14. Daniels TJ, Falco RC, Curran KL, Fish D. Timing of *Ixodes scapularis* (Acari: Ixodidae) oviposition and larval activity in southern New York. J Med Entomol. 1996;33:140–7.
15. Padgett KA. Lane RS life cycle of *Ixodes pacificus* (Acari: Ixodidae): timing of developmental processes under field and laboratory conditions. J Med Entomol. 2001;38:684–93.
16. Gray JS. The development and seasonal activity of the tick, *Ixodes ricinus*: a vector of Lyme borreliosis. Rev Med Vet Entomol. 1991;79:323–33.
17. Dautel H, Dippel C, Kämmer D, Werkhausen A, Kahl O. Winter activity of *Ixodes ricinus* in a Berlin forest. Int J Med Microbiol. 2008;298(Supplement 1):50–4.
18. Yousfi-Monod R, Aeschlimann A. Studies on ticks (Acarina, Ixodidae), parasites of cattle in West Algeria. I. Systematic survey and seasonal activity. Ann Parasitol Hum Comp. 1986;61:341–58. In French
19. Vahedi-Noori N, Rahbari S, Bokaei S. The seasonal activity of *Ixodes ricinus* tick in Amol, Mazandaran Province, Northern Iran. J Arthropod Borne Dis. 2012;6:129–35.
20. Gray JS. The ecology of Lyme borreliosis vectors. Exp Appl Acarol. 1998;22:249–58.
21. Dennis DT, Hayes EB. Epidemiology of Lyme borreliosis. In: "Lyme Borreliosis: biology, epidemiology and control J.S. Gray, O. Kahl, R.S. Lane, G. Stanek. CABI, Oxford 2002, pp. 251–280.
22. Jaenson TG, Tälleklint L. Incompetence of roe deer as reservoirs of the Lyme borreliosis spirochete. J Med Entomol. 1992;29:813–7.
23. Tälleklint L, Jaenson TG. Infestation of mammals by *Ixodes ricinus* ticks (Acari: Ixodidae) in south-Central Sweden. Exp Appl Acarol. 1997;21:755–71.
24. Gilbert L, Jones LD, Hudson PJ, Gould EA, Reid HW. Role of small mammals in the persistence of Louping-ill virus: field survey and tick co-feeding studies. Med Vet Entomol. 2000;14:277–82.
25. Telford SR 3rd, Mather TN, Moore S. Incompetence of deer as reservoirs of the Lyme disease spirochete. Am J Trop Med Hyg. 1988;39:105–9.
26. LoGiudice K, Ostfeld RS, Schmidt KA, Keesing F. The ecology of infectious disease: effects of host diversity and community composition on Lyme disease risk. Proc Natl Acad Sci U S A. 2003;100:567–71.
27. Huang CI, Kay SC, Davis S, Tufts DM, Gaffett K, Tefft B, Diuk-Wasser MA. High burdens of *Ixodes scapularis* larval ticks on white-tailed deer may limit Lyme disease risk in a low biodiversity setting. Ticks Tick Borne Dis. 2019;10:258–8.
28. Dautel H, Kämmer D, Kahl O. How an extreme weather spell in winter can influence vector tick abundance and tick-borne disease incidence. In: Braks MAH, Van Wierer SE, Takken W, Sprong H, editors. Ecology and prevention of Lyme Borreliosis. Wageningen: Wageningen Academic Publishers; 2016. p. 335–50.
29. Jaenson TG, Lindgren E. The range of *Ixodes ricinus* and the risk of contracting Lyme borreliosis will increase northwards when the vegetation period becomes longer. Ticks Tick Borne Dis. 2011;2:44–9.
30. Clow KM, Leighton PA, Ogden NH, Lindsay LR, Michel P, Pearl DL, Jardine CM. Northward range expansion of *Ixodes scapularis* evident over a short timescale in Ontario. Canada PLoS One. 2017;12:e0189393.
31. Hvidsten D, Frafjord K, Gray JS, Henningsson AJ, Jenkins A, Kristiansen BE, Lager M, Rognerud B, Slåtsve AM, Stordal F, Stuen S, Wilhelmsson P. The distribution limit of the common tick, *Ixodes ricinus,* and some associated pathogens in North-Western Europe. Ticks Tick Borne Dis. 2020;11:101388.
32. Gray JS, Kahl O, Janetzki C, Stein J. Studies on the ecology of Lyme disease in a deer forest in county Galway. Ireland J Med Entomol. 1992;29:915–20.
33. Deblinger RD, Wilson ML, Rimmer DW, Spielman A. Reduced abundance of immature *Ixodes dammini* (Acari: Ixodidae) following incremental removal of deer. J Med Entomol. 1993;30:144–50.

34. Rand PW, Lubelczyk C, Holman MS, Lacombe EH, Smith RP Jr. Abundance of *Ixodes scapularis* (Acari: Ixodidae) after the complete removal of deer from an isolated offshore island, endemic for Lyme disease. J Med Entomol. 2004;41:779–84.
35. Gilbert L, Maffey GL, Ramsay SL, Hester AJ. The effect of deer management on the abundance of *Ixodes ricinus* in Scotland. Ecol Appl. 2012;22:658–67.
36. Hofmeester TR, Sprong H, Jansen PA, Prins HHT, van Wieren SE. Deer presence rather than abundance determines the population density of the sheep tick, *Ixodes ricinus*, in Dutch forests. Parasit Vectors. 2017;10:433.
37. Hansson L. Mast seeding and population dynamics of rodents: one factor is not enough. Oikos. 1998;82:591–4.
38. Jones CG, Ostfeld RS, Richard MP, Schauber EM, Wolff JO. Chain reactions linking acorns to gypsy moth outbreaks and Lyme disease risk. Science. 1998;279:1023–6.
39. Bregnard C, Rais O, Voordouw MJ. Climate and tree seed production predict the abundance of the European Lyme disease vector over a 15-year period. Parasit Vectors. 2020;13:408.
40. Gern L, Schaible UE, Simon MM. Mode of inoculation of the Lyme disease agent *Borrelia burgdorferi* influences infection and immune responses in inbred strains of mice. J Infect Dis. 1993;167:971–5.
41. Fingerle V, Goettner G, Gern L, Wilske B, Schulte-Spechtel U. Complementation of a *Borrelia afzelii* OspC mutant highlights the crucial role of OspC for dissemination of *Borrelia afzelii* in *Ixodes ricinus*. Int J Med Microbiol. 2007;297:97–107.
42. Radolf JD, Caimano MJ. The long strange trip of *Borrelia burgdorferi* outer-surface protein C. Mol Microbiol. 2008;69:1–4.
43. Richter D, Debski A, Hubalek Z, Matuschka FR. Absence of Lyme disease spirochetes in larval *Ixodes ricinus* ticks. Vector Borne Zoonotic Dis. 2012;12:21–7.
44. Rollend L, Fish D, Childs JE. Transovarial transmission of *Borrelia* spirochetes by *Ixodes scapularis*: a summary of the literature and recent observations. Ticks Tick Borne Dis. 2013;4:46–51.
45. Gern L, Rais O. Efficient transmission of *Borrelia burgdorferi* between cofeeding *Ixodes ricinus* ticks (Acari: Ixodidae). J Med Entomol. 1996;33:189–92.
46. Patrican LA. Acquisition of Lyme disease spirochetes by cofeeding *Ixodes scapularis* ticks. Am J Trop Med Hyg. 1997;57:589–93.
47. Pérez D, Kneubühler Y, Rais O, Jouda F, Gern L. *Borrelia afzelii* ospC genotype diversity in *Ixodes ricinus* questing ticks and ticks from rodents in two Lyme borreliosis endemic areas: contribution of co-feeding ticks. Ticks Tick Borne Dis. 2011;2:137–42.
48. States SL, Huang CI, Davis S, Tufts DM, Diuk-Wasser MA. Co-feeding transmission facilitates strain coexistence in *Borrelia burgdorferi*, the Lyme disease agent. Epidemics. 2017;19:33–42.
49. Kurtenbach K, De Michelis S, Etti S, Schäfer SM, Sewell HS, Brade V, Kraiczy P. Host association of *Borrelia burgdorferi* sensu lato - the key role of host complement. Trends Microbiol. 2002;10:74–9.
50. Richter D, Schlee DB, Matuschka FR. Reservoir competence of various rodents for the Lyme disease spirochete *Borrelia spielmanii*. Appl Environ Microbiol. 2011;77:3565–70.
51. Johnson TL, Graham CB, Hojgaard A, Breuner NE, Maes SE, Boegler KA, Replogle AJ, Kingry LC, Petersen JM, Eisen L, Eisen RJ. Isolation of the Lyme disease spirochete *Borrelia mayonii* from naturally infected rodents in Minnesota. J Med Entomol. 2017;54:1088–92.
52. Kurtenbach K, Kampen H, Dizij A, Arndt S, Seitz HM, Schaible UE, Simon MM. Infestation of rodents with larval *Ixodes ricinus* (Acari: Ixodidae) is an important factor in the transmission cycle of *Borrelia burgdorferi* s.l. in German woodlands. J Med Entomol. 1995;32:807–17.
53. Gray JS, Kahl O, Janetzki C, Stein J, Guy E. The spatial distribution of *Borrelia burgdorferi*-infected *Ixodes ricinus* in the Connemara region of county Galway. Ireland Exp Appl Acarol. 1995;19:163–72.
54. Matuschka FR, Heiler M, Eiffert H, Fischer P, Lotter H, Spielman A. Diversionary role of hoofed game in the transmission of Lyme disease spirochetes. Am J Trop Med Hyg. 1993;48:693–9.

55. Eisen L, Gray JS. Lyme borreliosis prevention strategies: United States versus Europe. In: Braks MAH, Van Wierer SE, Takken W, Sprong H, editors. Ecology and prevention of Lyme Borreliosis. Wageningen: Wageningen Academic Publishers; 2016. p. 429–50.
56. Gray JS, Kahl O, Robertson JN, Daniel M, Estrada-Peña A, Gettinby G, Jaenson TG, Jensen P, Jongejan F, Korenberg E, Kurtenbach K, Zeman P. Lyme borreliosis habitat assessment. Zentralbl Bakteriol. 1998;287:211–28.
57. Piesman J. Response of nymphal *Ixodes scapularis*, the primary tick vector of Lyme disease spirochetes in North America, to barriers derived from wood products or related home and garden items. J Vector Ecol. 2006;31:412–7.
58. Aenishaenslin C, Michel P, Ravel A, Gern L, Waaub JP, Milord F, Bélanger D. Acceptability of tick control interventions to prevent Lyme disease in Switzerland and Canada: a mixed-method study. BMC Public Health. 2016;16:12.
59. Beaujean DJ, Bults M, van Steenbergen JE, Voeten HA. Study on public perceptions and protective behaviors regarding Lyme disease among the general public in the Netherlands: implications for prevention programs. BMC Public Health. 2013;13:225.
60. Balashov YS. Blood sucking ticks (Ixodoidea), vectors of diseases of man, and animals. Misc Publ Entomol Soc Am. 1972;8:161–376.

Pathogenesis and Immune Defense

3

Catherine Brissette and Peter Kraiczy

3.1 Introduction

Like other zoonotic pathogens affecting humans, Lyme disease (LD) spirochetes belonging to the *Borrelia burgdorferi* sensu lato [s.l.] complex primarily alternate in nature between arthropods and diverse vertebrates while humans are incidental and dead-end hosts [1]. LD spirochetes are capable of persistently infecting multiple tissues resulting in disease progression over months and years if the infection is not appropriately treated with antibiotics. In contrast to other extracellular pathogens, *Borrelia* do not produce their own toxins or proteases for invading deeper tissues and organs. Thus, the pathobiology of LD spirochetes is certainly complex and involves an arsenal of host-acquiring factors and virulence determinants that allows *Borrelia* to perfectly adapt to different environments they encounter and to survive in their hosts despite the expanded inflammatory reactions they cause, in particular in the human host. *Borrelia* reside exclusively inside their hosts are incapable of living in an external environment and become pathogenic when infecting humans. The route of infection involves a number of key steps described in more detail below including (1) the transmission of the pathogen during feeding of an infected tick, (2) adaptation to the human host, (3) dissemination and hematogenous spread of spirochetes, (4) tissue colonization, and (5) establishment of organ-specific manifestations (reviewed in [2]). A simplified view of the complex scenario of a *Borrelia*-induced infection in the human host is demonstrated in Fig. 3.1.

C. Brissette
Department of Biomedical Sciences, School of Medicine and Health Sciences,
University of North Dakota, Grand Forks, ND, USA
e-mail: catherine.brissette@und.edu

P. Kraiczy (✉)
Institute of Medical Microbiology and Infection Control, University Hospital Frankfurt,
Goethe University Frankfurt, Frankfurt, Germany
e-mail: Kraiczy@uni-frankfurt.de

K.-P. Hunfeld, J. Gray (eds.), *Lyme Borreliosis*,
https://doi.org/10.1007/978-3-030-93680-8_3

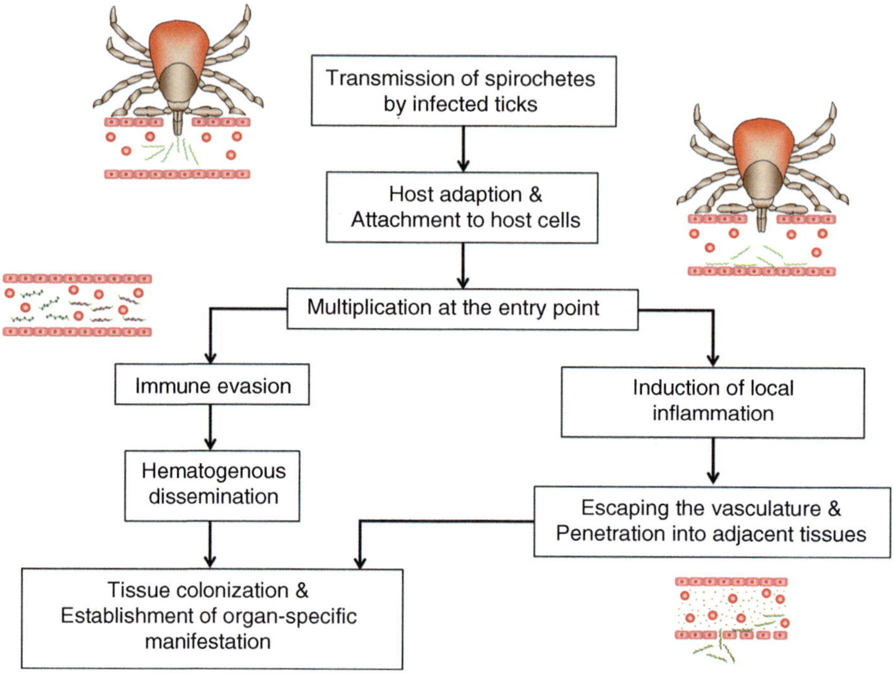

Fig. 3.1 Schematic overview of the infection routes of *Borrelia burgdorferi* s.l. infection in the mammalian host

The infection is always accomplished by the transmission of spirochetes during feeding of an infected tick on the human host that is accompanied by dramatic changes in bacterial gene expression preparing the incoming pathogens to immediately adapt to the host environment. LD spirochetes are also protected by a cocktail of salivary factors from the tick, consisting of immunomodulatory, immunosuppressive, vasodilatory, and complement-inhibitory proteins that are simultaneously injected into the dermis to prevent tick recognition by the human immune system (reviewed in [3–5]. A well-studied example is the interaction of the *Borrelia*-derived OspC (Outer surface protein C) protein with the tick Salp15 protein known to facilitate colonization of LD spirochetes in the murine host [6, 7]. Confronted with the host defense system, LD spirochetes have to develop different means of adapting to the new microenvironment and to combat innate immunity. In the initial phase of infection, upregulation of genes encoding for a range of surface-exposed determinants, all of which play a central role in host adaptation and tissue colonization, takes place including adhesins and proteins that interact with extracellular matrix components (see Sect. 3.2.1). Once adapted to the host, *Borrelia* cells multiply in the dermis and induce strong inflammatory responses (see Sects. 3.3.1.3 and 3.3.1.4) by moving away from the port of entry to distant sites often resulting initially in a circular red rash with central clearing also described as erythema migrans. At this stage of infection, motility plays a major role in the dissemination of LD spirochetes to distant tissues or organs [8]. Interaction with the host vasculature and transmigration through the endothelium by an intercellular (between junctions of neighboring cells) or intracellular (traversing the endothelial cells) route [9, 10] allows the spreading spirochetes to leave the bloodstream and penetrate deep into connective tissues and reach compartments known as immunoprivileged sites, where they are protected from the destructive properties of the host innate immune system. Particularly, the avascular connective tissue appears to be not very well penetrated by complement, phagocytes, antibodies, or antibiotics.

Like other blood-borne pathogens, LD spirochetes employ elaborate strategies to hide, combat, inhibit, or overcome the innate and adaptive immunity of the human host and thereby avoid clearance by the immune system, e.g., by changing their surface composition (antigenic variation) or by preventing complement activation (CRASP proteins or the production of a slime layer) (reviewed in [11–15]). The major factors involved in immune evasion are described in more detail in Sect. 3.2.3 and summarized in Table 3.1.

Table 3.1 Outer surface proteins involved in the pathogenesis of *Borrelia burdorferi* s.l. infection of humans

Description	Synonym	*Borrelia* species	Function[a]	Role in pathogenesis
BBK32		Bb	Binding to fibronectin, GAG, C1r	Adherence Immune evasion (Termination of CP)
BAD16		Ba	Binding to C1r	Termination of CP
BGD19		Bg	Binding to C1r	Termination of CP (reduced complement-inhibitory capacity)
DbpA/DbpB		Bb, Ba,	Binding to decorin, dermatan sulfate	Adherence
Bgp		Bb	Binding to glycosamino-glycans (GAGs)	Adherence
P66		Bb	Porin, Binding to $\alpha_{IIb}\beta_3$ and $\alpha_V\beta_3$ integrin	Adherence Establishment of infection (mice)
RevA		Bb	Binding to fibronectin	Adherence
RevB		Bb	Binding to fribronectin	Adherence
ErpX		Bb	Binding to laminin	Adherence
BmpA		Bb	Binding to laminin	Adherence Potential role in arthritis (mice)
BB0406		Bb, Ba, Bg, Bba	Binding to laminin	Adherence Establishment of infection (mice)
BB0347		Bb	Binding to fibronectin	Adherence

(continued)

Table 3.1 (continued)

Description	Synonym	*Borrelia* species	Function[a]	Role in pathogenesis
OspC		Bb, Ba, Bg	Binding of plasminogen Binding to fibronectin Restricted binding to dermatan sulfate	Adherence Host adaption and tissue tropism, immune evasion (Termination of the CP and LP) Inter and intra species-specific variation
VlsE		Bb	Antigenic variation	Immune evasion Establishment of infection
CspA	CRASP-1, BbCRASP-1, BBA68, ZS7.A68, FHBP	Bb, Ba, Bs, Bm	Binding of FH, FHL-1, C7, C8, C9, TCC, plasminogen, collagen, fibronectin	Immune evasion (Termination of AP and TP) Adherence Host specificity
CspZ	CRASP-2 BbCRASP-2 BBH06	Bb	Binding of FH, FHL-1, plasminogen, laminin, collagen, fibronectin	Immune evasion (Termination of AP) Adherence Host specificity
ErpA	CRASP-3, BbCRASP-3, BBN38	Bb	Binding of FH, FHR-1, FHR-2, FHR-5, plasminogen	Immune evasion (Termination AP)[b]
ErpC	CRASP-4, BbCRASP-4	Bb	Binding of FH, FHR-1, FHR-2, plasminogen	Immune evasion (Termination AP)[b] Adherence[b]
ErpP	CRASP-5, BbCRASP-5, ErpI, ErpN, BBP38, BBL39, OspE	Bb	Binding of FH, FHR-1, FHR-2, FHR-5, plasminogen	Immune evasion (Termination AP)[b]
Erp ortholog	Erp63	Bs	Binding of FH, FHR-1, plasminogen	Immune evasion (Termination AP)[b]
BGA66		Bba	Binding of C7, C8, C9, TCC	Immune evasion (Termination of TP)
BGA71		Bba	Binding of C7, C8, C9, TCC	Immune evasion (Termination of TP)
pncA		Bb		Infectivity

Abbreviations: *CRASP* complement-regulator acquiring surface protein, *Erp* OspE/F-like protein, *Dbp* decorin-binding protein, *Bmp Borrelia* membrane protein, *Bb B. burgdorferi*, *Bba B. bavariensis*, *Ba B. afzelii*, *Bs B. spielmanii*, *Bg B. garinii*, *Bm B. mayonii*, *FH* Factor H, *FHL* factor H-like protein, *FHR* FH-related protein, *TCC* terminal complement complex, *GAG* glycosaminoglycan, *AP* alternative pathway, *CP* classical pathway, *LP* lectin pathway, *TP* terminal pathway, *pncA* plasmid-encoded nicotinamidase

[a]Proteins mentioned in the table are of human origins (proteins of animal sources have been excluded due to simplification)

[b]The indicated function of the respective protein and the relevance for pathogenesis is unclear

It has been shown that LD spirochetes are able to colonize collagenous tissues and survive in multiple organs for at least 1 year of experimentally infected mice suggesting that similar mechanisms of persistence might also occur in patients with a late manifestation such as acrodermatitis chronica atrophicans, even though these patients with late manifestations elicit robust antibody responses to the pathogen. It is thought that the spirochetes "hide in plain sight" as concluded by Cabello et al. [16] in protective niches but the exact mechanism(s) of persistence and the prolonged survival in a minority of patients is far from being completely understood and warrants further clinical investigations. The genetic disposition of patients with late or chronic manifestations might also play a critical role in the establishment and the development of the disease, as in patients with antibiotic-refractory arthritis who carry the HLA-DRB1*04 and HLA-DRB1*0101 alleles [17]. How *Borrelia* as an obligate extracellular pathogen can persist in the human host is an unsolved mystery, and the stage of latency might be explained in part by the fact that this pathogen is shielded by host-acquired proteins or by changing its surface to diminish recognition by the host immune system.

The aim of this chapter is to provide an understanding of the molecular mechanisms and the determinants, factors, and molecules known to participate in the central steps of a spirochetal infection, as well as the dynamics of the host responses provoked during an infection with *B. burgdorferi* s.l. It would be overambitious to attempt to describe all the findings that have emerged within the last decades of intensive research and have led to our understanding of the fundamental aspects of pathobiology of LD. Nevertheless, this chapter will focus on the most widely studied factors known to participate in the major steps of infection, namely host adaptation, tissue colonization, dissemination, immune evasion, persistence, and host response. References provided will direct the readers to the original literature and state-of-the-art review articles.

3.2 Pathogenesis

3.2.1 Factors Involved in Host Adaptation and Tissue Colonization of *B. burgdorferi* s.l.

LD spirochetes elicit a robust humoral immune response that is critical for controlling infection [18, 19]. However, *B. burgdorferi* s.l. are quite adept at evading the host humoral response, primarily through variation of surface-exposed proteins. Lyme disease spirochetes utilize diverse strategies, e.g., antigenic variation, immune evasion, sequestration, penetrating immune-protective niches, motility, chemotaxis as well as modulation of outer surface proteins influenced by an environmental-induced gene expression at different time points in the infectious cycle to outmaneuver the hostile immune system. These traits combine to form an efficient strategy utilized by LD spirochetes to adapt to and to successfully survive in the human host for a prolonged time despite eliciting robust antibody and cellular responses. Owing to the limited space, the most prominent mechanisms and the factors participating in these processes are described in more detail below and summarized in Table 3.1.

Shortly after transmission to the human host, *B. burgdorferi* s.l. either attach to the dense extracellular matrix of multiple host tissues or disseminate hematogenously by the dynamics of blood circulation to distant tissues and organs [9, 10]. The ability of spirochetes to adhere to and to colonize different tissues is a key step for establishing an initial or later on a chronic infection.

To exit the bloodstream/vasculature following colonization, spirochetes produce an arsenal of surface-exposed proteins displaying adhesive functions [11, 20, 21] or that bind to cell receptors following induction of specific signals for internalization (reviewed by [22]). Numerous factors involved in tissue adhesion and in binding to extracellular matrix components such as collagen, fibronectin, laminin, decorin, integrins, and glycosaminoglycans have predominantly been described for *B. burgdorferi,* including well-characterized outer surface proteins such as BBK32, DbpA, DbpB, OspC, p66, RevA, RevB, Bgp, CspA, CspZ, BB0347, ErpX, and BB0406 [2, 11, 23] (see Table 3.1). Several adhesins possess multifunctional properties, e.g., to circumvent innate immunity and therefore display redundant roles in the pathobiology of Lyme borreliosis. Reflecting the attribute of *B. burgdorferi* sensu stricto (henceforward *B. burgdorferi*) to colonize specific tissues, certain adhesins, e.g., BBK32, DbpA, and DbpB selectively bind to diverse glycosaminoglycans (GAGs) produced by different cell types [22, 24] leading to the assumption of a tissue-specific tropism of *B. burgdorferi*. Furthermore, variable expression of multiple GAG-binding adhesins might also account for a species-specific as well as strain-specific attachment to different mammalian cells [25]. The characteristics of the above-mentioned proteins are described in more detail in the following subsections.

3.2.1.1 The GAG-Binding and Complement-Targeting Surface Protein BBK32

BBK32, a 47 kDa outer surface protein encoded on linear plasmid 36 (lp36), binds the glycosaminoglycans heparin sulfate and dermatan sulfate, in addition to fibronectin [26–28]. BBK32 has sequence similarities with fibronectin-binding adhesins of Gram-positive pathogens such as *Staphylococcus aureus* and the streptococci [29, 30]. BBK32 deletion mutants demonstrate a slight, but significant, defect in infectivity in the mouse [31–33], and demonstrate that this adhesin is important in the earlier stages of infection and contributes to colonization of the joints [28]. BBK32 plays an important role in the adhesion to the vasculature [34] and possesses complement-inhibitory activity [35, 36]. This multifunctional protein specifically terminates the activation of the classical pathway by interacting with complement component C1r of the initiated C1q complex [35]. Similar complement inhibitory potential on the classical pathway has also been elucidated for the BBK32 orthologous proteins BAD16 of *B. afzelii* and BGD19 of *B. garinii* but the latter appears to display a reduced inhibitory activity compared to BBK32 of *B. burgdorferi* and BAD16 [36]. Consistent with its main function as an adhesin, BBK32 expression is induced during tick feeding and is continuously produced in the mammalian host [37, 38].

3.2.1.2 The Decorin-Binding Proteins DbpA and DbpB

Decorin is a small leucine-rich proteoglycan that associates with collagen; it possesses a collagen-binding core protein and single GAG chain, either dermatan sulfate or chondroitin-6 sulfate [39–41]. *B. burgdorferi* has two decorin-binding proteins that recognize decorin and other proteoglycans with GAG chains [24, 42–44]. The genes encoding decorin-binding proteins A and B (*dbpA/B*) are composed in a bicistronic operon on lp54. Both proteins are exposed to the spirochetal surface and differ in their specificity to bind to decorin. Compared to DbpB (18-kDa), DbpA (20-kDa) binds to decorin with more affinity, suggesting that while DbpA primarily mediates attachment of spirochetes to the ECM, both adhesins are required for optimal binding of decorin [42, 43]. Mutants deficient in decorin-binding proteins are still infectious; however, *dbpA/B* deficient bacteria are impaired in both colonization of various tissues and in persistent infection [45–48]. Decorin-deficient mice are resistant to *B. burgdorferi* infection, exhibiting fewer bacteria in joints upon infection as well as less severe arthritis than that induced in wild-type mice [49]. These data highlight the importance of decorin interactions to the establishment of disseminated infections by *B. burgdorferi*. Despite a strong allelic variation among DbpA and DbpB among the pathogenic genospecies, all these proteins display GAG-binding activity [44, 50]. Moreover, borrelial strains exhibiting different GAG-binding specificities are able to bind to different cell types indicating that *Borrelia* produce diverse GAG-binding adhesins for colonization of particular cells/organs (tissue tropism) [24, 51]. By comparative sequence analysis, five major groups of DbpA proteins have been delineated, of which DbpA orthologs comprising groups I to IV were used as valuable discriminating antigens for the serodiagnosis of Lyme disease and have been thought to serve as promising antigens for vaccine development [52].

3.2.1.3 The Glycosaminoglycan-Binding Protein Bgp

In addition to DbpA, DbpB, and BBK32, Bgp was the first described binding adhesin of *B. burgdorferi* and is a 5′ methylthioadenosine/S-adenosyl homocysteine nucleosidase [53, 54]. This secreted protein exhibits binding specificities to GAG but in the absence of other adhesins, Bgp does not promote attachment of spirochetes to eukaryotic cells [55] making its adhesive function in vivo highly questionable.

3.2.1.4 The Pore-Forming and Integrin-Binding Protein P66

The 66-kDa P66 or Oms66 protein is unique among the genus *Borrelia* and was initially identified as a ligand for β_3 integrins ($\alpha_{IIb}\beta_3$ integrin) [56, 57]. In vivo studies showed that integrin binding mediated by P66 is important for vascular transmigration and an efficient dissemination of spirochetes in infected mice [58, 59]. In addition, the P66 protein also serves as an adhesin for endothelial cells [60]. Structural and functional analyses revealed that P66 is an outer membrane-spanning protein that functions as a porin of *B. burgdorferi* [61]. Although P66 of *B. burgdorferi* elicits a robust immune response in humans directed against the surface-exposed domain, sera collected from patients with early disseminated and persistent Lyme borreliosis failed to recognize orthologs of *B. afzelii* and *B. garinii* [62] suggesting that P66 is not an appropriate serologic candidate for an in vitro diagnostic test for Lyme disease and a second-generation vaccine.

3.2.1.5 The Fibronectin-Binding Proteins RevA and RevB

RevA is a surface protein encoded on the circular plasmid 32 (cp32) family of plasmids of many, but not all, Lyme disease borreliae. RevB is encoded on cp9 and shares 28% overall amino acid sequence identity with RevA. This plasmid is missing from many infectious Lyme disease spirochetes, and its biological significance is uncertain. Both RevA and RevB were shown to bind fibronectin in vitro [63]. RevA has the potential to play an important role in disease. Its expression is upregulated in the mammal compared to the tick vector and its expression pattern and surface exposure suggest a potential role in *B. burgdorferi* pathogenesis [63–66]. Patients with various manifestations of Lyme disease, including patients with erythema migrans, make antibodies to this protein [67]. Studies in mice demonstrated that *revA* mutants are deficient in colonization of the heart, suggesting this protein may play a role in tissue tropism [68]. In addition, the absence of RevA induces more severe joint pathology and inflammation [68].

3.2.1.6 The Laminin-Binding Proteins ErpX, BmpA, and BB0406

Laminin is a glycoprotein component of the ECM that serves a scaffolding function [69]. The outer surface protein ErpX binds laminin [70] through a unstructured hydrophilic domain. The biological significance of this protein is largely unknown but more recently it has been hypothesized that ErpX along with other Erp proteins, e.g., ErpL and ErpY might be a target for a second-generation vaccine employing a proteomic-conducted approach of the interactome of human and borrelial proteins [71].

BmpA (*Borrelia* membrane protein A) originally described as P39 antigen [72] as well as the three paralogous proteins BmpB, BmpC, and BmpD exhibit a restricted binding property to mammalian laminin but did not bind to type I or type IV collagens or fibronectin [73]. The *bmpA* gene is located on the main chromosome of *B. burgdorferi* and forms a gene cluster together with the three paralogous genes *bmpB*, *bmpC*, and *bmpD*. Although BmpA and BmpB are co-transcribed, BmpA appears to be expressed in higher amounts [7]. In addition, borrelial cells lacking the BmpA or BmpB encoding gene are unable to persist in the murine joint tissue suggesting that these proteins play an important role in maintaining mammalian infection [74]. Of note, humans frequently produce a robust immune response to this particular antigen in the early course of infection, and thus, BmpA along with OspC and the FlaB protein was used as a marker for the recommended two-tiered IgM testing of acute or early Lyme disease [75, 76].

Recently, a novel laminin-binding protein, BB0406 has been identified that is capable of supporting spirochete colonization and survival in the mammalian host by interacting with extracellular matrix components [77]. The chromosomally encoded *bb0406* gene is co-transcribed with the *bb0404* and *bb0405* genes all of which are grouped in the same paralogous gene family. BB0405 and BB0406 are also highly conserved paralogous proteins in other human pathogenic species such as *B. garinii, B. bavariensis,* and *B. afzelii* as well as being immunogenic during mammalian infection [78]. Antibodies specific for BB0405 and BB0406 elicited during murine infection possess a high borreliacidal activity of >95% [78].

3.2.2 Factors Involved in Dissemination and Persistence of *B. burgdorferi*

3.2.2.1 OspC, a Multi-Functional Protein Involved in Early Dissemination

OspC has diverse roles, many of which are essential for transmission from *Ixodes* ticks and establishing infection in the mammalian host. The timing of OspC expression is incredibly important for the whole life cycle of *Borrelia* and its survival in different hosts: the *ospC* gene is upregulated during the early stages of infection and downregulated after infection has been established [79, 80]. Importantly, the expression of OspC is lost rapidly after infection due to the development of bactericidal antibodies generated against this antigen and thus, a constitutive expression of the protein prevents the persistence of the bacterium. Conversely, deletion or overexpression of *ospC* results in a rapid clearance of spirochetes from the murine host [81–83]. However, unlike VlsE, each OspC is present as a single-copy locus; therefore, any genetic variation is seen at the population level. That is, excluding random mutation or horizontal gene transfer events, a single spirochete cannot produce different OspC types in situ.

More recently, it has been shown that inter- and intraspecies variations of the OspC protein contribute to strain-specific differences in binding to diverse extracellular matrix components, in particular fibronectin and dermatan sulfate [84]. Sequence variations of OspC enable *B. burgdorferi* to colonize diverse tissues including the skin, heart, bladder, and the joints, whereas OspC of *B. garinii* was incapable of binding dermatan sulfate and also did not promote joint colonization. These findings underpin the role of OspC in adherence, tissue tropism, and higher invasiveness observed for certain *Borrelia* strains. OspC functions as an immune-evasion molecule through several different mechanisms. It protects *B. burgdorferi* from antibody-mediated killing by binding Salp15, a tick salivary protein [7] at the very early steps of infection and also prevents phagocytosis by macrophages [85] and binds host complement component C4b [86]. Binding to C4b and inhibition of the classical and lectin pathway appears to be important for short-term bloodstream survival of *B. burgdorferi* [86]. Finally, OspC also binds plasminogen from the host, which can be activated to form active protease plasmin and can help facilitate the dissemination of the bacterium [87]. The multifunctional nature of OspC is not unusual in *B. burgdorferi*; with a limited genome, the bacterium has myriad outer surface proteins that harbor more than one binding partner or function. The combined effect of the multi-interacting properties of OspC finally leads to immune evasion of spirochetes. It is worth noting that different OspC types are correlated with a strain's ability to establish infection in different vertebrate hosts [88, 89], thus influencing the range of animals *B. burgdorferi* is able to infect in nature. In addition, OspC proteins serve as important serological markers for the detection of early and early-disseminated manifestation of Lyme disease.

3.2.2.2 Host-Derived Factors Involved in Dissemination of *B. burgdorferi*

Invasion of deeper tissues depends on the pathogen ability to secrete proteases for degradation of the extracellular matrix, the most important structural component of connective tissues. This fibrous network is composed of different molecules including collagen, decorin, laminin, and fibronectin. In contrast to other invading pathogens such as Gram-positive *Staphylococcus aureus* or *Streptococcus pyogenes*, *B. burgdorferi* completely lacks proteolytic proteins capable of degrading extracellular matrix components. To overcome the obvious limitations for penetrating host barriers, *B. burgdorferi* utilizes host-derived proteases by producing a number of plasmin(ogen)-binding proteins (for review see [2, 11]) or induces the expression of different matrix metalloproteinases (MMPs) [90–95]. Recruitment of serum-derived plasminogen from the circulation and subsequent activation of surface-bound plasmin would allow *B. burgdorferi* to traverse the endothelial layers of the vasculature and break down extracellular matrix components to escape host adaptive immunity and to reside in a protective environment [16, 96]. Plasmin is an unspecific serine protease displaying broad-spectrum enzymatic activity and degrades laminin (12), fibronectin (13), vitronectin (14,15), heparan sulfate proteoglycans (16) as well as elastin and is able to inactivate complement components C3 and C5 [97, 98]. It is noteworthy that plasmin also plays an important role in the activation of diverse MMPs including MMP-1, -3, -9, and -13, synthesized as inactive proenzymes by macrophages [97]. In vivo studies with plasminogen-deficient mice revealed that plasmin is necessary for an efficient migration of spirochetes from the tick midgut to the salivary glands and for the establishment of a higher spirochetemia in mice [99]. Certainly, plasmin did not influence the dissemination of *B. burgdorferi* to distant sites suggesting that other matrix-degrading proteases such as MMPs might play a role in these processes. Although multiple cell types including keratinocytes, fibroblasts, astrocytes, chondrocytes, and PBMCs respond to infection by *B. burgdorferi* by the induction of certain MMPs in vitro [91, 93, 94, 100–102], in vivo studies with knockout mice deficient in MMP-9 showed that this particular protease was not required for the dissemination of the spirochetes to distant sites [103], suggesting that other MMPs possessing similar substrate specificities might compensate for the deficiency of the respective protease. In patients with Lyme arthritis, elevated levels of MMP-1, -3, -9, and -13 could be detected in the synovial fluids and the activation of MMPs might also account for the irreparable damage of the cartilage after infection with *B. burgdorferi* in prolonged cases of Lyme borreliosis. Of note, animal studies do not completely reflect what has been seen in humans as specific MMPs are differentially induced in animals and in human tissues making it somewhat difficult to extrapolate the findings obtained in animal studies to the situation in humans.

A large number of proteins have been detected in *B. burgdorferi* that may serve as ligands for host-derived plasminogen [104]. Among these molecules, the surface-exposed proteins OspA [105], OspC [106], the 70-kDa plasminogen-binding protein BPBP [107], ErpA, ErpC, and ErpP [108, 109]; Erp63 [110]; CspA [109]; CspZ [109]; BBA70 [111] as well as the "moonlighting" cytoplasmic protein enolase [112] have been identified as ligands for the serine protease. The multifunctional properties of these proteins (see Table 3.1) enabling *B. burgdorferi* s.l. to quickly adapting to the human host, colonize specific tissue, and disseminate through the human body to infect distant organs and, thus play a crucial role in the pathogenesis of Lyme borreliosis.

3.2.3 Immune Evasion Factors of *B. burgdorferi*

3.2.3.1 Antigenic Variation and the VlsE System *of B. burgdorferi* s.l.

Antigenic variation is the mechanism by which an infectious agent such as a bacterium alters its composition of the outer surface in order to overcome a host immune response. For *B. burgdorferi* s.l., antigenic recombination of the outer surface protein VlsE is important in maintaining infection in mammals through evasion of the humoral immune response [113–119]. The Vls system can change the expressed surface antigen in situ. The Vls system is composed of approximately 16 *vls* cassettes with the exact number varying by strain, and one expression locus, *vlsE*. All of the identified *vls* cassettes are located on the same plasmid (lp28–1) in close proximity to but situated in the opposite direction of *vlsE*. Random recombination of segments of multiple *vls* cassettes, rather than recombination of an entire, single *vls* cassette, results in a novel *vls* sequence in the *vlsE* expression locus. Thus, recombination events result in thousands of unique expressed VlsE variants, all approximately 36 kDa.

VlsE is highly antigenic; in fact, diagnostic tests utilizing the "C6" peptide, a 23 amino acid segment of VlsE, are in wide use. How then does variation in this protein help borreliae evade host immune responses [120–123]? Antibodies against the C6 peptide and other invariant regions of VlsE are present in infected humans and animals, yet antibodies against these regions do not kill the Lyme disease spirochete [120]. The invariable regions of VlsE are inaccessible to host antibody, whereas the variable regions are accessible [124, 125]. Therefore, antigenic variation of the VlsE surface protein allows the bacterium to stay one step ahead of the host antibody response.

3.2.3.2 Complement Evasion and Complement Regulator-Acquiring Surface Proteins (CRASP)

It is well-known that *Borrelia* species substantially differ in their susceptibility to human serum leading to classification into three main categories based on their phenotypical appearance after serum treatment into serum-resistant, intermediate serum-resistant (or partial resistant), and serum-sensitive strains. Among Lyme disease spirochetes, *B. burgdorferi, B. afzelii, B. spielmanii, B. bavariensis, B. mayonii,* and *B. japonica* are classified as resistant to complement-mediated killing, *B. bissettiae* represents an intermediate serum-resistant phenotype, and *B. garinii, B. valaisiana,* and *B. lusitaniae* comprise the group of highly susceptible spirochetes. With the exception of *B. garinii,* known to be one of the predominant causative agents of Lyme disease in Europe, the serum susceptibility pattern of all other genospecies almost matches their pathogenicity for humans. How *B. garinii* overcome complement-mediated killing and which factors contribute to its survival in the human host is still a matter of controversy.

To overcome the first line of immune defense, in particular the human complement system, borreliae possess a number of diverse outer surface molecules, collectively termed *C*omplement *R*egulator-*A*cquiring *S*urface *P*rotein(s) or CRASP that bind complement regulators or interact with certain complement components to affect the complement system at different activation levels (Table 3.1) (reviewed in [2, 12–15, 126]). Termination of human complement mainly includes recruitment of complement regulators of the alternative pathway Factor H and Factor H-like protein 1 (FHL-1) [12, 127–129] or the complement regulator of the classical pathway, C4b-binding protein C4BP [130], and binding of complement regulatory proteins Factor H-related protein FHR-1, FHR-2, and FHR-5 [131, 132], component C1r[35], C4b [86] or components of the terminal pathway including C7, C8, and C9 [133–135]. While the C4BP-interacting borrelial protein provisionally named p43 and a CD59-like molecule found in *B. burgdorferi* has not been identified so far, all other proteins interacting with diverse complement components have been functionally characterized in in vitro studies including CspA, CspZ, ErpA, ErpC, ErpP, BGA66, BGA71, BBK32, and OspC [35, 36, 86, 131, 133–144]. An overview of the species origin and the binding and inhibitory properties of these outer surface proteins are presented in Table 3.1.

The physiological importance of CspA, CspZ, BGA66, BGA71, BBK32, OspC for complement evasion has been demonstrated by mouse and avian infection models and by using genetically modified borrelial strains producing the respective complement-interacting protein on the cell surface [35, 36, 86, 126, 133–135, 137, 141, 142, 145–148]. The role of Factor H/FHR-binding ErpA, ErpC, and ErpP proteins for complement evasion is controversial and therefore further investigations are required to confirm the participation of these in vivo-expressed molecules in immune evasion and pathogenesis of *Borrelia* [132, 140].

Although most of these proteins investigated so far have been detected in *B. burgdorferi*, orthologous proteins from *B. afzelii*, *B. spielmanii*, *B. bavariensis*, and *B. mayonii* have also been characterized (see Table 3.1) supporting the hypothesis that these human pathogenic species utilize similar or even identical mechanisms to combat the innate immune system of the human host [134, 135, 149–152]. More recent studies revealed a selective function of CspA orthologs concerning host specificity as CspA from different *Borrelia* genospecies specifically bind to Factor H from distinct hosts, allowing spirochetes to survive within the blood meal in the midgut of a feeding tick [126, 146]. Thus, host specificity of certain *Borrelia* species directly correlates with the Factor H binding capabilities of CspA variants and underpin the concept of a complement-driven, selective transmission of spirochetes to diverse mammalian hosts facilitated by a specific molecule.

3.3 Immune Defense and Host Response

3.3.1 Adaptive Immunity to *B. burgdorferi* s.l.

3.3.1.1 Role of B Cells and Antibody Responses in Lyme Disease

B. burgdorferi induces a strong antibody response, and SCID mice as well as B cell-deficient mice have high spirochete loads [19]. These data suggest that the adaptive immune system is critical for controlling the growth of *B. burgdorferi* s.l. However, *B. burgdorferi* s.l. has evolved strategies to subvert those normal immune responses and make them less effective.

For instance, while *B. burgdorferi* s.l. induces antibody production in the host, the quality of those antibodies is subpar in their specificity for *B. burgdorferi* antigens; inappropriate isotype profiles; and poor binding avidity. Thus, while antibody production is high in response to a *B. burgdorferi* s.l. infection, those antibodies are ineffective at clearing the pathogen. Variable expression of targeting antigens might also enable *B. burgdorferi* s.l. to hide and to escape the adaptive immunity of the host [96, 116, 153, 154].

Normally, antibodies undergo class switching from the initial IgM antibody isotype to the IgG form. Although class switching occurs in a *B. burgdorferi* s.l. infection, there is also a continual production of low-affinity IgM [155–157]. As an antibody response matures, the initial binding avidity of antibodies increase. However, during infection with *B. burgdorferi*, this binding avidity initially increases as expected, but then drops off [158], resulting in a population of antibodies that are less efficient at recognizing *B. burgdorferi* antigens.

Activated B cells in draining lymph nodes proliferate rapidly and form extrafollicular foci and become plasmablasts. Germinal centers consisting of B cells, CD4+ T cells, follicular dendritic cells form and are necessary for affinity maturation of antibodies and immunological memory. However, germinal centers collapse in a *B. burgdorferi* infection, along with a loss of T and B cell zones in secondary lymphoid tissues [156–159]. The end result is that long-lived memory responses are not induced, meaning that a person can become infected again and again with the Lyme disease spirochete. This lack of long-lived immunity also has particular implications for vaccine development.

3.3.1.2 Role of T Cells in Lyme Disease

Innate T cell subsets such as γδ T cells and NKT cells respond to lipoproteins or lipid antigens, respectively, whereas γδ T cells induce maturation of dendritic cells [160–162]. Activation of γδ T cells is indirect and depends on Toll-like receptor (TLR) signaling [162]. The absence of NKT cells leads to higher *B. burgdorferi* burdens [163]. Both subsets contribute to local defenses whereby the responsiveness to *Borrelia* antigens seems to be largely restricted to Vδ1 γδ T cells at least to synovial fluid-derived cells [164]. The roles of αβ T cells are less clear. The fact that SCID and rag$^{-/-}$ mice develop persistent arthritis and carditis demonstrates that adaptive immunity is critically important for disease resolution. Adoptive transfer experiments suggest that B cells and pathogen-specific antibody are necessary for control of *B. burgdorferi* and disease remission [165]. Different subsets of αβ T cells (e.g., CD4+ vs. CD8+) are recruited to sites of infection and activated, and certainly influence the disease outcome. However, the balance of local Th1/Th2 responses does not impact arthritis severity [166–169]. There may be a role for Th17 and Treg cells; balance may play a role in disease severity or resolution [170–174]. An important consideration is the expression of certain HLA (human leukocyte antigen) molecules (MHC Class II) that present antigens to T cells. Some of these HLA alleles have been associated with predisposition to more severe Lyme arthritis and other disease manifestations. HLA-DRB1*04 (DR4) is associated with refractory Lyme arthritis [175–177], while a recent study on Latvian patients found an association with the DRB1*07 allele with Lyme neuroborreliosis [178]. Patients with the HLA-DRB1*11 (DR11) allele tended to resolve their arthritis more quickly. Studies using transgenic mice showed that the DR11 allele is associated with higher titers of anti-*Borrelia* antibodies and a lower spirochete burden, while the DR4 allele mice showed a more inflammatory Th1 response [179]. These data again demonstrate the importance of adaptive immunity, particularly the B cell response, to disease resolution and control of infection.

3.3.1.3 Induction of Cytokines and Other Mediators

During the infection process, spirochetes induced a strong host response resulting in a massive release of cytokines and pro-inflammatory mediators such as TNF-α, IFN-γ, IL-1β, IL-6, IL-12, IL-17, IL-22, and GM-CSF as well as chemoattractants CXCL1, CXCL2, CXCL5, and CXCL10 in vitro and in vivo [180–185]. Induction of these pro-inflammatory cytokines is mainly attributed to the recognition of spirochetal-derived lipoproteins due to the pattern recognition receptors (PRRs) on monocytes or macrophages, in particular Toll-like receptor 2 (TLR2) and the nucleotide-binding oligomerization domain 2 (NOD2) [185–188]. Although paradoxically, different cell types or tissues including synovia, skin, lymph node cells, splenocytes, glial cells, macrophages, lymphocytes, and dendritic cells elicit the anti-inflammatory cytokine, IL-10 in response to stimulation by live, heat-inactivated, or cell lysates of spirochetes [184, 189, 190]. A proteome-conducted analysis revealed that *Borrelia*-induced stimulation of IL-10 simultaneously modulates pro-inflammatory responses of TNF-α, IFN-γ, IL-1β, IL-6, IL-12, IL-18, CCL2, CCL4, and G-CSF in order to control inflammation [191, 192]. It has been thought that spirochetes control the inflammatory process they themselves induced by stimulation of IL-10 production and thereby impair the burden of infection and the outcome of the disease [193]. The inflammatory response/process to a *Borrelia* infection in vitro most likely mirrors what can be seen in skin lesions of patients with erythema migrans, synovial fluid of Lyme arthritis patients, or inflammation in the CNS of patients with neuroborreliosis. Apparently, IL-6 and IFN-γ are the dominant cytokines released by certain cell types in response to a borrelial infection.

3.3.1.4 Recognition of *Borrelia* by Human Host Cells

Recognition of spirochetes by the host innate immune system plays a critical role at the very early stage of the infection to eliminate the bacteria from the blood/circulation and infected tissues [18, 194, 195]. It has been shown that *Borrelia* are recognized by diverse cell types of the innate immune system including monocytes, macrophages, dendritic cells, polymorphonuclear cells (PMNs), natural killer cells (NK-cells), and NK-T cells mainly via Toll-like receptors (TLR) activated through specific pathogen-associated molecular patterns (PAMPS) that are released, e.g., during phagocytosis (reviewed in [196, 197]). The interplay between microbial PAMPS and TLRs is accompanied by the induction of specific inflammatory signaling pathways resulting in the release of various cytokines (see Sect. 3.3.1.4) (Fig. 3.2). Among TLRs, heterodimeric complexes formed by TLR1 and TLR2 are activated by borrelial lipoproteins, while TLR7 and TLR8 play a central role in the recognition of ssRNA and dsDNA, and TLR5 acts as a receptor for flagellin. Of note, lipoprotein-mediated stimulation of TLR2 causes downregulation of TLR5 indicating that diverse stimuli affect the expression of different TLRs [198].

Hematogenous dissemination by the pathogen via the circulation also involves the activation of certain adhesion molecules such as E-selectin, VCAM-1, ICAM-1, and VLA-4 by endothelial cells and the upregulation of IL-8 necessary for the transmigration of macrophages, monocytes, neutrophils, and T-cells to combat the incoming spirochetes as shown by in vitro assays applying human umbilical vein endothelial cells (HUVEC) as a model system [199, 200]. Compared to Th2 cells,

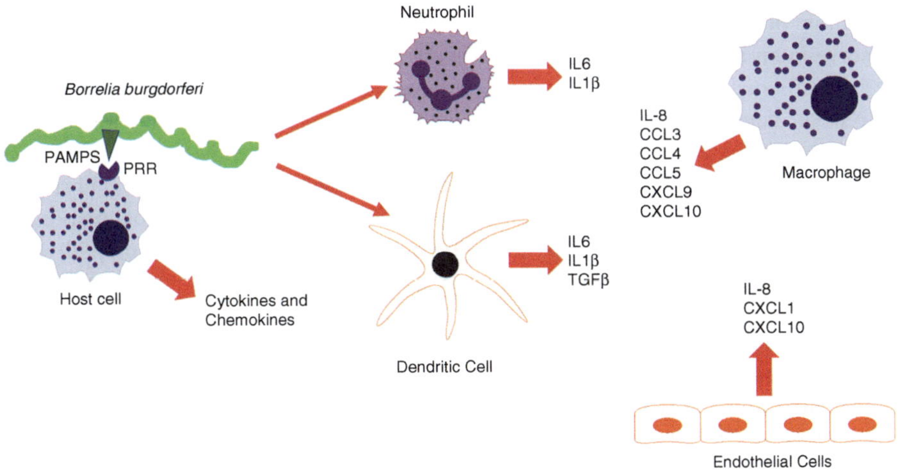

Fig. 3.2 Innate immune responses to *Borrelia burgdorferi* s.l. infections. *IL* interleukin, *PAMP* pathogen-associated molecular pattern, *PRR* pattern recognition receptors, *TGF* transforming growth factor, *TLR* toll-like receptor

Th1 cells releasing IFN-γ are preferentially transferred but the simultaneous production of IL-10 might affect this process as mentioned above. Despite the data available, it is not entirely clear how strong host-adapted spirochetes activate the endothelium in vivo but it is thought that recognition by TLRs appears to play a central role in activating the inflammatory response/signaling. Moreover, additional TLR-independent pathways should recognize incoming spirochetes but they are insufficient for the eradication of spirochetes when they are activated alone.

In addition, primary human microglia treated with *B. burgdorferi* showed an increased expression of pattern recognition receptors and genes known to be involved with cytoskeletal rearrangement and phagocytosis including MARCO, SCARB1, PLA2, PLD2, CD14, and TLR3. These data also indicate that *B. burgdorferi* interacts with the cell surface of primary human microglia and may be internalized following this initial interaction. Furthermore, cell lysates of *B. burgdorferi* induce a significantly larger inflammatory response than live bacteria [181].

It is noteworthy to mention that the majority of the studies investigated were conducted in murine hosts and in mice deficient in certain genes involved in pathogen recognition (TLR2, CD14, MyD88, CD1), and B-cell deficient mice, e.g., SCID mice. Although these studies provided plenty of information about the immune responses and the signaling pathways involved, many clinical aspects of human Lyme borreliosis cannot be explained. For example, mice never develop skin manifestations such as an erythema migrans or acrodermatitis chronica atrophicans and also do not develop peripheral or central system involvement accompanied with meningoradiculoneuritis (Garin–Bujadoux–Bannwarth syndrome), cranial nerve palsies, or progressive neuroborreliosis. Also, the pathology of Lyme arthritis differs between humans and mice, late manifestations of the joints being more common in humans than mice. In humans, Lyme arthritis can be distinguished in two forms: acute and a protracted form that looks like a rheumatoid arthritis [201]. Infection of the heart resulting in the development of a carditis is more often observed in mice while in humans, internistic manifestations including endocarditis or hepatitis occur very rarely and infection of the eye (chorioretinitis, uveitis) has also never been observed in the murine host. In contrast, disseminated spirochetes frequently colonize the spleen, kidney, and ears within a short period of time in infected mice. Despite the obvious drawbacks, the mouse model of Lyme borreliosis has provided important information about the complexity of the host responses and the magnitude of factors, activators, ligands, receptors, and signaling pathways involved in a spirochetal infection.

3.3.1.5 Persistent Infection of *Borrelia* and Post-Lyme Disease Syndrome

Persistence implicates an active process of infection, reinfection, and subsequent invasion of target tissues where spirochetes are able to survive, despite the innate and adaptive immune systems, in an uncontrolled manner. In fact, *Borrelia* have developed sophisticated means to successfully overcome innate and acquired immunity (as discussed in Sect. 3.2.3) while host cells simultaneously activate manifold tools to control and eliminate the spirochetes. In vitro and infection studies revealed that a spirochetal infection is well controlled by both the innate and acquired host defenses. Neither phagocytosis nor complement nor specific antibodies alone are able to completely eliminate the pathogen from the circulation and reduce tissue burden to an undetectable level. From the murine model, it has been shown that a strong antibody response failed to clear the spirochetes from circulation and did not prevent colonization of tissues, most likely due to intrinsic mechanisms developed by *Borrelia*, e.g., antigenic variation and variable expression of antigens, respectively, or by an active mechanism involving suppression and alteration of the host's immune response and immunoseclusion to suppress recruitment of inflammatory cells and recognition of the pathogen [202]. In contrast to what has been observed in infection studies with mice-administered antibiotics, long-term follow-up clinical studies showed that there is no evidence, with exception of reinfections, for a relapse by bacteria that survived the antibiotic treatment [203–207].

3.3.1.6 Candidates for Lyme Disease Vaccine Development

Since the first licensed OspA-based vaccine for Lyme disease, LYMERrix, was officially withdrawn from the commercial market by the manufacturer SmithKline Beecham in February 2002 in the United States, no further vaccine has been released so far, although there is compelling justification for the development of a safer and efficient formulation. Due to the phylogenetic diversity of the six genospecies (*B. burgdorferi*, *B. afzelii*, *B. garinii*, *B. bavariensis*, *B. spielmanii*, and *B. mayonii*) causing Lyme disease in humans and the heterogeneity of the most promising candidates (e.g., OspA, OspC, DbpA, OspE, BBK32), the development of a second-generation vaccine tends to be a big challenge. Investigations have focused on either combination of recombinant proteins (a dual combination of OspA and DbpA or a triple combination comprising OspC, BBK32, and DbpA) to synergize the protective effect of a single protein [208–210] or a chimeric OspA- and OspC-based vaccine [211, 212]. Preclinical studies demonstrated broad protection of these second-generation vaccines but there is no phase III multicenter trial reported so far. Furthermore, the biggest challenge in terms of a high-risk investment and the risk of unforeseen side effects, as known from LYMErix, the first-generation OspA-based vaccine, would be to bring such a vaccine to the global market.

References

1. Radolf JD, Caimano MJ, Stevenson B, Hu LT. Of ticks, mice and men: understanding the dual-host lifestyle of Lyme disease spirochaetes. Nat Rev Microbiol. 2012;10(2):87–99. https://doi.org/10.1038/nrmicro2714.
2. Coburn J, Garcia B, Hu LT, Jewett MW, Kraiczy P, Norris SJ, et al. Lyme disease pathogenesis. Curr Issues Mol Biol. 2021;42:473–518. https://doi.org/10.21775/cimb.042.473.
3. de Taeye SW, Kreuk L, van Dam AP, Hovius JW, Schuijt TJ. Complement evasion by *Borrelia burgdorferi*: it takes three to tango. Trends Parasitol. 2013;29(3):119–28. https://doi.org/10.1016/j.pt.2012.12.001.

4. Mason LM, Veerman CC, Geijtenbeek TB, Hovius JW. Menage a trois: *Borrelia*, dendritic cells, and tick saliva interactions. Trends Parasitol. 2014;30(2):95–103. https://doi.org/10.1016/j.pt.2013.12.003.
5. de la Fuente J, Antunes S, Bonnet S, Cabezas-Cruz A, Domingos AG, Estrada-Pena A, et al. Tick-pathogen interactions and vector competence: identification of molecular drivers for tick-borne diseases. Front Cell Infect Microbiol. 2017;7:114. https://doi.org/10.3389/fcimb.2017.00114.
6. Hovius JW, Levi M, Fikrig E. Salivating for knowledge: potential pharmacological agents in tick saliva. PLoS Med. 2008;5(2):e43.
7. Ramamoorthi N, Narasimhan S, Pal U, Bao F, Yang XF, Fish D, et al. The Lyme disease agent exploits a tick protein to infect the mammalian host. Nature. 2005;436(7050):573–7.
8. Charon NW, Goldstein SF. Genetics of motility and chemotaxis of a fascinating group of bacteria: the spirochetes. Annu Rev Genet. 2002;36:47–73.
9. Moriarty TJ, Norman MU, Colarusso P, Bankhead T, Kubes P, Chaconas G. Real-time high resolution 3D imaging of the Lyme disease spirochete adhering to and escaping from the vasculature of a living host. PLoS Pathog. 2008;4(6):e1000090.
10. Norman MU, Moriarty TJ, Dresser AR, Millen B, Kubes P, Chaconas G. Molecular mechanisms involved in vascular interactions of the Lyme disease pathogen in a living host. PLoS Pathog. 2008;4(10):e1000169.
11. Brissette CA, Gaultney RA. That's my story, and I'm sticking to it--an update on *B. burgdorferi* adhesins. Front Cell Infect Microbiol. 2014;4:41. https://doi.org/10.3389/fcimb.2014.00041.
12. Kraiczy P. Hide and seek: how Lyme disease spirochetes overcome complement attack. Front Immunol. 2016;7:385. https://doi.org/10.3389/fimmu.2016.00385.
13. Skare JT, Garcia BL. Complement evasion by Lyme disease spirochetes. Trends Microbiol. 2020;28(11):889–99. https://doi.org/10.1016/j.tim.2020.05.004.
14. Anderson C, Brissette CA. The brilliance of *Borrelia*: mechanisms of host immune evasion by Lyme disease-causing spirochetes. Pathogens. 2021;10(3) https://doi.org/10.3390/pathogens10030281.
15. Dulipati V, Meri S, Panelius J. Complement evasion strategies of *Borrelia burgdorferi* sensu lato. FEBS Lett. 2020;594(16):2645–56. https://doi.org/10.1002/1873-3468.13894.
16. Cabello FC, Godfrey HP, Newman SA. Hidden in plain sight: *Borrelia burgdorferi* and the extracellular matrix. Trends Microbiol. 2007;15(8):350–4. https://doi.org/10.1016/j.tim.2007.06.003.
17. Steere AC, Klitz W, Drouin EE, Falk BA, Kwok WW, Nepom GT, et al. Antibiotic-refractory Lyme arthritis is associated with HLA-DR molecules that bind a *Borrelia burgdorferi* peptide. J Exp Med. 2006;203(4):961–71. https://doi.org/10.1084/jem.20052471.
18. Barthold SW, Sidman CL, Smith AL. Lyme borreliosis in genetically resistant and susceptible mice with severe combined immunodeficiency. Am J Trop Med Hyg. 1992;47:605–13.
19. McKisic MD, Barthold SW. T-cell-independent responses to *Borrelia burgdorferi* are critical for protective immunity and resolution of Lyme disease. Infect Immun. 2000;68(9):5190–7.
20. Caine JA, Coburn J. Multifunctional and redundant roles of *Borrelia burgdorferi* outer surface proteins in tissue adhesion, colonization, and complement evasion. Front Immunol. 2016;7:442. https://doi.org/10.3389/fimmu.2016.00442.
21. Norris SJ, Coburn J, Leong JM, Hu LT, Höök M. Pathobiology of Lyme disease *Borrelia*. In: Samuels DS, Radolf JD, editors. *Borrelia*: molecular biology, host interaction and pathogenesis. Norfolk: Caister Academic Press; 2010. p. 299–331.
22. Coburn J, Fischer JR, Leong JM. Solving a sticky problem: new genetic approaches to host cell adhesion by the Lyme disease spirochete. Mol Microbiol. 2005;57(5):1182–95. https://doi.org/10.1111/j.1365-2958.2005.04759.x.
23. Coburn J, Leong J, Chaconas G. Illuminating the roles of the *Borrelia burgdorferi* adhesins. Trends Microbiol. 2013;21(8):372–9. https://doi.org/10.1016/j.tim.2013.06.005.
24. Parveen N, Robbins D, Leong JM. Strain variation in glycosaminoglycan recognition influences cell-type-specific binding by Lyme disease spirochetes. Infect Immun. 1999;67(4):1743–9.

25. Leong JM, Robbins D, Rosenfeld L, Lahiri B, Parveen N. Structural requirements for glycosaminoglycan recognition by the Lyme disease spirochete, *Borrelia burgdorferi*. Infect Immun. 1998;66(12):6045–8.
26. Probert WS, Johnson BJ. Identification of a 47 kDa fibronectin-binding protein expressed by *Borrelia burgdorferi* isolate B31. Mol Microbiol. 1998;30(5):1003–15.
27. Probert WS, Kim JH, Hook M, Johnson BJ. Mapping the ligand-binding region of *Borrelia burgdorferi* fibronectin-binding protein BBK32. Infect Immun. 2001;69(6):4129–33. https://doi.org/10.1128/IAI.69.6.4129-4133.2001.
28. Lin YP, Chen Q, Ritchie JA, Dufour NP, Fischer JR, Coburn J, et al. Glycosaminoglycan binding by *Borrelia burgdorferi* adhesin BBK32 specifically and uniquely promotes joint colonization. Cell Microbiol. 2015;17(6):860–75. https://doi.org/10.1111/cmi.12407.
29. Raibaud S, Schwarz-Linek U, Kim JH, Jenkins HT, Baines ER, Gurusiddappa S, et al. *Borrelia burgdorferi* binds fibronectin through a tandem beta-zipper, a common mechanism of fibronectin binding in staphylococci, streptococci, and spirochetes. J Biol Chem. 2005;280(19):18803–9. https://doi.org/10.1074/jbc.M501731200.
30. Kim JH, Singvall J, Schwarz-Linek U, Johnson BJ, Potts JR, Hook M. BBK32, a fibronectin binding MSCRAMM from *Borrelia burgdorferi*, contains a disordered region that undergoes a conformational change on ligand binding. J Biol Chem. 2004;279(40):41706–14. https://doi.org/10.1074/jbc.M401691200.
31. Li X, Liu X, Beck DS, Kantor FS, Fikrig E. *Borrelia burgdorferi* lacking BBK32, a fibronectin-binding protein, retains full pathogenicity. Infect Immun. 2006;74(6):3305–13. https://doi.org/10.1128/IAI.02035-05.
32. Seshu J, Esteve-Gassent MD, Labandeira-Rey M, Kim JH, Trzeciakowski JP, Hook M, et al. Inactivation of the fibronectin-binding adhesin gene bbk32 significantly attenuates the infectivity potential of *Borrelia burgdorferi*. Mol Microbiol. 2006;59(5):1591–601. https://doi.org/10.1111/j.1365-2958.2005.05042.x.
33. Hyde JA, Weening EH, Chang M, Trzeciakowski JP, Hook M, Cirillo JD, et al. Bioluminescent imaging of *Borrelia burgdorferi* in vivo demonstrates that the fibronectin-binding protein BBK32 is required for optimal infectivity. Mol Microbiol. 2011;82(1):99–113. https://doi.org/10.1111/j.1365-2958.2011.07801.x.
34. Moriarty TJ, Shi M, Lin YP, Ebady R, Zhou H, Odisho T, et al. Vascular binding of a pathogen under shear force through mechanistically distinct sequential interactions with host macromolecules. Mol Microbiol. 2012;86(5):1116–31. https://doi.org/10.1111/mmi.12045.
35. Garcia BL, Zhi H, Wager B, Hook M, Skare JT. *Borrelia burgdorferi* BBK32 inhibits the classical pathway by blocking activation of the C1 complement complex. PLoS Pathog. 2016;12(1):e1005404. https://doi.org/10.1371/journal.ppat.1005404.
36. Xie J, Zhi H, Garrigues RJ, Keightley A, Garcia BL, Skare JT. Structural determination of the complement inhibitory domain of *Borrelia burgdorferi* BBK32 provides insight into classical pathway complement evasion by Lyme disease spirochetes. PLoS Pathog. 2019;15(3):e1007659. https://doi.org/10.1371/journal.ppat.1007659.
37. Fikrig E, Feng W, Barthold SW, Telford SR 3rd, Flavell RA. Arthropod- and host-specific *Borrelia burgdorferi* bbk32 expression and the inhibition of spirochete transmission. J Immunol. 2000;164(10):5344–51.
38. Suk K, Das S, Sun W, Jwang B, Barthold SW, Flavell RA, et al. *Borrelia burgdorferi* genes selectively expressed in the infected host. Proc Natl Acad Sci U S A. 1995;92(10):4269–73.
39. Danielson KG, Baribault H, Holmes DF, Graham H, Kadler KE, Iozzo RV. Targeted disruption of decorin leads to abnormal collagen fibril morphology and skin fragility. J Cell Biol. 1997;136(3):729–43.
40. Keene DR, San Antonio JD, Mayne R, McQuillan DJ, Sarris G, Santoro SA, et al. Decorin binds near the C terminus of type I collagen. J Biol Chem. 2000;275(29):21801–4. https://doi.org/10.1074/jbc.C000278200.
41. Zhang G, Ezura Y, Chervoneva I, Robinson PS, Beason DP, Carine ET, et al. Decorin regulates assembly of collagen fibrils and acquisition of biomechanical properties during tendon development. J Cell Biochem. 2006;98(6):1436–49. https://doi.org/10.1002/jcb.20776.

42. Guo BP, Norris SJ, Rosenberg LC, Hook M. Adherence of *Borrelia burgdorferi* to the proteoglycan decorin. Infect Immun. 1995;63(9):3467–72.
43. Guo BP, Brown EL, Dorward DW, Rosenberg LC, Hook M. Decorin-binding adhesins from *Borrelia burgdorferi*. Mol Microbiol. 1998;30(4):711–23.
44. Leong JM, Wang H, Magoun L, Field JA, Morrissey PE, Robbins D, et al. Different classes of proteoglycans contribute to the attachment of *Borrelia burgdorferi* to cultured endothelial and brain cells. Infect Immun. 1998;66(3):994–9.
45. Shi Y, Xu Q, Seemanapalli SV, McShan K, Liang FT. The dbpBA locus of *Borrelia burgdorferi* is not essential for infection of mice. Infect Immun. 2006;74(11):6509–12. https://doi.org/10.1128/IAI.00740-06.
46. Shi Y, Xu Q, Seemanaplli SV, McShan K, Liang FT. Common and unique contributions of decorin-binding proteins a and B to the overall virulence of *Borrelia burgdorferi*. PLoS One. 2008;3(10):e3340. https://doi.org/10.1371/journal.pone.0003340.
47. Shi Y, Xu Q, McShan K, Liang FT. Both decorin-binding proteins a and B are critical for the overall virulence of *Borrelia burgdorferi*. Infect Immun. 2008;76(3):1239–46. https://doi.org/10.1128/IAI.00897-07.
48. Weening EH, Parveen N, Trzeciakowski JP, Leong JM, Hook M, Skare JT. *Borrelia burgdorferi* lacking DbpBA exhibits an early survival defect during experimental infection. Infect Immun. 2008;76(12):5694–705. https://doi.org/10.1128/IAI.00690-08.
49. Blaho VA, Zhang Y, Hughes-Hanks JM, Brown CR. 5-lipoxygenase-deficient mice infected with *Borrelia burgdorferi* develop persistent arthritis. J Immunol. 2011;186(5):3076–84. https://doi.org/10.4049/jimmunol.1003473.
50. Benoit VM, Fischer JR, Lin YP, Parveen N, Leong JM. Allelic variation of the Lyme disease spirochete adhesin DbpA influences spirochetal binding to decorin, dermatan sulfate, and mammalian cells. Infect Immun. 2011;79(9):3501–9. https://doi.org/10.1128/IAI.00163-11.
51. Lin T, Troy EB, Hu LT, Gao L, Norris SJ. Transposon mutagenesis as an approach to improved understanding of *Borrelia* pathogenesis and biology. Front Cell Infect Microbiol. 2014;4:63. https://doi.org/10.3389/fcimb.2014.00063.
52. Schulte-Spechtel U, Fingerle V, Goettner G, Rogge S, Wilske B. Molecular analysis of decorin-binding protein A (DbpA) reveals five major groups among European *Borrelia burgdorferi* sensu lato strains with impact for the development of serological assays and indicates lateral gene transfer of the *dbpA* gene. Int J Med Microbiol. 2006;296(Suppl 40):250–66. https://doi.org/10.1016/j.ijmm.2006.01.006.
53. Leong JM, Morrissey PE, Ortega-Barria E, Pereira ME, Coburn J. Hemagglutination and proteoglycan binding by the Lyme disease spirochete, *Borrelia burgdorferi*. Infect Immun. 1995;63(3):874–83.
54. Parveen N, Leong JM. Identification of a candidate glycosaminoglycan-binding adhesin of the Lyme disease spirochete *Borrelia burgdorferi*. Mol Microbiol. 2000;35(5):1220–34.
55. Parveen N, Cornell KA, Bono JL, Chamberland C, Rosa P, Leong JM. Bgp, a secreted glycosaminoglycan-binding protein of *Borrelia burgdorferi* strain N40, displays nucleosidase activity and is not essential for infection of immunodeficient mice. Infect Immun. 2006;74(5):3016–20. https://doi.org/10.1128/IAI.74.5.3016-3020.2006.
56. Coburn J, Leong JM, Erban JK. Integrin alpha IIb beta 3 mediates binding of the Lyme disease agent *Borrelia burgdorferi* to human platelets. Proc Natl Acad Sci U S A. 1993;90(15):7059–63.
57. Coburn J, Cugini C. Targeted mutation of the outer membrane protein P66 disrupts attachment of the Lyme disease agent, *Borrelia burgdorferi*, to integrin alphavbeta3. Proc Natl Acad Sci U S A. 2003;100(12):7301–6. https://doi.org/10.1073/pnas.1131117100.
58. Ristow LC, Bonde M, Lin YP, Sato H, Curtis M, Wesley E, et al. Integrin binding by *Borrelia burgdorferi* P66 facilitates dissemination but is not required for infectivity. Cell Microbiol. 2015;17(7):1021–36. https://doi.org/10.1111/cmi.12418.
59. Kumar D, Ristow LC, Shi M, Mukherjee P, Caine JA, Lee WY, et al. Intravital imaging of vascular transmigration by the Lyme spirochete: requirement for the integrin binding residues of the *B. burgdorferi* P66 protein. PLoS Pathog. 2015;11(12):e1005333. https://doi.org/10.1371/journal.ppat.1005333.

60. Antonara S, Chafel RM, LaFrance M, Coburn J. *Borrelia burgdorferi* adhesins identified using in vivo phage display. Mol Microbiol. 2007;66(1):262–76. https://doi.org/10.1111/j.1365-2958.2007.05924.x.
61. Skare JT, Mirzabekov TA, Shang ES, Blanco DR, Erdjument-Bromage H, Bunikis J, et al. The Oms66 (p66) protein is a *Borrelia burgdorferi* porin. Infect Immun. 1997;65(9):3654–61.
62. Bunikis J, Noppa L, Ostberg Y, Barbour AG, Bergstrom S. Surface exposure and species specificity of an immunoreactive domain of a 66-kilodalton outer membrane protein (P66) of the *Borrelia* spp. that cause Lyme disease. Infect Immun. 1996;64(12):5111–6.
63. Brissette CA, Bykowski T, Cooley AE, Bowman A, Stevenson B. *Borrelia burgdorferi* RevA antigen binds host fibronectin. Infect Immun. 2009;77(7):2802–12. https://doi.org/10.1128/IAI.00227-09.
64. Carroll JA, El-Hage N, Miller JC, Babb K, Stevenson B. *Borrelia burgdorferi* RevA antigen is a surface-exposed outer membrane protein whose expression is regulated in response to environmental temperature and pH. Infect Immun. 2001;69:5286–93.
65. Gilmore RD Jr, Mbow ML. A monoclonal antibody generated by antigen inoculation via tick bite is reactive to the *Borrelia burgdorferi* rev protein, a member of the 2.9 gene family locus. Infect Immun. 1998;66:980–6.
66. Mbow ML, Gilmore RD, Jr., , Stevenson B, Golde WT, Piesman J, Johnson BJB. *Borrelia burgdorferi*-specific monoclonal antibodies derived from mice primed with Lyme disease spirochete-infected *Ixodes scapularis* ticks. Hybrid Hybridomics 2002;21:179–182.
67. Brissette CA, Rossmann E, Bowman A, Cooley AE, Riley SP, Hunfeld KP, et al. The borrelial fibronectin-binding protein RevA is an early antigen of human Lyme disease. Clin Vaccine Immunol. 2010;17(2):274–80. https://doi.org/10.1128/CVI.00437-09.
68. Byram R, Gaultney RA, Floden AM, Hellekson C, Stone BL, Bowman A, et al. *Borrelia burgdorferi* RevA significantly affects pathogenicity and host response in the mouse model of Lyme disease. Infect Immun. 2015;83(9):3675–83. https://doi.org/10.1128/IAI.00530-15.
69. Colognato H, Yurchenco PD. Form and function: the laminin family of heterotrimers. Dev Dyn. 2000;218(2):213–34. https://doi.org/10.1002/(SICI)1097-0177(200006)218:2<213::AID-DVDY1>3.0.CO;2-R.
70. Brissette CA, Verma A, Bowman A, Cooley AE, Stevenson B. The *Borrelia burgdorferi* outer-surface protein ErpX binds mammalian laminin. Microbiology. 2009;155(Pt 3):863–72. https://doi.org/10.1099/mic.0.024604-0.
71. Bencurova E, Gupta SK, Oskoueian E, Bhide M, Dandekar T. Omics and bioinformatics applied to vaccine development against *Borrelia*. Mol Omics. 2018;14(5):330–40. https://doi.org/10.1039/c8mo00130h.
72. Simpson WJ, Schrumpf ME, Schwan TG. Reactivity of human Lyme borreliosis sera with a 39-kilodalton antigen specific to *Borrelia burgdorferi*. J Clin Microbiol. 1990;28(6):1329–37.
73. Verma A, Brissette CA, Bowman A, Stevenson B. *Borrelia burgdorferi* BmpA is a laminin-binding protein. Infect Immun. 2009;77(11):4940–6. https://doi.org/10.1128/IAI.01420-08.
74. Pal U, Wang P, Bao F, Yang X, Samanta S, Schoen R, et al. *Borrelia burgdorferi* basic membrane proteins a and B participate in the genesis of Lyme arthritis. J Exp Med. 2008;205(1):133–41. https://doi.org/10.1084/jem.20070962.
75. Aguero-Rosenfeld ME, Nowakowski J, McKenna DF, Carbonaro CA, Wormser GP. Serodiagnosis in early Lyme disease. J Clin Microbiol. 1993;31(12):3090–5.
76. Wormser GP. Clinical practice. Early Lyme disease. N Engl J Med. 2006;354(26):2794–801. https://doi.org/10.1056/NEJMcp061181.
77. Bista S, Singh P, Bernard Q, Yang X, Hart T, Lin YP, et al. A novel laminin-binding protein mediates microbial-endothelial cell interactions and facilitates dissemination of Lyme disease pathogens. J Infect Dis. 2020;221(9):1438–47. https://doi.org/10.1093/infdis/jiz626.
78. Shrestha B, Kenedy MR, Akins DR. Outer membrane proteins BB0405 and BB0406 are immunogenic, but only BB0405 is required for *Borrelia burgdorferi* infection. Infect Immun. 2017;85(2) https://doi.org/10.1128/IAI.00803-16.

79. Stewart PE, Wang X, Bueschel DM, Clifton DR, Grimm D, Tilly K, et al. Delineating the requirement for the *Borrelia burgdorferi* virulence factor OspC in the mammalian host. Infect Immun. 2006;74(6):3547–53.
80. Mbow ML, Gilmore RD Jr, Titus RG. An OspC-specific monoclonal antibody passively protects mice from tick-transmitted infection by *Borrelia burgdorferi* B31. Infect Immun. 1999;67(10):5470–2.
81. Tilly K, Bestor A, Jewett MW, Rosa P. Rapid clearance of Lyme disease spirochetes lacking OspC from skin. Infect Immun. 2007;75(3):1517–9. https://doi.org/10.1128/IAI.01725-06.
82. Embers ME, Alvarez X, Ooms T, Philipp MT. The failure of immune response evasion by linear plasmid 28-1-deficient *Borrelia burgdorferi* is attributable to persistent expression of an outer surface protein. Infect Immun. 2008;76(9):3984–91. https://doi.org/10.1128/IAI.00387-08.
83. Liang FT, Nelson FK, Fikrig E. Molecular adaptation of *Borrelia burgdorferi* in the murine host. J Exp Med. 2002;196(2):275–80.
84. Lin YP, Tan X, Caine JA, Castellanos M, Chaconas G, Coburn J, et al. Strain-specific joint invasion and colonization by Lyme disease spirochetes is promoted by outer surface protein C. PLoS Pathog. 2020;16(5):e1008516. https://doi.org/10.1371/journal.ppat.1008516.
85. Carrasco SE, Troxell B, Yang Y, Brandt SL, Li H, Sandusky GE, et al. Outer surface protein OspC is an antiphagocytic factor that protects *Borrelia burgdorferi* from phagocytosis by macrophages. Infect Immun. 2015;83(12):4848–60. https://doi.org/10.1128/IAI.01215-15.
86. Caine JA, Lin YP, Kessler JR, Sato H, Leong JM, Coburn J. *Borrelia burgdorferi* outer surface protein C (OspC) binds complement component C4b and confers bloodstream survival. Cell Microbiol. 2017; https://doi.org/10.1111/cmi.12786.
87. Onder O, Humphrey PT, McOmber B, Korobova F, Francella N, Greenbaum DC, et al. OspC is potent plasminogen receptor on surface of *Borrelia burgdorferi*. J Biol Chem. 2012;287(20):16860–8. https://doi.org/10.1074/jbc.M111.290775.
88. Vuong HB, Canham CD, Fonseca DM, Brisson D, Morin PJ, Smouse PE, et al. Occurrence and transmission efficiencies of *Borrelia burgdorferi ospC* types in avian and mammalian wildlife. Infect Genet Evol. 2014;27:594–600. https://doi.org/10.1016/j.meegid.2013.12.011.
89. Barbour AG, Travinsky B. Evolution and distribution of the ospC gene, a transferable serotype determinant of *Borrelia burgdorferi*. MBio. 2010;1(4) https://doi.org/10.1128/mBio.00153-10.
90. Coleman JL, Gebbia JA, Benach JL. *Borrelia burgdorferi* and other bacterial products induce expression and release of the urokinase receptor (CD87). J Immunol. 2001;166(1):473–80.
91. Gebbia JA, Coleman JL, Benach JL. *Borrelia spirochetes* upregulate release and activation of matrix metalloproteinase gelatinase B (MMP-9) and collagenase 1 (MMP-1) in human cells. Infect Immun. 2001;69(1):456–62. https://doi.org/10.1128/IAI.69.1.456-462.2001.
92. Klempner MS, Noring R, Epstein MP, McCloud B, Hu R, Limentani SA, et al. Binding of human plasminogen and urokinase-type plasminogen activator to the Lyme disease spirochete, *Borrelia burgdorferi*. J Infect Dis. 1995;171(5):1258–65.
93. Behera AK, Hildebrand E, Scagliotti J, Steere AC, Hu LT. Induction of host matrix metalloproteinases by *Borrelia burgdorferi* differs in human and murine Lyme arthritis. Infect Immun. 2005;73(1):126–34. https://doi.org/10.1128/IAI.73.1.126-134.2005.
94. Zhao Z, Chang H, Trevino RP, Whren K, Bhawan J, Klempner MS. Selective up-regulation of matrix metalloproteinase-9 expression in human erythema migrans skin lesions of acute Lyme disease. J Infect Dis. 2003;188(8):1098–104. https://doi.org/10.1086/379039.
95. Grab DJ, Perides G, Dumler JS, Kim KJ, Park J, Kim YV, et al. *Borrelia burgdorferi*, host-derived proteases, and the blood-brain barrier. Infect Immun. 2005;73(2):1014–22. https://doi.org/10.1128/IAI.73.2.1014-1022.2005.
96. Liang FT, Brown EL, Wang T, Iozzo RV, Fikrig E. Protective niche for *Borrelia burgdorferi* to evade humoral immunity. Am J Pathol. 2004;165(3):977–85. https://doi.org/10.1016/S0002-9440(10)63359-7.
97. Lijnen HR. Plasmin and matrix metalloproteinases in vascular remodeling. Thromb Haemost. 2001;86(1):324–33.

98. Barthel D, Schindler S, Zipfel PF. Plasminogen is a complement inhibitor. J Biol Chem. 2012;287(22):18831–42. https://doi.org/10.1074/jbc.M111.323287.
99. Coleman JL, Gebbia JA, Piesman J, Degen JL, Bugge TH, Benach JL. Plasminogen is required for efficient dissemination of *Borrelia burgdorferi* in ticks and for enhancement of spirochetemia in mice. Cell. 1997;89(7):1111–9.
100. Perides G, Tanner-Brown LM, Eskildsen MA, Klempner MS. *Borrelia burgdorferi* induces matrix metalloproteinases by neural cultures. J Neurosci Res. 1999;58(6):779–90.
101. Hu LT, Eskildsen MA, Masgala C, Steere AC, Arner EC, Pratta MA, et al. Host metalloproteinases in Lyme arthritis. Arthritis Rheum. 2001;44(6):1401–10. https://doi.org/10.1002/1529-0131(200106)44:6<1401::AID-ART234>3.0.CO;2-S.
102. Lin B, Kidder JM, Noring R, Steere AC, Klempner MS, Hu LT. Differences in synovial fluid levels of matrix metalloproteinases suggest separate mechanisms of pathogenesis in Lyme arthritis before and after antibiotic treatment. J Infect Dis. 2001;184(2):174–80. https://doi.org/10.1086/322000.
103. Heilpern AJ, Wertheim W, He J, Perides G, Bronson RT, Hu LT. Matrix metalloproteinase 9 plays a key role in Lyme arthritis but not in dissemination of *Borrelia burgdorferi*. Infect Immun. 2009;77(7):2643–9. https://doi.org/10.1128/IAI.00214-09.
104. Coleman JL, Sellati TJ, Testa JE, Kew RR, Furie MB, Benach JL. *Borrelia burgdorfer*i binds plasminogen, resulting in enhanced penetration of endothelial monolayers. Infect Immun. 1995;63(7):2478–84.
105. Fuchs H, Wallich R, Simon MM, Kramer MD. The outer surface protein a of the spirochete *Borrelia burgdorferi* is a plasmin(ogen) receptor. Proc Natl Acad Sci U S A. 1994;91(26):12594–8.
106. Lagal V, Portnoi D, Faure G, Postic D, Baranton G. *Borrelia burgdorferi* sensu stricto invasiveness is correlated with OspC-plasminogen affinity. Microbes Infect. 2006;8(3):645–52.
107. Hu LT, Pratt SD, Perides G, Katz L, Rogers RA, Klempner MS. Isolation, cloning, and expression of a 70-kilodalton plasminogen binding protein of *Borrelia burgdorferi*. Infect Immun. 1997;65(12):4989–95.
108. Brissette CA, Haupt K, Barthel D, Cooley AE, Bowman A, Skerka C, et al. *Borrelia burgdorferi* infection-associated surface proteins ErpP, ErpA, and ErpC bind human plasminogen. Infect Immun. 2009;77(1):300–6. https://doi.org/10.1128/IAI.01133-08.
109. Hallström T, Haupt K, Kraiczy P, Hortschansky P, Wallich R, Skerka C, et al. Complement regulator-acquiring surface protein 1 of *Borrelia burgdorferi* binds to human bone morphogenic protein 2, several extracellular matrix proteins, and plasminogen. J Infect Dis. 2010;202(3):490–8.
110. Seling A, Siegel C, Fingerle V, Jutras BL, Brissette CA, Skerka C, et al. Functional characterization of *Borrelia spielmanii* outer surface proteins that interact with distinct members of the human factor H protein family and with plasminogen. Infect Immun. 2010;78(1):39–48.
111. Koenigs A, Hammerschmidt C, Jutras BL, Pogoryelov D, Barthel D, Skerka C, et al. BBA70 of *Borrelia burgdorferi* is a novel plasminogen-binding protein. J Biol Chem. 2013;288(35):25229–43. https://doi.org/10.1074/jbc.M112.413872.
112. Floden AM, Watt JA, Brissette CA. *Borrelia burgdorferi* enolase is a surface-exposed plasminogen binding protein. PLoS One. 2011;6(11):e27502. https://doi.org/10.1371/journal.pone.0027502.
113. Hudson CR, Frye JG, Quinn FD, Gherardini FC. Increased expression of *Borrelia burgdorferi vlsE* in response to human endothelial cell membranes. Mol Microbiol. 2001;41:229–39.
114. Lawrenz MB, Hardham JM, Owens RT, Nowakowski J, Steere AC, Wormser GP, et al. Human antibody responses to VlsE antigenic variation protein of *Borrelia burgdorferi*. J Clin Microbiol. 1999;37:3997–4004.
115. Anguita J, Thomas V, Samanta S, Persinski R, Hernanz C, Barthold SW, et al. *Borrelia burgdorferi*-induced inflammation facilitates spirochete adaptation and variable major protein-like sequence locus recombination. J Immunol. 2001;167(6):3383–90.

116. Coutte L, Botkin DJ, Gao L, Norris SJ. Detailed analysis of sequence changes occurring during vlsE antigenic variation in the mouse model of *Borrelia burgdorferi* infection. PLoS Pathog. 2009;5(2):e1000293. https://doi.org/10.1371/journal.ppat.1000293.
117. Jacek E, Tang KS, Komorowski L, Ajamian M, Probst C, Stevenson B, et al. Epitope-specific evolution of human B cell responses to *Borrelia burgdorferi* VlsE protein from early to late stages of Lyme disease. J Immunol. 2016;196(3):1036–43. https://doi.org/10.4049/jimmunol.1501861.
118. Liang FT, Jacobs MB, Bowers LC, Philipp MT. An immune evasion mechanism for spirochetal persistence in Lyme borreliosis. J Exp Med. 2002;195(4):415–22.
119. Norris SJ. Vls antigenic variation systems of Lyme disease *Borrelia*: eluding host immunity through both random, segmental gene conversion and framework heterogeneity. Microbiol Spectr. 2014;2(6) https://doi.org/10.1128/microbiolspec.MDNA3-0038-2014.
120. Liang FT, Alvarez AL, Gu Y, Nowling JM, Ramamoorthy R, Philipp MT. An immunodominant conserved region within the variable domain of VlsE, the variable surface antigen of *Borrelia burgdorferi*. J Immunol. 1999;163:5566–73.
121. Liang FT, Aberer E, Cinco M, Gern L, Hu CM, Lobet YN, et al. Antigenic conservation of an immunodominant invariable region of the VlsE lipoprotein among European pathogenic genospecies of *Borrelia burgdorferi* SL. J Infect Dis. 2000;182:1455–62.
122. Bacon RM, Biggerstaff BJ, Schriefer ME, Gilmore RD Jr, Philipp MT, Steere AC, et al. Serodiagnosis of Lyme disease by kinetic enzyme-linked immunosorbent assay using recombinant VlsE1 or peptide antigens of *Borrelia burgdorferi* compared with 2-tiered testing using whole-cell lysates. J Infect Dis. 2003;187(8):1187–99. https://doi.org/10.1086/374395.
123. Schulte-Spechtel U, Lehnert G, Liegl G, Fingerle V, Heimerl C, Johnson BJ, et al. Significant improvement of the recombinant *Borrelia*-specific immunoglobulin G immunoblot test by addition of VlsE and a DbpA homologue derived from *Borrelia garinii* for diagnosis of early neuroborreliosis. J Clin Microbiol. 2003;41(3):1299–303.
124. Eicken C, Sharma V, Klabunde T, Lawrenz MB, Hardham JM, Norris SJ, et al. Crystal structure of Lyme disease variable surface antigen VlsE of *Borrelia burgdorferi*. J Biol Chem. 2002;277:21691–6.
125. McDowell JV, Sung S-Y, Hu LT, Marconi RT. Evidence that the variable regions of the central domain of VlsE are antigenic during infection with Lyme disease spirochetes. Infect Immun. 2002;70:4196–203.
126. Lin YP, Frye AM, Nowak TA, Kraiczy P. New insights into CRASP-mediated complement evasion in the Lyme disease enzootic cycle. Front Cell Infect Microbiol. 2020;10:1. https://doi.org/10.3389/fcimb.2020.00001.
127. Alitalo A, Meri T, Ramo L, Jokiranta TS, Heikkila T, Seppala IJT, et al. Complement evasion by *Borrelia burgdorferi*: serum-resistant strains promote C3b inactivation. Infect Immun. 2001;69(6):3685–91. https://doi.org/10.1128/iai.69.6.3685-3691.2001.
128. Kraiczy P, Skerka C, Brade V, Zipfel PF. Further characterization of complement regulator-acquiring surface proteins of *Borrelia burgdorferi*. Infect Immun. 2001;69(12):7800–9. https://doi.org/10.1128/iai.69.12.7800-7809.2001.
129. Kraiczy P, Skerka C, Kirschfink M, Brade V, Zipfel PF. Immune evasion of *Borrelia burgdorferi* by acquisition of human complement regulators FHL-1/reconectin and factor H. Eur J Immunol. 2001;31(6):1674–84.
130. Pietikainen J, Meri T, Blom AM, Meri S. Binding of the complement inhibitor C4b-binding protein to Lyme disease *Borreliae*. Mol Immunol. 2010;47(6):1299–305.
131. Haupt K, Kraiczy P, Wallich R, Brade V, Skerka C, Zipfel P. Binding of human factor H-related protein 1 to serum-resistant *Borrelia burgdorferi* is mediated by borrelial complement regulator-acquiring surface proteins. J Infect Dis. 2007;196(1):124–33. https://doi.org/10.1086/518509.
132. Siegel C, Hallström T, Skerka C, Eberhardt H, Uzonyi B, Beckhaus T, et al. Complement factor H-related proteins CFHR2 and CFHR5 represent novel ligands for the infection-associated CRASP proteins of *Borrelia burgdorferi*. PLoS One. 2010;5(10):e13519.

133. Hallström T, Siegel C, Morgelin M, Kraiczy P, Skerka C, Zipfel PF. CspA from *Borrelia burgdorferi* inhibits the terminal complement pathway. MBio. 2013;4(4) https://doi.org/10.1128/mBio.00481-13.
134. Hammerschmidt C, Klevenhaus Y, Koenigs A, Hallstrom T, Fingerle V, Skerka C, et al. BGA66 and BGA71 facilitate complement resistance of *Borrelia bavariensis* by inhibiting assembly of the membrane attack complex. Mol Microbiol. 2016;99(2):407–24. https://doi.org/10.1111/mmi.13239.
135. Hammerschmidt C, Koenigs A, Siegel C, Hallstrom T, Skerka C, Wallich R, et al. Versatile roles of CspA orthologs in complement inactivation of serum-resistant Lyme disease spirochetes. Infect Immun. 2014;82(1):380–92. https://doi.org/10.1128/IAI.01094-13.
136. Alitalo A, Meri T, Lankinen H, Seppala I, Lahdenne P, Hefty PS, et al. Complement inhibitor factor H binding to Lyme disease spirochetes is mediated by inducible expression of multiple plasmid-encoded outer surface protein E paralogs. J Immunol. 2002;169(7):3847–53.
137. Hartmann K, Corvey C, Skerka C, Kirschfink M, Karas M, Brade V, et al. Functional characterization of BbCRASP-2, a distinct outer membrane protein of *Borrelia burgdorferi* that binds host complement regulators factor H and FHL-1. Mol Microbiol. 2006;61(5):1220–36. https://doi.org/10.1111/j.1365-2958.2006.05318.x.
138. Hellwage J, Meri T, Heikkila T, Alitalo A, Panelius J, Lahdenne P, et al. The complement regulator factor H binds to the surface protein OspE of *Borrelia burgdorferi*. J Biol Chem. 2001;276(11):8427–35. https://doi.org/10.1074/jbc.M007994200.
139. Hovis KM, Tran E, Sundy CM, Buckles E, McDowell JV, Marconi RT. Selective binding of *Borrelia burgdorferi* OspE paralogs to factor H and serum proteins from diverse animals: possible expansion of the role of OspE in Lyme disease pathogenesis. Infect Immun. 2006;74(3):1967–72. https://doi.org/10.1128/iai.74.3.1967-1972.2006.
140. Kenedy MR, Akins DR. The OspE-related proteins inhibit complement deposition and enhance serum resistance of *Borrelia burgdorferi*, the Lyme disease spirochete. Infect Immun. 2011;79(4):1451–7.
141. Kenedy MR, Vuppala SR, Siegel C, Kraiczy P, Akins DR. CspA-mediated binding of human factor H inhibits complement deposition and confers serum resistance in *Borrelia burgdorferi*. Infect Immun. 2009;77(7):2773–82. https://doi.org/10.1128/IAI.00318-09.
142. Siegel C, Schreiber J, Haupt K, Skerka C, Brade V, Simon MM, et al. Deciphering the ligand-binding sites in the *Borrelia burgdorferi* complement regulator-acquiring surface protein 2 required for interactions with the human immune regulators factor H and factor H-like protein 1. J Biol Chem. 2008;283(50):34855–63. https://doi.org/10.1074/jbc.M805844200.
143. Stevenson B, El-Hage N, Hines MA, Miller JC, Babb K. Differential binding of host complement inhibitor factor H by *Borrelia burgdorferi* Erp surface proteins: a possible mechanism underlying the expansive host range of Lyme disease spirochetes. Infect Immun. 2002;70(2):491–7. https://doi.org/10.1128/iai.70.2.491-497.2002.
144. Pausa M, Pellis V, Cinco M, Giulianini PG, Presani G, Perticarari S, et al. Serum-resistant strains of *Borrelia burgdorferi* evade complement-mediated killing by expressing a CD59-like complement inhibitory molecule. J Immunol. 2003;170(6):3214–22.
145. Brooks CS, Vuppala SR, Jett AM, Alitalo A, Meri S, Akins DR. Complement regulator-acquiring surface protein 1 imparts resistance to human serum in *Borrelia burgdorferi*. J Immunol. 2005;175(5):3299–308.
146. Hart T, Nguyen NTT, Nowak NA, Zhang F, Linhardt RJ, Diuk-Wasser M, et al. Polymorphic factor H-binding activity of CspA protects Lyme borreliae from the host complement in feeding ticks to facilitate tick-to-host transmission. PLoS Pathog. 2018;14(5):e1007106. https://doi.org/10.1371/journal.ppat.1007106.
147. Bykowski T, Woodman ME, Cooley AE, Brissette CA, Brade V, Wallich R, et al. Coordinated expression of *Borrelia burgdorferi* complement regulator-acquiring surface proteins during the Lyme disease spirochete's mammal-tick infection cycle. Infect Immun. 2007;75(9):4227–36. https://doi.org/10.1128/iai.00604-07.
148. von Lackum K, Miller JC, Bykowski T, Riley SP, Woodman ME, Brade V, et al. *Borrelia burgdorferi* regulates expression of complement regulator-acquiring surface protein 1 dur-

ing the mammal-tick infection cycle. Infect Immun. 2005;73(11):7398–405. https://doi.org/10.1128/iai.73.11.7398-7405.2005.
149. Bhide MR, Escudero R, Camafeita E, Gil H, Jado I, Anda P. Complement factor H binding by different Lyme disease and relapsing fever *Borrelia* in animals and human. BMC Res Notes. 2009;2:134. https://doi.org/10.1186/1756-0500-2-134.
150. Herzberger P, Siegel C, Skerka C, Fingerle V, Schulte-Spechtel U, van Dam A, et al. Human pathogenic *Borrelia spielmanii* sp. nov. resists complement-mediated killing by direct binding of immune regulators factor H and factor H-like protein 1. Infect Immun. 2007;75(10):4817–25. https://doi.org/10.1128/iai.00532-07.
151. McDowell JV, Wolfgang J, Tran E, Metts MS, Hamilton D, Marconi RT. Comprehensive analysis of the factor H binding capabilities of *Borrelia* species associated with Lyme disease: delineation of two distinct classes of factor H binding proteins. Infect Immun. 2003;71(6):3597–602. https://doi.org/10.1128/iai.71.6.3597-3602.2003.
152. Walter L, Sürth V, Röttgerding F, Zipfel PF, Fritz-Wolf K, Kraiczy P. Elucidating the immune evasion mechanisms of *Borrelia mayonii*, the causative agent of Lyme disease. Front Immunol. 2019;10:2722. https://doi.org/10.3389/fimmu.2019.02722.
153. Liang FT, Yan J, Mbow ML, Sviat SL, Gilmore RD, Mamula M, et al. *Borrelia burgdorferi* changes its surface antigenic expression in response to host immune responses. Infect Immun. 2004;72(10):5759–67. https://doi.org/10.1128/IAI.72.10.5759-5767.2004.
154. Miller J, Stevenson B. Increased expression of *Borrelia burgdorferi* factor H-binding surface proteins during transmission from ticks to mice. Int J Med Microbiol. 2004;293(37):120–5.
155. Elsner RA, Hastey CJ, Olsen KJ, Baumgarth N. Suppression of long-lived humoral immunity following *Borrelia burgdorferi* infection. PLoS Pathog. 2015;11(7):e1004976. https://doi.org/10.1371/journal.ppat.1004976.
156. Hastey CJ, Elsner RA, Barthold SW, Baumgarth N. Delays and diversions mark the development of B cell responses to *Borrelia burgdorferi* infection. J Immunol. 2012;188(11):5612–22. https://doi.org/10.4049/jimmunol.1103735.
157. Tunev SS, Hastey CJ, Hodzic E, Feng S, Barthold SW, Baumgarth N. Lymphoadenopathy during Lyme borreliosis is caused by spirochete migration-induced specific B cell activation. PLoS Pathog. 2011;7(5):e1002066. https://doi.org/10.1371/journal.ppat.1002066.
158. Elsner RA, Hastey CJ, Baumgarth N. CD4+ T cells promote antibody production but not sustained affinity maturation during *Borrelia burgdorferi* infection. Infect Immun. 2015;83(1):48–56. https://doi.org/10.1128/IAI.02471-14.
159. Hastey CJ, Ochoa J, Olsen KJ, Barthold SW, Baumgarth N. MyD88- and TRIF-independent induction of type I interferon drives naive B cell accumulation but not loss of lymph node architecture in Lyme disease. Infect Immun. 2014;82(4):1548–58. https://doi.org/10.1128/IAI.00969-13.
160. Divan A, Budd RC, Tobin RP, Newell-Rogers MK. Gammadelta T cells and dendritic cells in refractory Lyme arthritis. J Leukoc Biol. 2015;97(4):653–63. https://doi.org/10.1189/jlb.2RU0714-343RR.
161. Verma A, Hellwage J, Artiushin S, Zipfel PF, Kraiczy P, Timoney JF, et al. LfhA, a novel factor H-binding protein of *Leptospira interrogans*. Infect Immun. 2006;74(5):2659–66. https://doi.org/10.1128/IAI.74.5.2659-2666.2006.
162. Collins C, Shi C, Russell JQ, Fortner KA, Budd RC. Activation of gamma delta T cells by *Borrelia burgdorferi* is indirect via a TLR- and caspase-dependent pathway. J Immunol. 2008;181(4):2392–8.
163. Kumar H, Belperron A, Barthold SW, Bockenstedt LK. Cutting edge: CD1d deficiency impairs murine host defense against the spirochete, *Borrelia burgdorferi*. J Immunol. 2000;165(9):4797–801.
164. Glatzel A, Entschladen F, Zollner TM, Kraiczy P, Brade V, Kaufmann R, et al. The responsiveness of human V delta 1 gamma delta T cells to *Borrelia burgdorferi* is largely restricted to synovial-fluid cells from patients with Lyme arthritis. J Infect Dis. 2002;186(7):1043–6.
165. Barthold SW, Feng S, Bockenstedt LK, Fikrig E, Feen K. Protective and arthritis-resolving activity in sera of mice infected with *Borrelia burgdorferi*. Clin Infect Dis. 1997;25(Suppl 1):S9–17.

166. Brown JP, Zachary JF, Teuscher C, Weis JJ, Wooten RM. Dual role of interleukin-10 in murine Lyme disease: regulation of arthritis severity and host defense. Infect Immun. 1999;67:5142–50.
167. Brown EL, Guo BP, O'Neal P, Hook M. Adherence of *Borrelia burgdorferi*. Identification of critical lysine residues in DbpA required for decorin binding. J Biol Chem. 1999;274(37):26272–8.
168. Glickstein L, Edelstein M, Dong JZ. Gamma interferon is not required for arthritis resistance in the murine Lyme disease model. Infect Immun. 2001;69(6):3737–43. https://doi.org/10.1128/IAI.69.6.3737-3743.2001.
169. Potter MR, Noben-Trauth N, Weis JH, Teuscher C, Weis JJ. Interleukin-4 (IL-4) and IL-13 signaling pathways do not regulate *Borrelia burgdorferi*-induced arthritis in mice: IgG1 is not required for host control of tissue spirochetes. Infect Immun. 2000;68(10):5603–9.
170. Nardelli DT, Warner TF, Callister SM, Schell RF. Anti-CD25 antibody treatment of mice vaccinated and challenged with *Borrelia* spp. does not exacerbate arthritis but inhibits borreliacidal antibody production. Clin Vaccine Immunol. 2006;13(8):884–91. https://doi.org/10.1128/CVI.00137-06.
171. Nardelli DT, Kevin Luk KH, Kotloski NJ, Warner TF, Torrealba JR, Callister SM, et al. Role of IL-17, transforming growth factor-beta, and IL-6 in the development of arthritis and production of anti-outer surface protein A borreliacidal antibodies in *Borrelia*-vaccinated and -challenged mice. FEMS Immunol Med Microbiol. 2008;53(2):265–74. https://doi.org/10.1111/j.1574-695X.2008.00431.x.
172. Nardelli DT, Cloute JP, Luk KH, Torrealba J, Warner TF, Callister SM, et al. CD4(+) CD25(+) T cells prevent arthritis associated with *Borrelia* vaccination and infection. Clin Diagn Lab Immunol. 2005;12(6):786–92. https://doi.org/10.1128/CDLI.12.6.786-792.2005.
173. Nardelli DT, Burchill MA, England DM, Torrealba J, Callister SM, Schell RF. Association of CD4+ CD25+ T cells with prevention of severe destructive arthritis in *Borrelia burgdorferi*-vaccinated and challenged gamma interferon-deficient mice treated with anti-interleukin-17 antibody. Clin Diagn Lab Immunol. 2004;11(6):1075–84. https://doi.org/10.1128/CDLI.11.6.1075-1084.2004.
174. Iliopoulou BP, Alroy J, Huber BT. CD28 deficiency exacerbates joint inflammation upon *Borrelia burgdorferi* infection, resulting in the development of chronic Lyme arthritis. J Immunol. 2007;179(12):8076–82.
175. Steere AC, Dwyer E, Winchester R. Association of chronic Lyme arthritis with HLA-DR4 and HLA-DR2 alleles. N Engl J Med. 1990;323(4):219–23. https://doi.org/10.1056/NEJM199007263230402.
176. Steere AC, Falk B, Drouin EE, Baxter-Lowe LA, Hammer J, Nepom GT. Binding of outer surface protein a and human lymphocyte function-associated antigen 1 peptides to HLA-DR molecules associated with antibiotic treatment-resistant Lyme arthritis. Arthritis Rheum. 2003;48(2):534–40. https://doi.org/10.1002/art.10772.
177. Kalish RA, Leong JM, Steere AC. Association of treatment-resistant chronic Lyme arthritis with HLA-DR4 and antibody reactivity to OspA and OspB of *Borrelia burgdorferi*. Infect Immun. 1993;61(7):2774–9.
178. Kovalchuka L, Cvetkova S, Trofimova J, Eglite J, Gintere S, Lucenko I, et al. Immunogenetic markers definition in Latvian patients with Lyme borreliosis and Lyme neuroborreliosis. Int J Environ Res Public Health. 2016;13(12) https://doi.org/10.3390/ijerph13121194.
179. Iliopoulou BP, Guerau-de-Arellano M, Huber BT. HLA-DR alleles determine responsiveness to *Borrelia burgdorferi* antigens in a mouse model of self-perpetuating arthritis. Arthritis Rheum. 2009;60(12):3831–40. https://doi.org/10.1002/art.25005.
180. Bachmann M, Horn K, Rudloff I, Goren I, Holdener M, Christen U, et al. Early production of IL-22 but not IL-17 by peripheral blood mononuclear cells exposed to live *Borrelia burgdorferi*: the role of monocytes and interleukin-1. PLoS Pathog. 2010;6(10):e1001144. https://doi.org/10.1371/journal.ppat.1001144.
181. Greenmyer JR, Gaultney RA, Brissette CA, Watt JA. Primary human microglia are phagocytically active and respond to *Borrelia burgdorferi* with upregulation of chemokines and cytokines. Front Microbiol. 2018;9:811. https://doi.org/10.3389/fmicb.2018.00811.

182. Mullegger RR, Means TK, Shin JJ, Lee M, Jones KL, Glickstein LJ, et al. Chemokine signatures in the skin disorders of Lyme borreliosis in Europe: predominance of CXCL9 and CXCL10 in erythema migrans and acrodermatitis and CXCL13 in lymphocytoma. Infect Immun. 2007;75(9):4621–8. https://doi.org/10.1128/IAI.00263-07.
183. Salazar JC, Pope CD, Moore MW, Pope J, Kiely TG, Radolf JD. Lipoprotein-dependent and -independent immune responses to spirochetal infection. Clin Diagn Lab Immunol. 2005;12(8):949–58. https://doi.org/10.1128/CDLI.12.8.949-958.2005.
184. Oosting M, Kerstholt M, Ter Horst R, Li Y, Deelen P, Smeekens S, et al. Functional and genomic architecture of *Borrelia burgdorferi*-induced cytokine responses in humans. Cell Host Microbe. 2016;20(6):822–33. https://doi.org/10.1016/j.chom.2016.10.006.
185. Oosting M, Buffen K, van der Meer JW, Netea MG, Joosten LA. Innate immunity networks during infection with *Borrelia burgdorferi*. Crit Rev Microbiol. 2016;42(2):233–44. https://doi.org/10.3109/1040841X.2014.929563.
186. Behera AK, Hildebrand E, Uematsu S, Akira S, Coburn J, Hu LT. Identification of a TLR-independent pathway for *Borrelia burgdorferi*-induced expression of matrix metalloproteinases and inflammatory mediators through binding to integrin alpha 3 beta 1. J Immunol. 2006;177(1):657–64.
187. Hirschfeld M, Kirschning CJ, Schwandner R, Wesche H, Weis JH, Wooten RM, et al. Cutting edge: inflammatory signaling by *Borrelia burgdorferi* lipoproteins is mediated by toll-like receptor 2. J Immunol. 1999;163(5):2382–6.
188. Oosting M, Berende A, Sturm P, Ter Hofstede HJ, de Jong DJ, Kanneganti TD, et al. Recognition of *Borrelia burgdorferi* by NOD2 is central for the induction of an inflammatory reaction. J Infect Dis. 2010;201(12):1849–58. https://doi.org/10.1086/652871.
189. Guerau-de-Arellano M, Alroy J, Huber BT. Beta2 integrins control the severity of murine Lyme carditis. Infect Immun. 2005;73(6):3242–50. https://doi.org/10.1128/IAI.73.6.3242-3250.2005.
190. Pohl-Koppe A, Balashov KE, Steere AC, Logigian EL, Hafler DA. Identification of a T cell subset capable of both IFN-gamma and IL-10 secretion in patients with chronic *Borrelia burgdorferi* infection. J Immunol. 1998;160(4):1804–10.
191. Murthy PK, Dennis VA, Lasater BL, Philipp MT. Interleukin-10 modulates proinflammatory cytokines in the human monocytic cell line THP-1 stimulated with *Borrelia burgdorferi* lipoproteins. Infect Immun. 2000;68(12):6663–9.
192. Gautam A, Dixit S, Philipp MT, Singh SR, Morici LA, Kaushal D, et al. Interleukin-10 alters effector functions of multiple genes induced by *Borrelia burgdorferi* in macrophages to regulate Lyme disease inflammation. Infect Immun. 2011;79(12):4876–92. https://doi.org/10.1128/IAI.05451-11.
193. Dame TM, Orenzoff BL, Palmer LE, Furie MB. IFN-gamma alters the response of *Borrelia burgdorferi*-activated endothelium to favor chronic inflammation. J Immunol. 2007;178(2):1172–9.
194. Sellati TJ, Bouis DA, Kitchens RL, Darveau RP, Pugin J, Ulevitch RJ, et al. *Treponema pallidum* and *Borrelia burgdorferi* lipoproteins and synthetic lipopeptides activate monocytic cells via a CD14-dependent pathway distinct from that used by lipopolysaccharide. J Immunol. 1998;160(11):5455–64.
195. Wooten RM, Morrison TB, Weis JH, Wright SD, Thieringer R, Weis JJ. The role of CD14 in signaling mediated by outer membrane lipoproteins of *Borrelia burgdorferi*. J Immunol. 1998;160(11):5485–92.
196. Cervantes JL, Hawley KL, Benjamin SJ, Weinerman B, Luu SM, Salazar JC. Phagosomal TLR signaling upon *Borrelia burgdorferi* infection. Front Cell Infect Microbiol. 2014;4:55. https://doi.org/10.3389/fcimb.2014.00055.
197. Salazar JC, Pope CD, Sellati TJ, Feder HM Jr, Kiely TG, Dardick KR, et al. Coevolution of markers of innate and adaptive immunity in skin and peripheral blood of patients with erythema migrans. J Immunol. 2003;171(5):2660–70.

198. Cabral ES, Gelderblom H, Hornung RL, Munson PJ, Martin R, Marques AR. *Borrelia burgdorferi* lipoprotein-mediated TLR2 stimulation causes the down-regulation of TLR5 in human monocytes. J Infect Dis. 2006;193(6):849–59. https://doi.org/10.1086/500467.
199. Burns MJ, Sellati TJ, Teng EI, Furie MB. Production of interleukin-8 (IL-8) by cultured endothelial cells in response to *Borrelia burgdorferi* occurs independently of secreted IL-1 and tumor necrosis factor alpha and is required for subsequent transendothelial migration of neutrophils. Infect Immun. 1997;65(4):1217–22.
200. Sellati TJ, Burns MJ, Ficazzola MA, Furie MB. *Borrelia burgdorferi* upregulates expression of adhesion molecules on endothelial cells and promotes transendothelial migration of neutrophils in vitro. Infect Immun. 1995;63(11):4439–47.
201. Steere AC, Angelis SM. Therapy for Lyme arthritis: strategies for the treatment of antibiotic-refractory arthritis. Arthritis Rheum. 2006;54(10):3079–86. https://doi.org/10.1002/art.22131.
202. Embers ME, Ramamoorthy R, Philipp MT. Survival strategies of *Borrelia burgdorferi*, the etiologic agent of Lyme disease. Microbes Infect. 2004;6(3):312–8.
203. Berger BW, Johnson RC, Kodner C, Coleman L. Failure of *Borrelia burgdorferi* to survive in the skin of patients with antibiotic-treated Lyme disease. J Am Acad Dermatol. 1992;27(1):34–7.
204. Dandache P, Nadelman RB. Erythema migrans. Infect Dis Clin N Am. 2008;22(2):235–60., vi. https://doi.org/10.1016/j.idc.2007.12.012.
205. Nadelman RB, Nowakowski J, Forseter G, Bittker S, Cooper D, Goldberg N, et al. Failure to isolate *Borrelia burgdorferi* after antimicrobial therapy in culture-documented Lyme borreliosis associated with erythema migrans: report of a prospective study. Am J Med. 1993;94(6):583–8.
206. Nowakowski J, Nadelman RB, Sell R, McKenna D, Cavaliere LF, Holmgren D, et al. Long-term follow-up of patients with culture-confirmed Lyme disease. Am J Med. 2003;115(2):91–6.
207. Wormser GP. Hematogenous dissemination in early Lyme disease. Wien Klin Wochenschr. 2006;118(21–22):634–7. https://doi.org/10.1007/s00508-006-0688-9.
208. Brown EL, Kim JH, Reisenbichler ES, Hook M. Multicomponent Lyme vaccine: three is not a crowd. Vaccine. 2005;23(28):3687–96. https://doi.org/10.1016/j.vaccine.2005.02.006.
209. Feng S, Hodzic E, Stevenson B, Barthold SW. Humoral immunity to *Borrelia burgdorferi* N40 decorin binding proteins during infection of laboratory mice. Infect Immun. 1998;66(6):2827–35.
210. Hanson MS, Cassatt DR, Guo BP, Patel NK, McCarthy MP, Dorward DW, et al. Active and passive immunity against *Borrelia burgdorferi* decorin binding protein a (DbpA) protects against infection. Infect Immun. 1998;66(5):2143–53.
211. Comstedt P, Schuler W, Meinke A, Lundberg U. The novel Lyme borreliosis vaccine VLA15 shows broad protection against *Borrelia* species expressing six different OspA serotypes. PLoS One. 2017;12(9):e0184357. https://doi.org/10.1371/journal.pone.0184357.
212. Earnhart CG, Marconi RT. An octavalent Lyme disease vaccine induces antibodies that recognize all incorporated OspC type-specific sequences. Hum Vaccin. 2007;3(6):281–9. https://doi.org/10.4161/Hv.4661.

4 The History, Epidemiology, Clinical Manifestations and Treatment of Lyme Borreliosis

Gerold Stanek and Franc Strle

4.1 Introduction

Lyme borreliosis is caused by certain genospecies of the *Borrelia burgdorferi* sensu lato (s.l.) complex. The disease presents with diverse clinical manifestations. A prerequisite for a correct diagnosis is that physicians should have the best possible knowledge of the clinical features of Lyme borreliosis, which should be acquired through clinical instruction and personal experience. The evidence-based knowledge of Lyme borreliosis is available from case definitions, guidelines, reviews and seminar articles in peer-reviewed publications [1–7]. However, great caution is advised when consulting the internet about the spectrum of clinical symptoms of Lyme borreliosis and approaches for diagnosing Lyme borreliosis. There are hundreds of sites available containing much misinformation [8].

The causative *Borrelia* species of Lyme borreliosis occur in natural foci in vertebrate reservoir hosts and in certain *Ixodes* tick species that transmit the pathogens to other vertebrates, including man. The seasonal occurrence of the main skin manifestation of infection, erythema migrans, is thus linked to tick seasonal activity. Disseminated or late disease shows little seasonality and may appear throughout the year. Reliable clinical diagnosis of Lyme borreliosis without laboratory confirmation is only possible for typical erythema migrans, whereas other manifestations clinically suspicious for Lyme borreliosis need laboratory confirmation. The emphasis in this chapter is on European Lyme borreliosis. It provides information on the

G. Stanek (✉)
Institute for Hygiene and Applied Immunology, Medical University of Vienna, Vienna, Austria
e-mail: Gerold.stanek@meduniwien.ac.at

F. Strle
Department of Infectious Diseases, University Medical Centre Ljubljana, Ljubljana, Slovenia
e-mail: franc.strle@kclj.si

K.-P. Hunfeld, J. Gray (eds.), *Lyme Borreliosis*,
https://doi.org/10.1007/978-3-030-93680-8_4

various clinical presentations of Lyme borreliosis with respect to diagnosis and treatment and is intended to provide an insight into the history and epidemiology of the disease.

4.2 History of Lyme Borreliosis

The history of this disease begins at the end of the nineteenth century when Alfred Buchwald from Breslau (today's Wroclaw) reported on a patient with a "diffuse idiopathic skin atrophy" [9]. It was the first description of a chronic skin disease later referred to as "acrodermatitis chronica atrophicans" [10]. European dermatology literature had described a relationship between joint and bone abnormalities and acrodermatitis chronica atrophicans, as emphasised by the term "akrodermatitis atrophicans arthropathica" [11]. In 1909, Arvid Afzelius reported to the Swedish Dermatological Academy on his observations of an expanding reddening of the skin, which he called "erythema migrans" [12]. In 1913, the Viennese dermatologist Benjamin Lipschütz reported that in one case he had observed a skin rash expanding over a period of 7 months [13]. The skin rash developed from a spot around a tick bite on the thigh and extended over time over the buttocks and the back up to the shoulder; then it healed spontaneously. Lipschütz called this rash "erythema chronicum migrans." Lipschütz recognised the connection with the tick bite and later suggested examination of tick saliva, which he assumed contains the cause of the observed skin disorder [14].

In 1922, Garin and Bujadoux from Lille described a paralysis that occurred after a tick bite [15], which Schaltenbrand clearly differentiated clinically from other arthropod-borne diseases of the nervous system in 1967 [16] and was named radiculo-myelo-meningitis following a tick bite, but the cause was still unknown. However, due to successful treatment with antibiotics [17], it had become very unlikely that a virus could cause this condition. Since the 1950s, dermatologists in Europe have successfully used penicillin for the treatment of acrodermatitis chronica atrophicans and erythema chronicum migrans. Hollström reported the successful treatment of erythema migrans in 16 cases including one with meningitis and found penicillin superior to other drugs [17]. In his article, he mentioned Carl Lennhoff of the dermatological hospital of Magdeburg University, Germany, and then the Karolinska Institute in Stockholm, Sweden, who demonstrated structures in a skin biopsy of erythema migrans that resembled spirochete-like elements, pointing to the possibility that this disease may be caused by tick-associated spirochetes [18]. The dermatologist Klaus Weber from Munich systematically went through all possible viral causes as well as the role of rickettsia and also the agent of tularemia, but had to rule out all of them as causative agents [19]. He also discussed borreliae, which he ruled out due to the prevailing opinion among acarologists at that time that only soft ticks and not hard ticks, such as *Ixodes ricinus,* are carriers of borrelia. The apparent effectiveness of antibiotics against the disorders suggests a bacterial cause, but what bacterial agent was responsible?

An important observation was made in the United States in 1975. Two mothers, Polly Murray and Judith Mensch, reported to the Connecticut State health department that many children in the neighbouring villages of Lyme, Old Lyme and East Haddam had joint problems. Doctors from the health authority and Allen Steere, then a rheumatologist at Yale University in New Haven, Connecticut, organised a monitoring program with the mothers, and the local and school doctors. They examined all children with inflammatory joint diseases from the region and did everything possible to track down the cause of the joint diseases. In a first report, they presented 39 children who suffered from a joint disease that was very similar to the so-called juvenile rheumatoid arthritis. However, the evaluation of the patient data revealed valid differences among the residents of the above-mentioned villages. A total of 4.3 in 1000 suffered from arthritis. Taking the children alone, 12.2 out of 1000 suffered from arthritis. This proportion was about a 100 times higher than the known incidence of juvenile rheumatoid arthritis. Arthritis cases were also found to be more frequent among the small population that lived on the left side of the Connecticut River in a forested area. Most of the patients also remembered that their illness began in summer or early autumn. The geographical and seasonal accumulation matched the picture of an arthropod-borne disease. In addition, about a quarter of the patients remembered a reddened papule on the skin, which they attributed to an insect bite, and that appeared on the skin about 4 weeks before the start of the joint inflammation. Some of these patients also reported that a reddening of the skin developed around the papule, which has been diagnosed as erythema chronicum migrans, for long known in Europe as a disorder following a tick bite [20–22]. In addition, the hard tick species *Ixodes scapularis* (then named *I. dammini*) was widespread in the Lyme area. *I. scapularis* is closely related to the hard tick *I. ricinus*, which is widespread in Europe and associated with erythema chronicum migrans. Thus the role of *I. scapularis* as a vector of an unknown etiological agent was almost beyond doubt [23].

The association of tick-borne erythema chronicum migrans with subsequent joint inflammation was named Lyme arthritis. The ongoing studies revealed other accompanying conditions or diseases following erythema chronicum migrans affecting the nervous system [24] and the heart [25]. Because of the broader spectrum of diseases, the term Lyme disease was then introduced.

The researchers from Yale, who initially considered a virus to be the cause of Lyme disease, nevertheless acted on the European experience of the beneficial effects of antibiotic treatment and treated erythema chronicum migrans cases in the summers of 1977 and 1979 with penicillin. They compared the results with untreated cases of 1976 and 1978 and found that when penicillin was administered at the beginning of the disease, erythema chronicum migrans quickly disappeared and prevented subsequent joint inflammation, or at least reduced its severity. This was another supporting fact for a penicillin-sensitive pathogen [25, 26].

A first-hand account of the discovery of the Lyme disease agent has recently been published by Alan Barbour and Jorge Benach [27]. This text illuminates the context of the discovery and stresses that "the discovery of the Lyme disease agent has threads originating in different places in the United States" and they conclude that the "discovery is actually the product of several threads coming together and is attributable to more people than appreciated." For the world of science it started with the Science paper "Lyme Disease—a Tick-Borne Spirochetosis?" [28] followed by reports on the isolation of cultivable spirochetes from *Ixodes* ticks [29, 30] and finally by the demonstration of the etiologic role of these spirochetes in Lyme disease by isolating them from blood, skin and other specimens from patients in the early 1980s [31, 32]. The "First International Symposium on Lyme Disease" was held at the Yale University School of Medicine in New Haven, Connecticut, November 16–18, 1983. The programme of this conference comprised the topics "clinical features, vector and causative agent, causative agent and host response, animal studies and epidemiological studies" and listed 36 speakers, 5 of them from Europe. The Lyme disease spirochete was described as a new species in the genus *Borrelia* [33] and a discussion on naming this new *Borrelia* species resulted in the name *Borrelia burgdorferi* [34]. Thanks to the activities of physicians and scientists in the United States, it was established that particular disorders of the skin and the nervous system—known in Europe for decades—form a nosological entity that is now summarised under the term Lyme borreliosis. Lyme borreliosis or Lyme disease occurs throughout regions of the northern hemisphere with moderate climates, where the pathogens are exclusively transmitted by hard ticks of the genus *Ixodes*. Although the disease was known before its discovery in Lyme, the terms Lyme disease and Lyme borreliosis have been used extensively and now remain as the accepted descriptors of this disorder.

It was the development of the Barbour–Stoenner–Kelly medium that allowed the cultivation of *B. burgdorferi* from ticks, animals and humans. For characterisation of *B. burgdorferi*, Barbour and Schrumpf raised monoclonal antibodies to the outer surface proteins OspA and OspB and to flagellin proteins [35]. Substantial differences in reactivity were found with isolates from Europe. An OspA typing system was developed by Bettina Wilske and colleagues in Munich and the resulting findings, in conjunction with molecular biological studies by Guy Baranton and colleagues in Paris, provided evidence for new *Borrelia* genospecies such as *B. afzelii* and *B. garinii* [36–39]. The number of genospecies of the *B. burgdorferi* s.l. complex has now increased to more than 20; only a small number of them have clinical significance [40–43]. The prevailing pathogens of Lyme borreliosis in Europe are the genospecies *B. afzelii*, *B. garinii*, *B. bavariensis* (formerly *B. garinii* OspA type 4) and *B. burgdorferi* sensu stricto (henceforward *B. burgdorferi*). *B. spielmanii*, *B. bissetiae*, *B. valaisiana* and *B. lusitaniae* have been identified as pathogens in single cases only. The US pathogenic genospecies are less diverse with only *B. burgdorferi* and *B. mayonii* (also refer Marques/Wormser chapter "Laboratory Diagnosis of Lyme Borreliosis").

The discovery of the causal agent of Lyme borreliosis sparked off a spate of activity in the field of borrelia and tick research. The need to exchange knowledge resulted in a series of biennial or triennial international conferences on Lyme borreliosis and other tick-borne diseases (ICLB), commencing in New Haven, USA in 1984 and then alternating between the United States and Europe. Fifteen such conferences have now been held so far. Additionally, many studies on Lyme borreliosis are presented periodically at other international conferences concerning tick-borne pathogens, such as the International Symposium on Ticks and Tick-borne Diseases (ISTTBD), Ticks and Tick-Borne Pathogens (TTP), and the International Symposium on Tick-Borne Pathogens and Disease (ITPD).

An activity with historical impact was the European Union Concerted Action on Risk Assessment in Lyme Borreliosis (EUCALB), a 3-year EU-funded project involving more than 30 scientists and physicians from 14 countries, which commenced in December 1993 and aimed to provide practical risk assessment criteria for Lyme borreliosis [44–54]. After a series of meetings, case definitions were agreed and published [55] and these were updated in 2011 [4]. Other publications concerned immunoblot serology [56], detection of borrelial infection in ticks, and habitat assessment for Lyme borreliosis risk. The latter study concluded that high risk was associated with highly heterogeneous recreational woodland, and case data from both high and low incidence countries suggested that most infections are acquired in recreational areas. In 2012 former EUCALB participants founded the ESCMID study group on Lyme borreliosis (ESGBOR), which remains active and publishing [57, 58].

Another relevant European project, NorthTick, is co-funded by the European Union through the European Regional Development Fund and the North Sea Region Programme 2014–2020. It addresses tick-borne diseases in general in the region and aims to provide a multidisciplinary and transnational approach in relation to risk assessment, preventive measures, diagnostic strategies and patient management. Eleven beneficiaries from seven different countries (Denmark, Sweden, Norway, Germany, Belgium, United Kingdom and the Netherlands) are involved.

4.3 Epidemiology

The main vector for the pathogens of Lyme borreliosis in Europe is *Ixodes ricinus*, overlapping in the north-eastern parts of Europe with *Ixodes persulcatus*, the principal vector further east. Mice, voles and other small mammals and certain species of birds are the principal vertebrate reservoirs for the agents of Lyme borreliosis. The feeding activity of *I. ricinus* nymphs is highest in late spring to early summer; however, depending on weather conditions and the nature of the habitat, questing ticks may be found throughout the year, even in wintertime. As stated previously, recreational areas are the predominant areas for risk of tick bites. Thus, humans are most frequently exposed to tick bites between April and October during the peak of tick activity, when people are most frequently outdoors and in direct contact with vegetation and tick habitats. Tick bites in children occur more often on the head, while in adults they are on the lower limbs and on the abdominal and gluteal region [59, 60].

A meta-analysis of studies from 23 European countries over the period 2010–2016, determined the prevalence of *Borrelia* strains in 115,028 questing *I. ricinus* ticks. This analysis revealed significantly higher infection rates in adult ticks compared to nymphal ticks (17.8% vs. 14.2%) and in female compared to male ticks (18.4% vs. 15.7%). The data also revealed significant differences between various European regions, with the highest infection rates in Central Europe (19.3% of ticks) and the lowest in the British Isles (3.6%). The most common genospecies found in ticks were *B. afzelii*, *B. garinii* and *B. valaisiana*. No statistically significant differences were found among the prevalence rates determined by conventional PCR, nested PCR, and real-time PCR [61]. Using the PCR-reverse line blot (RLB) method to screen for pathogens in a total of 554 *I. ricinus* ticks collected from all provinces of Austria, *B. burgdorferi* s.l. was found in 25.6% of ticks. Again, *B. afzelii* was the most frequently detected species, followed by *B. burgdorferi* and *B. valaisiana* [62].

Three genospecies, *B. afzelii*, *B. garinii*, and *B. burgdorferi*, are the important human pathogens for Lyme borreliosis in Europe. This is substantiated by the analysis of more than 1000 isolates obtained in prospective studies from Slovenian patients with Lyme borreliosis. Of the 780 *Borrelia* strains isolated from the skin of patients with solitary erythema migrans, 89.5% were *B. afzelii*, 9.4% *B. garinii* and only 1.1% *B. burgdorferi* [63–66]. A similar predominance of *B. afzelii* was shown for isolates from the skin and blood of patients with multiple erythema migrans and borrelial lymphocytoma. However, there have also been isolates of *B. garinii*, *B. burgdorferi*, and *B. bisettii* from patients presenting with these manifestations, suggesting that several species may cause erythema migrans or borrelial lymphocytoma. Isolates from acrodermatitis chronica atrophicans skin lesions were in 92.8% *B. afzelii*, in 3.6% each *B. garinii* and *B. burgdorferi* [67]. In contrast, over 75% of isolates from cerebrospinal fluid (CSF) of patients with Lyme neuroborreliosis were *B. garinii* [65, 68–70]. Of interest is that the frequency distribution of borrelial isolates from patients does not correspond with that found in ticks.

Lyme borreliosis is the most common tick-borne infection in humans throughout the moderate climates of the northern hemisphere. However, the actual incidence of this disease in Europe is very variable. This is well documented in the number of reported cases from countries with a history of mandatory reporting. The overall incidence in Slovenia for example ranged in a 10-year period (2009–2018) between 183 and 365 cases per 100,000 inhabitants, mean 257 (Strle personal comm. 2021). Incidence determined over the same period in Bulgaria ranged from 4.1 to 11.9 cases per 100,000 inhabitants, mean 6.9. Figure 4.1 displays the variation of overall incidence from year to year and also the difference in the disease burden between the two countries. However, a high variation of incidence was also observed in different regions of Bulgaria, varying from 0.30 to 30.9 per 100,000 inhabitants [71].

A population-based retrospective cohort study aimed to estimate the annual incidence of Lyme borreliosis over the years 2001–2012 in the United Kingdom. The results indicate a constant increase of incidence from 1.6 to 12.1, with a high variation of incidence rates across different parts of a region [72]. A database search again ascertained the large variance in the incidence rates of Lyme borreliosis in western countries of Europe, between the countries and in regions within the countries with a calculated mean incidence of 56.3 cases per 100,000 inhabitants per year [73]. The incidence of Lyme borreliosis in six eastern states of Germany varied

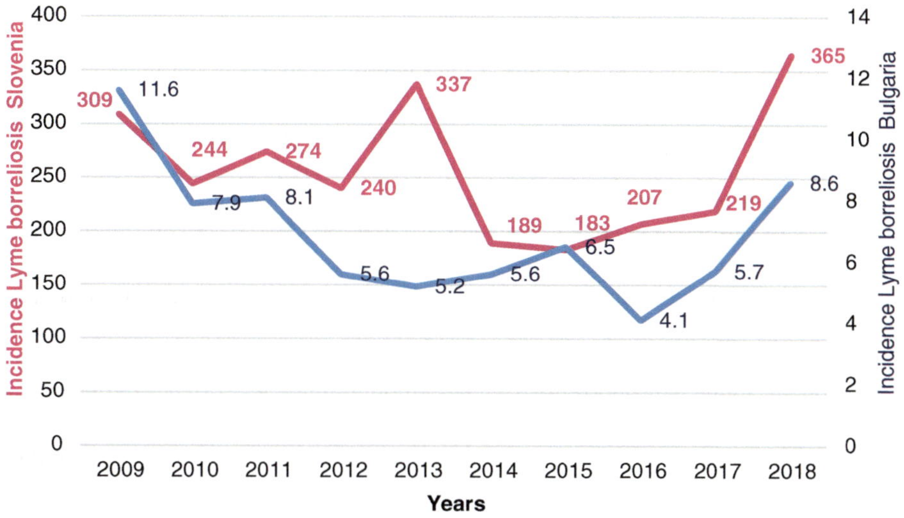

Fig. 4.1 Overall incidence of Lyme borreliosis (n cases per 100,000 inhabitants) per year in Bulgaria and Slovenia. Average population: BG 7.28 and SI 2.05 million people

between 35 cases in 2009 and 20 cases per 100,000 inhabitants in 2012 [74]. Another study from Germany used cases notified in the years 2013–2017 and calculated an incidence ranging from 41 per 100,00 in 2013 to 26 in 2015 with a mean 2013–2017 annual incidence on district level between 0.5 and 138 cases per 100,000 [75]. In France, the average incidence of Lyme borreliosis for the years 2004–2009 was 42 ranging from 0 to 184 per 100,000 inhabitants [76]. Another study from France found a mean yearly incidence of Lyme borreliosis of 53 cases per 100,000 inhabitants, ranging from 41 in 2011 to 84 in 2016. The incidence of patients hospitalised for Lyme borreliosis ranged from 1.1 cases per 100,000 in 2005 to 1.5 in 2016 [77]. In the Netherlands, a decrease of tick bite consultations and stabilisation of early Lyme borreliosis cases, erythema migrans, was observed in 2014. The incidence of erythema migrans retained at 140 per 100,000 [78]. The mean annual incidence of Lyme borreliosis in the Veneto area, Italy, for the period 2015–2019 was 0.999 cases per 100,000 inhabitants with a peak of 2 per 100,000 in 2018 [79]. Although overall incidence can vary widely incidences of districts particularly allow to identify areas of higher risk for tick-borne borrelia infection.

A surprisingly constant finding is the risk of acquiring a borrelia infection (Lyme borreliosis diagnosis and/or seroconversion) after a tick bite. A prospective study carried out in the years 2008–2009 in Sweden and on the Åland Islands showed that the risk of borrelia infection after a tick bite is 5% [80]. The same figure of 5% was obtained in a prospective study on the same topic in Austria in 2015–2018 [81].

More than 75% of all Lyme borreliosis cases are diagnosed between June and October, with erythema migrans being the most frequently diagnosed clinical manifestation, accounting for about 90% of all cases in central Europe, ranging between 95.4% [74] and 95%, 89% and 77% [59, 75, 82]. Another skin disorder, acrodermatitis chronica atrophicans occurs in about 3% of cases of Lyme borreliosis. The third skin disorder, borrelial lymphocytoma is seen in 2% [82], but more frequently in children than in adults. Lyme neuroborreliosis is the most common extracutaneous manifestation of Lyme borreliosis in Europe; its proportion ranges between 16.7% and 2.7% as reported in studies from southern Sweden in the 1990s and from Germany in the years 2013–2017, respectively [59, 75]. Lyme arthritis is apparently a less common manifestation in Europe than in the United States. Its frequency in European studies is between 2% and 7% [59, 74]. Heart involvement appears to be very rare. A bimodal age distribution of Lyme borreliosis is reported from several European countries, with incidence peaks reported in children 5–9 years old and in adults from 50 to 74 years [59, 75, 83]. Female patients are more frequently affected than males [59, 84]. The most common reasons for hospitalisation are Lyme neuroborreliosis and—although much less often—Lyme arthritis [75]. Erythema migrans occurs soon after the tick bite and is thus linked to the level of tick activity, which is seasonal, in contrast to other manifestations that may present at any time of the year [2, 59].

4.4 Clinical Manifestations of Lyme Borreliosis

The clinically most characteristic presentation of Lyme borreliosis in Europe is the skin infection, erythema migrans. Erythema migrans manifests in about 90% of patients with Lyme borreliosis; in the remaining 10%, the disease presents with disseminated or later manifestations of the illness, such as Lyme neuroborreliosis or arthritis [2, 7].

4.4.1 Skin Manifestations

Erythema migrans, borrelial lymphocytoma and acrodermatitis chronica atrophicans are characteristic manifestations of Lyme borreliosis. Other skin manifestations such as scleroderma circumscripta, lichen sclerosus et atrophicus and cutaneous B-cell lymphoma have also been associated with Lyme borreliosis, but these associations are questionable.

4.4.1.1 Erythema Migrans

Erythema migrans is defined as an erythematous skin lesion that develops days to weeks at the site of a bite where a borrelia-infected tick has transmitted borreliae into the skin during the course of its blood meal. The lesion typically begins as a red macula or papule and expands over days to weeks, with or without central clearing. For a reliable diagnosis, a single primary lesion must reach ≥5 cm in diameter. A lesion of <5 cm qualifies for the diagnosis of erythema migrans only if it develops at the site of a tick bite, if its onset has a delay of at least 2 days, and if the lesion is enlarging. Multiple erythema migrans is defined as the presence of two or more skin lesions, one of which must fulfil the size criteria for solitary erythema migrans [2, 4].

Untreated erythema migrans may persist and expand over weeks to several months, their diameter ranging from a few centimetres to more than a meter. Erythema migrans is most often located on the lower extremities in adult patients; in children, the upper part of the body is more often involved [2–6, 59, 60]. Local symptoms such as mild itching, burning or pain at the site of erythema migrans may be experienced in about half of European patients. Systemic symptoms, such as fatigue and malaise, headache, myalgia and arthralgia may only be experienced by about one-third of European patients. These symptoms are usually intermittent and often vary in intensity and location. Fever is only recorded exceptionally in adult European patients, whereas in the United States it occurs more frequently in erythema migrans patients. In multiple erythema migrans, the secondary lesions are similar in morphology to the initial solitary lesion, are usually smaller and are only exceptionally associated with local itching or pain. In Europe, multiple erythema migrans is more frequently seen in children than in adults. Differential diagnoses comprise tick- or insect-bite hypersensitivity reaction, fungal infection, erysipelas, urticaria, contact eczema, folliculitis, cellulitis, granuloma annulare and fixed drug eruption [2, 5, 69, 85–95].

4.4.1.2 Borrelial Lymphocytoma

Borrelial lymphocytoma presents as a solitary swelling up to a few centimetres in diameter and consists of a dense lymphocytic infiltration of dermis and subcutaneous tissue due to the borrelial infection. B-lymphocytes predominate in this polyclonal infiltration and germinal centres may be seen. The predominance of B cells contrasts with the findings in erythema migrans and acrodermatitis chronica atrophicans skin lesions where T cells prevail. High levels of the B-cell active chemokine CXCL13 are found in this skin manifestation in contrast to erythema migrans and acrodermatitis chronica atrophicans. Borrelial lymphocytoma is more frequently seen in children than in adults and most frequently located on the ear lobe. In adults it is mostly located in the region of the areola mammae, rarely on the nose, arm, shoulder or scrotum. Borrelial lymphocytoma, like erythema migrans, also resolves eventually without treatment. The isolation rate of borreliae is about 1/3; *B. afzelii* is most frequently identified. Differential diagnosis requires histological examination, particularly in patients with breast lymphocytoma or lymphocytoma at other (atypical) locations especially if an association with borrelial infection cannot be established and B-cell lymphoma and pseudolymphoma are considered [96–99].

4.4.1.3 Acrodermatitis Chronica Atrophicans

Acrodermatitis chronica atrophicans is a chronic skin manifestation of Lyme borreliosis. It is almost exclusively seen in Europe. Unlike erythema migrans and borrelial lymphocytoma, acrodermatitis chronica atrophicans does not heal spontaneously. The lesion is most often located on acral parts of the body, usually on the extensor part of the hands or feet. Initially it is usually unilateral, but later on it may become more or less symmetrical. Acrodermatitis chronica atrophicans is more often diagnosed in women than in men and occurs only very exceptionally in children. Patients are usually over 40 years old. It is most frequently caused by *B. afzelii*. A history of tick bites is not diagnostically supportive because of the long incubation time and the long duration of the skin lesions prior to diagnosis. Clinically, the involved region is initially usually edematous; erythema and swelling may vary in intensity. After the initial months to years, the edema slowly vanishes and gradually atrophy becomes more and more prominent. The skin becomes increasingly vulnerable, thin and wrinkling, with prominently visible underlying vessels. When exposed to a cold environment, the skin becomes pronouncedly bluish. Band-like fibrous indurations may occur in the involved regions, usually in ulnar or tibial regions, or they may be nodular, preferably localised prepatellarly or next to the olecranon. In some cases, sclerotic lesions are clinically and histologically indistinguishable from localised scleroderma (morphea) or lichen sclerosus et atrophicus. In typical inflammatory acrodermatitis chronica atrophicans every tenth patient may also have a lichen sclerosus et atrophicus-like lesion [63, 67, 84, 99–103].

Patients with long-lasting untreated acrodermatitis chronica atrophicans may suffer from some kind of mild or moderate neuropathy [104]. Sensory and motor mononeuropathy or polyneuropathy or patchy dysesthesia may develop at the site of the cutaneous lesions. Patients with acrodermatitis chronica atrophicans may complain of hyperesthesia, dysesthesia, muscle cramps, muscle weakness and/or sensations of heaviness, mainly in the affected limb(s) [105]. In long-lasting cases, subluxation and/or luxation of the small joints of hands or feet may occur. Periosteal thickening of bones similar to dactylitis syphilitica in the late phase of syphilis may also occur in a small proportion of patients. Preceding or accompanying inflammations may occur, such as bursitis of the knee or elbow, epicondylitis, retro- or subcalcaneal bursitis and Achilles tendinitis.

A proper diagnosis is based on clinical, serological and histological criteria. IgG antibodies to *B. burgdorferi* s.l. are a prerequisite; IgG-negative acrodermatitis chronica atrophicans patients are almost non-existent. Further consolidation of the diagnosis is achieved by histological examination of the involved skin. The diagnosis can be further supported by the isolation of *B. burgdorferi* s.l. from lesional skin, successful in about one-third of patients [67]. Differential diagnoses or more often false interpretation of acrodermatitis chronica atrophicans skin lesions on the lower extremities are vascular insufficiency such as chronic venous insufficiency, superficial thrombophlebitis, hypostatic eczema, arterial obliterative disease, acrocyanosis, livedo reticularis, lymphedema, "old skin," or chilblains. Fibrous nodules may be misinterpreted as rheumatoid nodules and gout or even as erythema nodosum.

4.4.2 Lyme Neuroborreliosis

Lyme neuroborreliosis appears during the first few weeks or months after the onset of infection. In adult patients, meningoradiculoneuritis is the most frequent clinical manifestation of Lyme neuroborreliosis in Europe. Its onset is gradual with increasing pain, later on accompanied by palsies and other neurological signs and symptoms that may, if untreated, persist for many weeks [106, 107]. Radicular pain, the most pronounced clinical symptom of meningoradiculoneuritis, is usually severe and most intense during the night. In children, isolated meningitis and peripheral facial palsy are more common than in adults [108–110]. Involvement of motor nerves may lead to paresis [107, 111, 112]. European patients with untreated meningopolyneuritis will develop signs and symptoms of disseminated encephalomyelitis in up to 10% that may in some respects resemble those seen in multiple sclerosis [111]. Dementia-like syndromes, diagnosed as definite Lyme neuroborreliosis according to the European guidelines, are rare manifestations of Lyme neuroborreliosis. It is essential to be aware of this manifestation of Lyme neuroborreliosis because antibiotic treatment will prevent permanent sequelae [113]. Patients with borrelial meningitis usually suffer from mild headache with intermittent improvements and deterioration. In adult patients, fever, nausea and vomiting and meningeal signs are usually absent [111, 112]. However, CSF findings display a lymphocytic pleocytosis up to several hundred million cells/l. Protein concentrations are normal or slightly elevated; glucose concentrations are usually normal or mildly depleted [111]. Any cranial nerve may be affected in Lyme neuroborreliosis but facial nerves are most frequently involved, resulting in unilateral or bilateral peripheral facial palsy [111]. This is due to *B. burgdorferi* s.l. infection in about 20% of adult patients and 25% of children in endemic regions [107, 109, 112, 114]. Lymphocytic pleocytosis is often seen in patients with borrelial peripheral facial palsy, although signs or symptoms of meningitis are absent [114]. Borrelial peripheral facial palsy responds very well to antibiotic treatment, but the prognosis is also good in untreated patients [112, 115]. However, in Sweden, mild sequelae were found in about every second child who had borrelial peripheral facial palsy 3–5 years ago [116]. Another Swedish study reported on about 20% of children with acute facial palsy who had permanent mild-to-moderate dysfunction of the facial nerve without other neurological symptoms or health problems, despite antibiotic treatment [117].

Intrathecal synthesis of antibodies may not be detectable and cerebrospinal fluid pleocytosis may be absent shortly after the onset of neurological symptoms, especially in children with isolated facial palsy [108]. Involvement of most other cranial nerves has been described, particularly nervus oculomotorius, n. abducens and n. vestibulocochlearis. Best support for a clinical diagnosis of Lyme neuroborreliosis is a preceding or accompanying erythema migrans, which is the case in 34–64% of patients with meningoradiculoneuritis [65]. In European patients, a close spatial relationship was found between the skin region of the tick bite, the subsequent erythema migrans, and the radicular lesion [118]. Pseudotumour cerebri is an unusual manifestation of Lyme neuroborreliosis which is seen primarily in children [119, 120].

Lyme neuroborreliosis in Europe is most often caused by *B. garinii*, less frequently by *B. afzelii* and *B. burgdorferi*, and only exceptionally by other genospecies [65, 68–70, 121–124]. Patients with a CSF culture-proven *B. garinii* Lyme neuroborreliosis have a different clinical course than patients with a *B. afzelii* Lyme neuroborreliosis. Painful meningoradiculoneuritis, Bannwarth syndrome, the typical early Lyme neuroborreliosis in Europe, is caused by *B. garinii*, whereas the clinical features of central nervous system (CNS) involvement associated with *B. afzelii* are much less specific and more difficult to diagnose since these patients rarely report radicular pains or express meningeal signs [65]. The European criteria for Lyme neuroborreliosis are not fulfilled by a large majority of *B. afzelii* Lyme neuroborreliosis cases, and the significance of these genospecies in Lyme neuroborreliosis remains to be elucidated. In peripheral neuropathy accompanying acrodermatitis chronica atrophicans, the most striking finding is axonal degeneration [104]. It occurs in more than half of patients with long-lasting acrodermatitis chronica atrophicans. Whether borrelial linked peripheral neuritis exists at all without acrodermatitis chronica atrophicans is doubtful.

The diagnosis of early Lyme neuroborreliosis should be based on clinical characteristics, the presence of lymphocytic pleocytosis and demonstration of intrathecal production of IgG antibodies against *B. burgdorferi* s.l. in order to prove borrelial infection of the CNS [3, 36, 65, 69, 70, 125–128]. Isolation of borreliae from the infection site would be the most reliable method of diagnosing Lyme neuroborreliosis, but unfortunately isolation from CSF or demonstration of borrelial DNA in CSF samples is limited by low sensitivity. Although the demonstration of intrathecally synthesised IgG antibodies to *B. burgdorferi* s.l. has been established for the diagnosis of Lyme neuroborreliosis, physicians should be aware that intrathecal antibodies may not be demonstrable shortly after the onset of Lyme neuroborreliosis. If there is strong clinical evidence, together with CSF pleocytosis and/or preceding erythema migrans, the clinician should stay with the clinical diagnosis, despite the absence of proof of intrathecal antibody production [69, 70]. Differential diagnosis comprises a list for each main manifestation of Lyme neuroborreliosis, such as meningitis, radiculoneuritis, cranial nerve involvement and others.

4.4.3 Lyme Carditis

Borrelial infection of the heart usually presents with acute onset of varying degrees of intermittent atrioventricular (A-V) heart block, often together with other manifestations of Lyme borreliosis such as erythema migrans, Lyme neuroborreliosis or arthritis. In most cases, it is a mild and self-limited event and the prognosis is usually favourable. Diagnosis of Lyme carditis is most reliable when occurring together with typical manifestation(s) of Lyme borreliosis such as erythema migrans or Lyme neuroborreliosis, and by the absence or exclusion of other explanations for cardiac abnormalities [2, 25, 129–132].

4.4.4 Lyme Arthritis

Arthritis due to a *B. burgdorferi* s.l. infection is mostly monoarticular or oligoarticular, typically involving the knee. The isolation rate of borreliae from joint fluid and synovia is very low; thus, data on the infecting agent are based predominantly on molecular detection of borrelial DNA in synovial fluid or synovial tissue. The genospecies identified in Lyme arthritis cases in Europe are *B. burgdorferi*, *B. afzelii* and *B. garinii* with a pronounced predominance of *B. burgdorferi* in some series [133–137]. *Borrelia bavariensis* was detected in the synovial fluid of the knee and ankle joint of an 11-year-old boy who suffered from intermittent arthritis over 5 years [138]. Acute arthritis results from *Borrelia*-induced infiltration of mononuclear cells into the synovial tissue and the accumulation of neutrophils, immune complexes, complement and cytokines in the synovial fluid [139].

For clinical diagnosis, it should be considered that Lyme arthritis usually consists of intermittent attacks of inflammation of one or a few large joints and is often preceded by intermittent migratory joint pain. Joint involvement is usually asymmetric, the onset of arthritis is acute and with effusion, and skin over the affected joint is warm but of normal colour. The knee is by far the most common joint involved, followed by ankle, wrist, finger, toe and elbow; heel swelling was found in 9% and dactylitis in as many as 23%. In the patients with knee involvement alone, Baker cysts were found in 50%. However, some patients with pronounced knee effusions have only mild pains. Joint inflammation usually lasts a few days to weeks, sometimes several months. The course of Lyme arthritis is usually recurring and may continue for several years. In the beginning, the attacks of arthritis are more frequent and short, later they may be more prolonged and about 10% of patients develop chronic arthritis with duration of a year or longer. Fatigue, malaise, low fever or night sweats may accompany Lyme arthritis in a small proportion of patients [140–143].

Diagnosis of Lyme arthritis is based on the medical history, history or the presence of other manifestations of Lyme borreliosis such as erythema migrans, Lyme neuroborreliosis or acrodermatitis chronica atrophicans, clinical features, laboratory findings, exclusion of other causes of arthritis and demonstration of serum IgG antibodies to *B. burgdorferi* s.l. Routine laboratory parameters such as C-reactive protein, rheumatoid factors and anti-nuclear antibodies are often within the normal range in Lyme arthritis. The pronounced elevation of laboratory inflammation parameters in a patient with arthritis argues strongly against a diagnosis of Lyme arthritis. Cryoglobulins and circulating immune complexes may be present. Synovial fluid shows elevated white cell counts with a predominance of polymorphonuclear leukocytes. Cryoglobulins and antigen–antibody complexes are commonly present in synovial fluid. Specific radiographic findings for Lyme arthritis have not been reported. Serum IgG antibodies to *B. burgdorferi* s.l. are almost always present in high titers in patients with Lyme arthritis. Negative IgG serology rules out the diagnosis of Lyme arthritis, but the detection of IgG antibodies alone is not diagnostic for Lyme borreliosis. Thus, detection of borrelial DNA in synovial tissue or synovial fluid should be attempted since its sensitivity is high [20, 21, 140–147].

The differential diagnosis of Lyme arthritis includes inflammatory rheumatic diseases, bacterial (septic) arthritis, viral arthritis and crystal-induced arthritis. Other differential diagnoses include psoriatic arthritis, early rheumatoid arthritis and systemic lupus erythematosus in patients who have borrelial antibodies in serum. Fibromyalgia in seropositive persons is often wrongly diagnosed as Lyme borreliosis [1, 6, 148, 149].

4.4.5 Eye Involvement

Eye involvement in the course of Lyme borreliosis appears to occur very rarely and is associated with erythema migrans, Lyme neuroborreliosis or Lyme arthritis, although it can be the sole manifestation of the disease. Diagnosis of borrelial eye involvement should be based on medical history, complete physical (not only ophthalmological) examination and demonstration of borrelial infection. The differential diagnosis is broad [150–154].

4.4.6 Lyme Borreliosis During Pregnancy

Information on this topic is limited. There is no substantial difference between pregnant and nonpregnant women, either in the presentation of Lyme borreliosis or in the outcome of treatment in the corresponding adult population, with the exception that in the second half of pregnancy the proportion of patients with erythema migrans having constitutional symptoms is lower than during the first months of pregnancy and in nonpregnant women of a comparable age. It seems that the outcome of pregnancies is similar to the outcome in pregnant women without Lyme borreliosis. With the exception of some individual reports that do not fulfill current diagnostic criteria, no causal relationship with borrelial infection has been established for unfavourable outcomes of pregnancies [155–159].

4.4.7 Lyme Borreliosis in Immunocompromised Patients

Information on this topic is also limited. However, the results of four studies revealed that all patients had a mild and uncomplicated erythema migrans, as well as a favourable outcome after treatment with the same antibiotic regimens as used for immunocompetent patients [160–163].

4.4.8 Chronic Lyme Borreliosis and "Chronic Lyme"

Chronic Lyme borreliosis exists in Europe. However, the designation should be reserved for patients with objective manifestations of late Lyme borreliosis. These patients typically present with acrodermatitis chronica atrophicans, chronic arthritis and very rarely with chronic Lyme neuroborreliosis. The term chronic Lyme borreliosis should not be misused or erroneously used for symptoms of unknown cause, nor for well-defined illness unrelated to borrelial infection but with antibodies against *B. burgdorferi* s.l., nor for symptoms of unknown cause with antibodies against *B. burgdorferi* s.l., but no reliable history of Lyme borreliosis, and not for post-Lyme borreliosis symptoms or syndrome [1, 164, 165].

4.4.9 Laboratory Support in the Diagnosis of Lyme Borreliosis

Table 4.1 summarises the essential and supporting laboratory evidence in relation to the various initial clinical diagnoses of Lyme borreliosis (also refer chapter "Prophylactic Measures Including Future Perspectives").

4.4.10 Treatment

It should be emphasised that early manifestations of Lyme borreliosis, both localised and disseminated, eventually heal spontaneously without antibiotic treatment. The main reason to treat such patients is to shorten the duration of the manifestation

Table 4.1 Laboratory support in the diagnosis of Lyme borreliosis; modified after Stanek et al. (2011) [4] and Stanek and Strle (2018) [7]

Initial clinical diagnosis	Essential laboratory evidence	Supporting laboratory evidence
Erythema migrans	None if typical	Culture from skin biopsy, Detection of borrelial DNA, significant change in levels of specific serum antibodies[a]
Borrelial lymphocytoma	Specific IgG antibodies	Histology, Culture from skin biopsy, Detection of borrelial DNA
Acrodermatitis chronica atrophicans	High level of specific serum IgG antibodies	Histology, Culture from skin biopsy, Detection of borrelial DNA
Early Lyme neuroborreliosis	Lymphocytic pleocytosis in CSF; Intrathecally produced specific antibodies[b]	Intrathecal total IgM and IgG, Specific oligoclonal bands in CSF, Significant change in levels of specific serum antibodies[a], Culture from CSF, detection of borrelial DNA
Late Lyme neuroborreliosis	Lymphocytic pleocytosis in CSF; intrathecally produced specific antibodies[b]; specific serum IgG	Specific oligoclonal bands in CSF
Lyme arthritis	High level of specific serum Antibodies	Detection of borrelial DNA in synovial fluid and/or tissue (culture from synovial Fluid and/or tissue)
Lyme carditis	Significant change in levels of specific IgG antibodies[a]	Culture from endomyocardial biopsy, Detection of borrelial DNA

[a] Specific antibody levels in serum may increase in response to progression of infection or treatment or may decrease due to abrogation of the infection process. Samples collected a minimum of 3 months apart may be required in order to detect a decrease in IgG levels
[b] Intrathecally produced specific antibodies are determined by investigating simultaneously drawn samples of CSF and serum

and to prevent the development of disseminated disease such as Lyme neuroborreliosis and Lyme arthritis. Doxycycline, amoxicillin, phenoxymethylpenicillin and cefuroxime axetil are highly effective and are the preferred antimicrobial agents for the treatment of early localised manifestations. Macrolides such as azithromycin seem to be clinically somewhat less effective than other oral antibiotics and are consequently used as second-line treatments [1, 5, 88, 90]. Roxithromycin should not be given due to commonly observed relapses after the administration of this drug. Quinolones are not used because *B. burgdorferi* s.l. showed resistance to these chemotherapeutics in in-vitro studies [166]. Early disseminated disease such as Lyme neuroborreliosis is usually treated with intravenous ceftriaxone or penicillin. However, results of more recent studies suggest that oral doxycycline treatment of Lyme neuroborreliosis is as effective as intravenous ceftriaxone for the treatment of European adults with Lyme neuroborreliosis [167, 168]. The shortest duration of effective treatment has never been assessed for any of the antimicrobial agents listed above. Today, it is recommended that antibiotics should be administered for 2 weeks in cases of early localised and early disseminated disease [1, 6, 93]. For chronic manifestations, a 4-week course is recommended. It has been shown that a 10-day regimen of oral doxycycline was not inferior to a 2 week-regimen for erythema migrans [92, 169]. However, there is no direct information on the shorter treatment for immunocompromised patients, nor for antibiotics other than doxycycline. Lyme arthritis typically responds to antibiotic treatment. Patients whose arthritis is improved but not resolved after an initial course of oral treatment can be re-treated with a second course of oral antibiotics, reserving parenteral antibiotic treatment for those without any substantial clinical response. After resolution of arthritis of the knee, physical therapy may be needed if quadriceps atrophy has developed [6]. Recommended antibiotic treatment for patients with Lyme borreliosis is shown in Table 4.2. Doxycycline should not be prescribed for pregnant and breast feeding women and has some restrictions also for children under the age of 8 years.

4.5 Concluding Statement

Lyme borreliosis is a common tick-borne disease in Europe. The identification of causative spirochetal agents, *Borrelia burgdorferi* sensu lato, in the 1980s allowed for specific diagnoses of diseases in several clinical disciplines and for causal antibiotic therapy. At the same time, misconception and speculation regarding links between borrelia infection and a variety of nonspecific symptoms and disorders resulted in overdiagnosis and overtreatment of suspected Lyme borreliosis. When chronic Lyme borreliosis is suspected, other potential causes of the clinical syndrome must be meticulously excluded. Particular caution is recommended when consulting the web for comprehensive information on the disease complex.

Table 4.2 Recommended antibiotic treatment for patients with Lyme borreliosis, modified after Stanek and Strle (2018) [7]

Clinical manifestation	Antibiotic	Mode of administration	Dosing: Adults	Dosing: Children[a]	Duration (days)	Contraindications
Erythema migrans, Borrelial lymphocytoma	Doxycycline or	Oral	100 mg bid	4.4 mg/kg: 2 (maximum, 100 mg per dose)	10–14	Children[b], pregnancy, lactation, allergy
	Amoxicillin or	Oral	500–1000 mg tid	25–50 mg/kg: 3 (maximum, 500 mg per dose)	14	Allergy
	Cefuroxime or	Oral	500 mg bid	28–40 mg/kg: 2 (maximum, 500 mg per dose)	14	Allergy
	Phenoxymethylpenicillin	Oral	0.5–1.0 × 10^6 IU tid	0.1–0.15 × 10^6 IE/kg: 3 (maximum, 1 × 10^6 IU per dose)	14	Allergy
	Azithromycin[c] or	Oral	500 mg bid	20 mg/kg: 2	1st day	Allergy
			500 mg od	10 mg/kg	4 days	
			or 500 mg od	10 mg/kg (maximum, 500 mg per day)	6 days	
	Erithromycin[c]	Oral	500 mg qid	28 mg/kg: 4 (maximum, 500 mg per dose)	14	Allergy
	Ceftriaxone[4] or	i.v.	2 g od	50–100 mg/kg (maximum, 2 g per dose)	14	Allergy
	Penicillin G[d]	i.v.	5 × 10^6 IU qid	0.25–0.5 × 10^6 IE/kg: 4 (maximum, 5 × 106 IU per dose)	14	Allergy

(continued)

Table 4.2 (continued)

Clinical manifestation		Antibiotic	Mode of administration	Dosing		Duration (days)	Contraindications
				Adults	Children[a]		
Lyme neuroborreliosis, Heart involvement		Ceftriaxone or	i.v.	2 g od	50–100 mg/kg (maximum, 2 g per dose)	14–28[e]	Allergy
		Penicillin G	i.v.	5×10^6 IU qid	0.25–0.5 × 10^6 IE/kg: 4 (maximum, 5 × 106 IU per dose)	14–28[e]	Allergy
		Doxycycline	Oral	100 mg bid or 200 mg od[f]	4.4 mg/kg: 2 (maximum, 100 mg per dose)	14–28[e]	children[b], pregnancy, lactation, allergy
Lyme arthritis	Initial treatment	Doxycycline or	Oral	100 mg bid	4.4 mg/kg: 2 (maximum, 100 mg per dose)	28	children[b], pregnancy, lactation, allergy
		Amoxicillin or	Oral	500–1000 mg tid	25–50 mg/kg: 3 (maximum, 500 mg per dose)	28	Allergy
		Cefuroxime	Oral	500 mg bid	28–40 mg/kg: 2 (maximum, 500 mg per dose)	28	Allergy
	Retreatment[g]	Doxycycline or	Oral	100 mg bid	4.4 mg/kg: 2 (maximum, 100 mg per dose)	28	children[b], pregnancy, lactation, allergy
		Amoxicillin or	Oral	500–1000 mg tid	25–50 mg/kg: 3 (maximum, 500 mg per dose)	28	Allergy
		Cefuroxime or	Oral	500 mg bid	28–40 mg/kg: 2 (maximum, 500 mg per dose)	28	Allergy
		Ceftriaxone[h]	i.v.	2 g od	50–100 mg/kg (maximum, 2 g per dose)	14–28	Allergy

Acrodermatitis chronica atrophicans	Doxycycline or	Oral	100 mg bid	4.4 mg/kg: 2 (maximum, 100 mg per dose)	21 (14–28)	children[b], pregnancy, lactation, allergy
	Amoxicillin or	Oral	500–1000 mg tid	25–50 mg/kg: 3 (maximum, 500 mg per dose)	21 (14–28)	Allergy
	Ceftriaxone[i]	i.v.	2 g od	50–100 mg/kg (maximum, 2 g per dose)	21 (14–28)	Allergy

od once daily, *bid* two times daily, *tid* three times daily, *qid* four times daily, *i.v.* intravenous, *IU* international units

[a] For children total daily dosage is given, divided into the number of doses per day

[b] Relative contraindication for age < 8 years

[c] Azithromycin and erythromycin are used in patients allergic to penicillin and tetracyclines

[d] Ceftriaxone and penicillin G are used for the treatment of erythema migrans and borrelial lymphocytoma very rarely (potentially for patients with severe immunodeficiency and for pregnant women)

[e] Early Lyme neuroborreliosis is as a rule treated for 2 weeks, heart involvement for 2–3 weeks, late Lyme neuroborreliosis for 4 weeks

[f] For treatment of early Lyme neuroborreliosis more information is available for 200 mg once daily than for 100 mg twice daily

[g] In case of recurrent Lyme arthritis or partial response to the initial treatment

[h] Ceftriaxone is most often used when there had been only a minimal response to previous oral antibiotics

[i] Cheaper and more patient-friendly oral treatment with doxycycline or amoxicillin is in general preferred to i.v. therapy with ceftriaxone

Lyme borreliosis has an excellent prognosis after adequate antibiotic therapy.
Clinical pictures of skin infection with *Borrelia burgdorferi* sensu lato

(a) *Ixodes ricinus* female tick almost fully engorged—a rare finding on human skin (©G. Stanek).
(b) Acrodermatitis chronica atrophicans on the dorsal side of both hands (©Hasel Druck & Verlag, 1090 Vienna, Austria).
(c) Borrelial lymphocytoma on the ear lobe (©Hasel Druck & Verlag, 1090 Vienna, Austria).
(d) Erythema migrans on left lower leg (©G. Stanek).
(e) Erythema migrans expanding from the scalp where the tick bite occurred (©Hasel Druck & Verlag, 1090 Vienna, Austria).
(f) Erythema migrans on the back of the knee (©G. Stanek).
(g) Erythema migrans on the right upper part of the shoulder (©Hasel Druck & Verlag, 1090 Vienna, Austria).
(h) Erythema migrans, intensively coloured, on the right side of the chest (©M. Markowicz).
(i) Erythema migrans expanding around the upper arm (©G. Stanek).

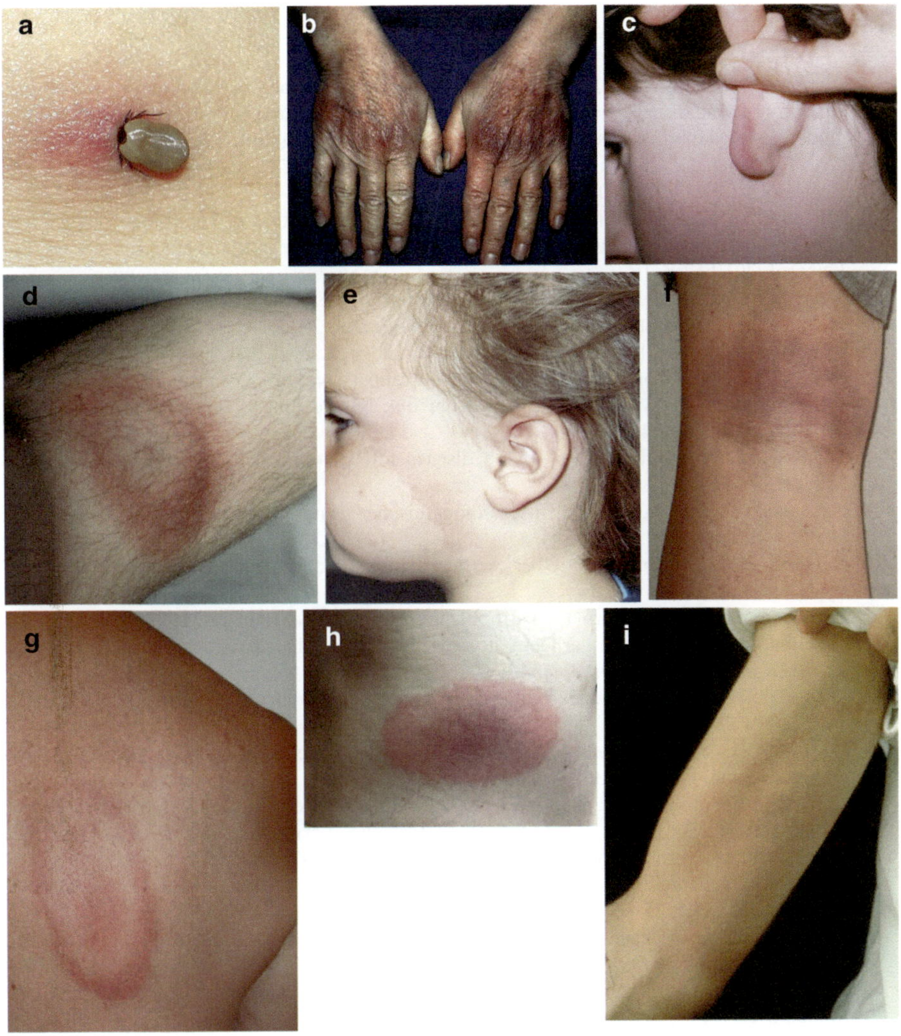
a
b
c
d
e
f
g
h
i

References

1. Wormser GP, Dattwyler RJ, Shapiro ED, et al. The clinical assessment, treatment, and prevention of Lyme disease, human granulocytic anaplasmosis, and babesiosis: clinical practice guidelines by the Infectious Diseases Society of America. Clin Infect Dis. 2006;43:1089–134.
2. Strle F, Stanek G. Clinical manifestations and diagnosis of Lyme borreliosis. Curr Probl Dermatol. 2009;37:51–110.
3. Mygland A, Ljøstad U, Fingerle V, et al. European Federation of Neurological Societies. EFNS guidelines on the diagnosis and management of European Lyme neuroborreliosis. Eur J Neurol. 2010;17:8–16.
4. Stanek G, Fingerle V, Hunfeld KP, et al. Lyme borreliosis: clinical case definitions for diagnosis and management in Europe. Clin Microbiol Infect. 2011;17:69–79.
5. Stanek G, Wormser GP, Gray J, et al. Lyme borreliosis. Lancet. 2012;379:461–73.
6. Steere AC, Strle F, Wormser GP, et al. Lyme borreliosis. Nat Rev Dis Primers. 2016;2:16090.
7. Stanek G, Strle F. Lyme borreliosis – from tick bite to diagnosis and treatment. FEMS Microbiol Rev. 2018;42:233–58.
8. Sood SK. Effective retrieval of Lyme disease information on the web. Clin Infect Dis. 2002;35:451–64.
9. Buchwald A. Ein Fall von diffuser idiopathischer Haut-Atrophie. Vierteljahresschrift f Dermatol u Syph. 1883;10:553–6.
10. Herxheimer K, Hartmann K. Uber Acrodermatitis chronica atrophicans. Arch Dermatol Syph. 1902;61:57–76.
11. Gans O, Landes E. Akrodermatitis atrophicans arthropathica. Hautarzt. 1952;3:151–5.
12. Afzelius A. Verhandlungen der Dermatologischen Gesellschaft zu Stockholm, 28 Oct 1909. Arch Dermatol Syph. 1909;101:404.
13. Lipschütz B. Über eine seltene Erythemform (Erythema chronicum migrans). Arch Dermatol Syph. 1913;118:349–56.
14. Lipschütz B. Weiterer Beitrag zur Kenntnis der "Erythema chronicum migrans". Arch Dermatol Syph. 1923;143:365–74.
15. Garin C, Bujadoux R. Paralysie par les tiques. Journal de Medicine de Lyon. 1922;71:765–7.
16. Schaltenbrand G. Durch Arthropoden übertragene Erkrankungen der Haut und des Nervensystems. Verh Dtsch Ges Kreislaufforsch. 1967;72:975–1006.
17. Hollström E. Penicillin treatment of erythema migrans Afzelius. Acta Derm Venereol (Stockh). 1957;31:235–43.
18. Lennhoff C. Spirochaetes in aetiologically obscure diseases. Acta Derm Venereol. 1948;28:295–324.
19. Weber K. Erythema-chronicum-migrans-Meningitis – eine bakterielle Infektionskrankheit? Munch Med Wochenschr. 1974;116:1993–8.
20. Steere AC, Malawista SE, Snydman DR, et al. Lyme arthritis: an epidemic of oligoarticular arthritis in children and adults in three Connecticut communities. Arthritis Rheum. 1977;20:7–17.
21. Steere AC, Malawista SE, Hardin JA. Erythema chronicum migrans and Lyme arthritis. The enlarging clinical spectrum. Ann Intern Med. 1977;86:685–98.
22. Steere AC, Broderick TF, Malawista SE. Erythema chronicum migrans and Lyme arthritis: epidemiologic evidence for a tick vector. Am J Epidemiol. 1978;108:312–21.
23. Steere AC, Malawista SE. Cases of Lyme disease in the United States: locations correlated with distribution of Ixodes dammini. Ann Intern Med. 1979;91:730–3.
24. Reik L, Steere AC, Bartenhagen NH, et al. Neurologic abnormalities of Lyme disease. Medicine (Baltimore). 1979;58:281–94.
25. Steere AC, Batsford WP, Weinberg M, et al. Lyme carditis: cardiac abnormalities of Lyme disease. Ann Intern Med. 1980;93:8–16.
26. Steere AC, Malawista SE, Newman JH, et al. Antibiotic therapy in Lyme disease. Ann Intern Med. 1980;93:1–8.

27. Barbour AG, Benach JL. Discovery of the Lyme disease agent. mBio. 2019;10:e02166–19. https://doi.org/10.1128/mBio.02166-19.
28. Burgdorfer W, Barbour AG, Hayes SF, et al. Lyme disease—a tickborne spirochetosis? Science. 1982;216:1317–9.
29. Barbour AG, Burgdorfer W, Hayes SF, et al. Isolation of a cultivable spirochete from *Ixodes ricinus* ticks of Switzerland. Curr Microbiol. 1983;8:123–1236.
30. Barbour AG. Isolation and cultivation of Lyme disease spirochetes. Yale J Biol Med. 1984;57:521–5.
31. Benach JL, Bosler EM, Hanrahan JP, et al. Spirochetes isolated from the blood of two patients with Lyme disease. New Engl J Med. 1983;308:740–2.
32. Steere AC, Grodzicki RL, Kornblatt AN, et al. The spirochetal etiology of Lyme disease. N Engl J Med. 1983;308:733–40.
33. Johnson RC, Hyde FW, Rumple CM. Taxonomy of the Lyme disease spirochetes. Yale J Biol Med. 1984;57:529–37.
34. Johnson RC, Schmid GP, Hyde FW, et al. *Borrelia burgdorferi* sp. nov.: etiologic agent of Lyme disease. Int J Syst Bacteriol. 1984;34:496–7.
35. Barbour AG, Schrumpf ME. Polymorphisms of major surface proteins of *Borrelia burgdorferi*. Zentralbl Bakteriol Mikrobiol Hyg. 1986;A263:83–91. https://doi.org/10.1016/s0176-6724(86)80107-9.
36. Wilske B, Schierz G, Preac-Mursic V, et al. Intrathecal production of specific antibodies against *Borrelia burgdorferi* in patients with lymphocytic meningoradiculitis (Bannwarth's syndrome). J Infect Dis. 1986;153:304–14.
37. Picken RN, Cheng Y, Strle F, et al. Patient isolates of *Borrelia burgdorferi* sensu lato with genotypic and phenotypic similarities to strain 25015. J Infect Dis. 1996;174:1112–5.
38. Baranton G, Marti Ras N, Postic D. Molecular epidemiology of the aetiological agents of Lyme borreliosis. Wien Klin Wochenschr. 1998;110:850–5.
39. Baranton G, Postic D, Saint Girons I, et al. Delineation of *Borrelia burgdorferi* sensu stricto, *Borrelia garinii* sp. nov., and group VS461 associated with Lyme borreliosis. Int J Syst Bacteriol. 1992;42:378–83.
40. Stanek G, Reiter M. The expanding Lyme borrelia complex— clinical significance of genomic species? Clin Microbiol Infect. 2011;17:487–93.
41. Maraspin V, Ruzic-Sabljic E, Strle F. Lyme borreliosis and *Borrelia spielmanii*. Emerg Infect Dis. 2006;12:1177.
42. Fingerle V, Schulte-Spechtel UC, Ruzic-Sabljic E, et al. Epidemiological aspects and molecular characterization of *Borrelia burgdorferi* s.l. from southern Germany with special respect to the new species *Borrelia spielmanii* sp. nov. Int J Med Microbiol. 2008;298:279–90.
43. Stupica D, Lusa L, Maraspin V, et al. Correlation of culture positivity, PCR positivity, and burden of *Borrelia burgdorferi* sensu lato in skin samples of erythema migrans patients with clinical findings. PLoS One. 2015;10(9):e0136600. https://doi.org/10.1371/journal.pone.0136600.
44. Gray JS, Kahl O, Robertson JN, et al. Lyme borreliosis habitat assessment. Zentralbl Bakteriol. 1998a;287:211–28.
45. Gray JS, Granström M, Cimmino M, et al. Lyme borreliosis awareness. Zentralbl Bakteriol. 1998;287:253–65.
46. Gray JS, Stanek G. Risk assessment in Lyme borreliosis. Zentralbl Bakteriol. 1998;287:175–6.
47. Gern L, Estrada-Peña A, Frandsen F, et al. European reservoir hosts of *Borrelia burgdorferi* sensu lato. Zentralbl Bakteriol. 1998;287:196–204.
48. Estrada-Peña A, Daniel M, Frandsen F, Gern L, et al. *Ixodes ricinus* strains in Europe. Zentralbl Bakteriol. 1998;287:185–9.
49. Smith M, Gettinby G, Granström M, et al. The European Union concerted action world wide web site for Lyme borreliosis. Zentralbl Bakteriol. 1998;287:266–9.
50. Cimmino M, Granström M, Gray JS, et al. European Lyme borreliosis clinical spectrum. Zentralbl Bakteriol. 1998;287:248–52.

51. O'Connell S, Granström M, Gray JS, et al. Epidemiology of European Lyme borreliosis. Zentralbl Bakteriol. 1998;287:229–40.
52. Kahl O, Gern L, Gray JS, et al. Detection of *Borrelia burgdorferi* sensu lato in ticks: immunofluorescence assay versus polymerase chain reaction. Zentralbl Bakteriol. 1998;287:205–10.
53. Saint Girons I, Gern L, Gray JS, et al. Identification of *Borrelia burgdorferi* sensu lato species in Europe. Zentralbl Bakteriol. 1998;287:190–5.
54. Gray J. Risk assessment in Lyme borreliosis. Wien Klin Wochenschr. 1999;111:990–3.
55. Stanek G, O'Connell S, Cimmino M, et al. European Union concerted action on risk assessment in Lyme borreliosis: clinical case definitions for Lyme borreliosis. Wien Klin Wochenschr. 1996;108:741–7.
56. Robertson J, Guy E, Andrews N, et al. A European multicenter study of immunoblotting in serodiagnosis of Lyme borreliosis. J Clin Microbiol. 2000;38:2097–102.
57. Dessau RB, van Dam AP, Fingerle V, et al. To test or not to test? Laboratory support for the diagnosis of Lyme borreliosis: a position paper of ESGBOR, the ESCMID study group for Lyme borreliosis. Clin Microbiol Infect Date. 2018;24:118–24.
58. Hillerdal H, Henningsson AJ. Serodiagnosis of Lyme borreliosis-is IgM in serum more harmful than helpful? Eur J Clin Microbiol Infect Dis. 2021;40(6):1161–8. https://doi.org/10.1007/s10096-020-04093-2.
59. Berglund J, Eitrem R, Ornstein K, et al. An epidemiologic study of Lyme disease in southern Sweden. New Engl J Med. 1995;333:1319–27.
60. Robertson JN, Gray JS, Stewart P. Tick bite and Lyme borreliosis risk at a recreational site in England. Eur J Epidemiol. 2000b;16:647–52.
61. Strnad M, Hönig V, Růžek D, et al. Europe-wide meta-analysis of *Borrelia burgdorferi* sensu lato prevalence in questing *Ixodes ricinus* ticks. Appl Environ Microbiol. 2017;83:e00609–17. https://doi.org/10.1128/AEM.00609-17.
62. Schötta AM, Wijnveld M, Stockinger H, et al. Approaches for reverse line blot-based detection of microbial pathogens in *Ixodes ricinus* ticks collected in Austria and impact of the chosen method. Appl Environ Microbiol. 2017;83:e00489–17. https://doi.org/10.1128/AEM.00489-17.
63. Ruzic-Sabljic E, Strle F, Cimperman J, et al. Characterisation of *Borrelia burgdorferi* sensu lato strains isolated from patients with skin manifestations of Lyme borreliosis residing in Slovenia. J Med Microbiol. 2000;49:47–53.
64. Ruzic-Sabljic E, Maraspin V, Lotric-Furlan S, et al. Characterization of *Borrelia burgdorferi* sensu lato strains isolated from human material in Slovenia. Wien Klin Wochenschr. 2002;114:544–50.
65. Strle F, Ruzic-Sabljic E, Cimperman J, et al. Comparison of findings for patients with *Borrelia garinii* and *Borrelia afzelii* isolated from cerebrospinal fluid. Clin Infect Dis. 2006;43:704–10.
66. O'Rourke M, Traweger A, Lusa L, et al. Quantitative detection of *Borrelia burgdorferi* sensu lato in erythema migrans skin lesions using internally controlled duplex real time PCR. PLoS One. 2013;16(8):e63968. https://doi.org/10.1371/journal.pone.0063968.
67. Ogrinc K, Maraspin V, Lusa L, et al. Acrodermatitis chronica atrophicans: clinical and microbiological characteristics of a cohort of 693 Slovenian patients. J Intern Med. 2021;290(2):335–48. https://doi.org/10.1111/joim.13266.
68. Ruzic-Sabljic E, Lotric-Furlan S, Maraspin V, et al. Analysis of *Borrelia burgdorferi* sensu lato isolated from cerebrospinal fluid. APMIS. 2001;109:707–13.
69. Ogrinc K, Lotric-Furlan S, Maraspin-Carman V, et al. Suspected early Lyme neuroborreliosis in patients with erythema migrans. Clin Infect Dis. 2013;57:501–9.
70. Ogrinc K, Lusa L, Lotric-Furlan S, et al. Course and outcome of early European Lyme neuroborreliosis (Bannwarth's syndrome) – clinical and laboratory findings. Clin Infect Dis. 2016;63:346–53.

71. Ermenlieva N, Tsankova G, Todorova TT. Epidemiological study of Lyme disease in Bulgaria. Cent Eur J Public Health. 2019;27:235–8. https://doi.org/10.21101/cejph.a5007.
72. Cairns V, Wallenhorst C, Rietbrock S, et al. Incidence of Lyme disease in the UK: a population-based cohort study. BMJ Open. 2019;31(9):e025916. https://doi.org/10.1136/bmjopen-2018-025916.
73. Sykes RA, Makiello P. An estimate of Lyme borreliosis incidence in Western Europe. J Public Health (Oxf). 2017;39:74–81. https://doi.org/10.1093/pubmed/fdw017.
74. Wilking H, Stark K. Trends in surveillance data of human Lyme borreliosis from six federal states in eastern Germany, 2009-2012. Ticks Tick Borne Dis. 2014;5:219–24. https://doi.org/10.1016/j.ttbdis.2013.10.010.
75. Enkelmann J, Böhmer M, Fingerle V, et al. Incidence of notified Lyme borreliosis in Germany, 2013-2017. Sci Rep. 2018;8:14976. https://doi.org/10.1038/s41598-018-33136-0.
76. Vandenesch A, Turbelin C, Couturier E, et al. Incidence and hospitalisation rates of Lyme borreliosis, France, 2004 to 2012. Eur Secur. 2014;19:20883. https://doi.org/10.2807/1560-7917.es2014.19.34.20883.
77. Septfons A, Goronflot T, Jaulhac B, et al. Epidemiology of Lyme borreliosis through two surveillance systems: the national Sentinelles GP network and the national hospital discharge database, France, 2005 to 2016. Euro Surveill. 2019;24:1800134. https://doi.org/10.2807/1560-7917.ES.2019.24.11.1800134.
78. Hofhuis A, Bennema S, Harms M, et al. Decrease in tick bite consultations and stabilization of early Lyme borreliosis in the Netherlands in 2014 after 15 years of continuous increase. BMC Public Health. 2016;16:425. https://doi.org/10.1186/s12889-016-3105-y.
79. Beltrame A, Rodari P, Mauroner L, et al. Emergence of Lyme borreliosis in the province of Verona, northern Italy: five-years of sentinel surveillance. Ticks Tick Borne Dis. 2021;12:101628. https://doi.org/10.1016/j.ttbdis.2020.101628.
80. Wilhelmsson P, Fryland L, Lindblom P, et al. A prospective study on the incidence of *Borrelia burgdorferi* sensu lato infection after a tick bite in Sweden and on the Åland Islands, Finland (2008-2009). Ticks Tick Borne Dis. 2016;7:71–9. https://doi.org/10.1016/j.ttbdis.2015.08.009.
81. Markowicz M, Schötta AM, Höss D, et al. Infections with tick-borne pathogens after tick bite, Austria, 2015-2018. Emerg Infect Dis. 2021;27:1048–56. https://doi.org/10.3201/eid2704.203366. PMID: 33755546
82. Huppertz HI, Böhme M, Standaert SM, Karch H, Plotkin SA. Incidence of Lyme borreliosis in the Würzburg region of Germany. Eur J Clin Microbiol Infect Dis. 1999;18:697–703.
83. Sajanti E, Virtanen M, Helve O, et al. Lyme borreliosis in Finland, 1995–2014. Emerg Infect Dis. 2017;23:1282–8.
84. Strle F, Wormser GP, Mead P, et al. Gender disparity between cutaneous and non-cutaneous manifestations of Lyme borreliosis. PLoS One. 2013;8(5):e64110. https://doi.org/10.1371/journal.pone.0064110.
85. Strle F, Nadelman RB, Cimperman J, et al. Comparison of culture confirmed erythema migrans caused by *Borrelia burgdorferi* sensu stricto in New York state and Borrelia afzelii in Slovenia. Ann Intern Med. 1999;130:32–6.
86. Logar M, Ruzic-Sabljić E, Maraspin V, et al. Comparison of erythema migrans caused by *Borrelia afzelii* and *Borrelia garinii*. Infection. 2004;32:15–9.
87. Strle F, Maraspin V, Furlan-Lortic S, et al. Epidemiologic study of a cohort of adult patients with erythema migrans registered in Slovenia in 1993. Eur J Epidemiol. 1996;12:503–7.
88. Strle F, Maraspin V, Pleterski-Rigler D, et al. Treatment of borrelial lymphocytoma. Infection. 1996;24:80–4.
89. Strle F, Nelson JA, Ruzic-Sabljic E, et al. European Lyme borreliosis: 231 culture-confirmed cases involving patients with erythema migrans. Clin Infect Dis. 1996;23:61–5.
90. Strle F. Principles of the diagnosis and antibiotic treatment of Lyme borreliosis. Wien Klin Wochenschr. 1999;111:911–5.

91. Cerar D, Cerar T, Ruzic-Sabljic E, et al. Subjective symptoms after treatment of early Lyme disease. Am J Med. 2010;123:79–86.
92. Stupica D, Lusa L, Ruzic-Sabljic E, et al. Treatment of erythema migrans with doxycycline for 10 days versus 15 days. Clin Infect Dis. 2012;55:343–50.
93. Stupica D, Maraspin V, Bogovic P, et al. Comparison of clinical course and treatment outcome for patients with early disseminated or early localized Lyme borreliosis. JAMA Dermatol. 2018;154:1050–6. https://doi.org/10.1001/jamadermatol.2018.2306.
94. Boršič K, Blagus R, Cerar T, et al. Clinical course, serologic response, and long-term outcome in elderly patients with early Lyme borreliosis. J Clin Med. 2018;2:506. https://doi.org/10.3390/jcm7120506.
95. Maraspin V, Bogovič P, Rojko T, et al. Erythema migrans: course and outcome in patients treated with rituximab. Open forum. Infect Dis. 2019;6:ofz292. https://doi.org/10.1093/ofid/ofz292.
96. Asbrink E, Hovmark A. Cutaneous manifestations in *Ixodes*-borne *Borrelia* spirochetosis. Int J Dermatol. 1987;26:215–25.
97. Strle F, Pleterski-Rigler D, Stanek G, et al. Solitary borrelial lymphocytoma: report of 36 cases. Infection. 1992;20:201–6.
98. Maraspin V, Nahtigal Klevisar M, Ruzic-Sabljic E, et al. Borrelial lymphocytoma in adult patients. Clin Infect Dis. 2016;63:914–21.
99. Mullegger RR, Means TK, Shin JJ, et al. Chemokine signatures in the skin disorders of Lyme borreliosis in Europe: predominance of CXCL9 and CXCL10 in erythema migrans and acrodermatitis and CXCL13 in lymphocytoma. Infect Immun. 2007;75:4621–8.
100. Asbrink E, Hovmark A, Olsson I. Clinical manifestations of acrodermatitis chronica atrophicans in 50 Swedish patients. Zbl Bakt Mik Hyg A. 1986;263:253–61.
101. Mullegger RR. Dermatological manifestations of Lyme borreliosis. Eur J Dermatol. 2004;14:296–309.
102. Ogrinc K, Wormser GP, Visintainer P, et al. Pathogenetic implications of the age at time of diagnosis and skin location for acrodermatitis chronica atrophicans. Ticks Tick Borne Dis. 2017;8:266–9.
103. Maraspin V, Mrvič T, Ružić-Sabljić E, et al. Acrodermatitis chronica atrophicans in children: report on two cases and review of the literature. Ticks Tick Borne Dis. 2019;10:180–5.
104. Kristoferitsch W, Sluga E, Graf M, et al. Neuropathy associated with acrodermatitis chronica atrophicans: clinical and morphological features. Ann N Y Acad Sci. 1988;539:35–45.
105. Kristoferitsch W. Neuropathien bei Lyme-Borreliose. Springer-Verlag, Wien/New York; 1989.
106. Kristoferitsch W, Spiel G, Wessely P. Meningopolyneuritis (Garin-Bujadoux-Bannwarth): clinical aspects and laboratory findings. Nervenarzt. 1983;54:640–6.
107. Hansen K, Crone C, Kristoferitsch W. Lyme neuroborreliosis. In: Said G, Krarup C, editors. Handbook of clinical neurology, peripheral nerve disorders, chapter 32. Elsevier B.V. Amsterdam: The Netherlands; 2013. p. 559–74. https://doi.org/10.1016/B978-0-444-52902-2.00032-1. PMID: 23931802.
108. Millner M, Schimek MG, Spork D, et al. Lyme borreliosis in children: a controlled clinical study based on ELISA values. Eur J Pediatr. 1989;148:527–30.
109. Christen HJ. Lyme neuroborreliosis in children. Ann Med. 1996;28:235–40.
110. Eiffert H, Karsten A, Schlott T, et al. Acute peripheral facial palsy in Lyme disease—a distal neuritis at the infection site. Neuropediatrics. 2004;35:267–73.
111. Kristoferitsch W. Neurological manifestations of Lyme borreliosis: clinical definition and differential diagnosis. Scand J Infect Dis. 1991;77S:64–73.
112. Hansen K. Lyme neuroborreliosis: improvements of the laboratory diagnosis and a survey of epidemiological and clinical features in Denmark 1985–1990. Acta Neurol Scand. 1994;89(S 151):7–44.

113. Kristoferitsch W, Aboulenein-Djamshidian F, Jecel J, et al. Secondary dementia due to Lyme neuroborreliosis. Wien Klin Wochenschr. 2018;130:468–78. https://doi.org/10.1007/s00508-018-1361-9.
114. Lotric-Furlan S, Cimperman J, Maraspin V, et al. Lyme borreliosis and peripheral facial palsy. Wien Klin Wochenschr. 1999;111:970–5.
115. Pachner AR, Steere AC. The triad of neurologic manifestations of Lyme disease: meningitis, cranial neuritis, and radiculoneuritis. Neurology. 1985;111:47–53.
116. Bagger-Sjoback D, Remahl S, Ericsson M. Long-term outcome of facial palsy in neuroborreliosis. Otol Neurotol. 2005;26:790–5.
117. Skogman BH, Croner S, Odkvist L. Acute facial palsy in children - a 2-year follow-up study with focus on Lyme neuroborreliosis. Int J Pediatr Otorhi. 2003;67:597–602.
118. Pfister HW, Kristoferitsch W. Early neurological involvement (Bannwarth's syndrome). In: Weber K, Burgdorfer W, editors. Aspects of Lyme borreliosis. Berlin Heidelberg/New York: Springer-Verlag; 1993. p. 152–67.
119. Steenhoff AP, Smith MJ, Shah SS, et al. Neuroborreliosis with progression from pseudotumor cerebri to aseptic meningitis. Pediatr Infect Dis J. 2006;25:91–2.
120. Feder HM Jr. Lyme disease in children. Infect Dis Clin N Am. 2008;22:315–26.
121. Peter O, Bretz AG, Postic D, et al. Association of distinct species of *Borrelia burgdorferi* sensu lato with neuroborreliosis in Switzerland. Clin Microbiol Infect. 1997;3:423–31.
122. Strle F, Picken RN, Cheng Y, et al. Clinical findings for patients with Lyme borreliosis caused by *Borrelia burgdorferi* sensu lato with genotypic and phenotypic similarities to strain 25015. Clin Infect Dis. 1997;25:273–80.
123. Ornstein K, Berglund J, Bergstrom S, et al. Three major Lyme borrelia genospecies (*Borrelia burgdorferi* sensu stricto, *B. afzelii* and *B. garinii*) identified by PCR in cerebrospinal fluid from patients with neuroborreliosis in Sweden. Scand J Infect Dis. 2002;34:341–6.
124. Rojko T, Bogovič P, Lotrič-Furlan S, et al. *Borrelia burgdorferi* sensu lato infection in patients with peripheral facial palsy. Ticks Tick Borne Dis. 2019;10:398–406.
125. Brouqui P, Bacellar F, Baranton G, et al. Guidelines for the diagnosis of tick-borne bacterial diseases in Europe. Clin Microbiol Infect. 2004;10:1108–32.
126. Aguero-Rosenfeld ME, Wang G, Schwartz I, et al. Diagnosis of Lyme borreliosis. Clin Microbiol Rev. 2005;18:484–509.
127. Ljøstad U, Mygland A. CSF B-lymphocyte chemoattractant (CXCL13) in the early diagnosis of acute Lyme neuroborreliosis. J Neurol. 2008;255:732–7.
128. Cerar T, Ogrinc K, Cimperman J, et al. Validation of cultivation and PCR methods for diagnosis of Lyme neuroborreliosis. J Clin Microbiol. 2008;46:3375–9.
129. McAlister HF, Klementowicz PT, Andrews C, et al. Lyme carditis: an important course of reversible heart block. Ann Intern Med. 1989;110:339–45.
130. van der Linde MR. Lyme carditis: clinical characteristics of 105 cases. Scand J Infect Dis. 1991;77:81–4.
131. Sigal LH. Early disseminated Lyme disease: cardiac manifestations. Am J Med. 1995;98:25S–8S.
132. Midttun M, Lebech AM, Hansen K, et al. Lyme carditis: a clinical presentation and long-time follow-up. Scand J Infect Dis. 1997;29:153–7.
133. Eiffert H, Karsten A, Thomssen R, et al. Characterization of *Borrelia burgdorferi* strains in Lyme arthritis. Scand J Infect Dis. 1998;30:265–8.
134. Vasiliu V, Herzer P, Rossler D, et al. Heterogeneity of *Borrelia burgdorferi* sensu lato demonstrated by an OspA-type-specific PCR in synovial fluid from patients with Lyme arthritis. Med Microbiol Immun. 1998;187:97–102.
135. van der Heijden IM, Wilbrink B, Rijpkema SG, et al. Detection of *Borrelia burgdorferi* sensu stricto by reverse line blot in the joints of Dutch patients with Lyme arthritis. Arthritis Rheum. 1999;42:1473–80.

136. Jaulhac B, Heller R, Limbach FX, et al. Direct molecular typing of *Borrelia burgdorferi* sensu lato species in synovial samples from patients with Lyme arthritis. J Clin Microbiol. 2000;38:1895–900.
137. Marlovits S, Khanakah G, Striessnig G, et al. Emergence of Lyme arthritis after autologous chondrocyte transplantation. Arthritis Rheum. 2004;50:259–64.
138. Markowicz M, Ladstatter S, Schotta AM, et al. Oligoarthritis caused by *Borrelia bavariensis*, Austria, 2014. Emerg Infect Dis. 2015;21:1052–4.
139. Grillon A, Scherlinger M, Boyer PH, et al. Characteristics and clinical outcomes after treatment of a national cohort of PCR-positive Lyme arthritis. Semin Arthritis Rheum. 2019;48:1105–12. https://doi.org/10.1016/j.semarthrit.2018.09.007.
140. Steere AC, Schoen RT, Taylor E. The clinical evolution of Lyme arthritis. Ann Intern Med. 1987;107:725–31.
141. Herzer P. Joint manifestations of Lyme borreliosis in Europe. Scand J Infect Dis. 1991;77:55–63.
142. Herzer P. Joint manifestations. In: Weber K, Burgdorfer W, editors. Aspects of Lyme Borreliosis. Berlin Heidelberg/New York: Springer-Verlag; 1993. p. 168–84.
143. Rees DH, Axford JS. Lyme arthritis. Ann Rheum Dis. 1994;53:553–6.
144. Hardin JA, Steere AC, Malawista SE. Immune complexes and the evolution of Lyme arthritis: dissemination and localization of abnormal C1q binding activity. N Engl J Med. 1979;301:1358–63.
145. Steere AC, Hardin JA, Ruddy S, et al. Lyme arthritis: correlation of serum and cryoglobulin IgM with activity, and serum IgG with remission. Arthritis Rheum. 1979;22:471–83.
146. Lawson JP, Steere AC. Lyme arthritis: radiologic findings. Radiology. 1985;154:37–43.
147. Snydman DR, Schenkein DP, Berardi VP, et al. *Borrelia burgdorferi* in joint fluid in chronic Lyme arthritis. Ann Intern Med. 1986;104:798–800.
148. Steere AC. Lyme disease. N Engl J Med. 2001;345:115–25.
149. Puius YA, Kalish RA. Lyme arthritis: pathogenesis, clinical presentation, and management. Infect Dis Clin N Am. 2008;22:289–300.
150. Kornmehl EW, Lesser RL, Jaros P, et al. Bilateral keratitis in Lyme disease. Ophthalmology. 1989;96:1194–7.
151. Schonherr U, Strle F. Ocular manifestations. In: Weber K, Burgdorfer W, editors. Aspects of Lyme Borreliosis. Berlin Heidelberg/New York: Springer-Verlag; 1993. p. 248–58.
152. Strle F. Ocular manifestations of Lyme borreliosis. Acta Dermatovenerol. 1994;1-2:1–6.
153. Mikkila HO, Seppala IJ, Viljanen MK, et al. The expanding clinical spectrum of ocular Lyme borreliosis. Ophthalmology. 2000;107:581–7.
154. Mahne J, Kranjc BS, Strle F, et al. Panuveitis caused by *Borrelia burgdorferi* sensu lato infection. Pediatr Infect Dis J. 2015;34:102–4.
155. Maraspin V, Cimperman J, Lotric-Furlan S, et al. Treatment of erythema migrans in pregnancy. Clin Infect Dis. 1996;22:788–93.
156. Maraspin V, Cimperman J, Lotric-Furlan S, et al. Erythema migrans in pregnancy. Wien Klin Wochenschr. 1999a;111:933–40.
157. Maraspin V, Ružič-Sabljić E, Pleterski-Rigler D, et al. Pregnant women with erythema migrans and isolation of borreliae from blood: course and outcome after treatment with ceftriaxone. Diagn Micr Infec Dis. 2011;71:446–8.
158. Maraspin V, Lusa L, Blejec T, et al. Course and outcome of erythema migrans in pregnant women. J Clin. 2020;9:2364. https://doi.org/10.3390/jcm9082364.
159. Maraspin V, Strle F. How do I manage tick bites and Lyme borreliosis in pregnant women? Curr Probl Dermatol. 2009;37:183–90.
160. Maraspin V, Lotric-Furlan S, Cimperman J, et al. Erythema migrans in the immunocompromised host. Wien Klin Wochenschr. 1999;111:923–32.

161. Maraspin V, Cimperman J, Lotric-Furlan S. Erythema migrans in solid-organ transplant recipients. Clin Infect Dis. 2006;42:1751–4.
162. Maraspin V, Ruzic-Sabljic E, Lusa L, et al. Course and outcome of early Lyme borreliosis in patients with hematological malignancies. Clin Infect Dis. 2015;61:427–31.
163. Furst B, Glatz M, Kerl H, et al. The impact of immunosuppression on erythema migrans: a retrospective study of clinical presentation, response to treatment and production of borrelia antibodies in 33 patients. Clin Exp Dermatol. 2006;31:509–14.
164. Feder HM Jr, Johnson BJ, O'Connell S, et al. A critical appraisal of 'chronic Lyme disease'. N Engl J Med. 2007;357:1422–30.
165. Marques A. Chronic Lyme disease: a review. Infect Dis Clin N Am. 2008;22:341–60.
166. Hunfeld KP, Brade V. Antimicrobial susceptibility of *Borrelia burgdorferi* sensu lato: what we know, what we don't know, and what we need to know. Wien Klin Wochenschr. 2006;118(21–22):659–68.
167. Borg R, Dotevall L, Hagberg L, et al. Intravenous ceftriaxone compared with oral doxycycline for the treatment of Lyme neuroborreliosis. Scand J Infect Dis. 2005;37:449–54.
168. Ljøstad U, Skogvoll E, Eikeland R, et al. Oral doxycycline versus intravenous ceftriaxone for European Lyme neuroborreliosis: a multicentre, non-inferiority, double-blind, randomised trial. Lancet Neurol. 2008;7:690–5.
169. Wormser GP, Ramanathan R, Nowakowski J, et al. Duration of antibiotic therapy for early Lyme disease. A randomized, double-blind, placebo-controlled trial. Ann Intern Med. 2003;138:697–704.

Special Aspects of Lyme Borreliosis in the United States

5

Adriana R. Marques and Gary P. Wormser

5.1 Introduction

Lyme borreliosis, or Lyme disease, is the most common vector-borne disease in the United States, with an estimate of 476,000 people treated for Lyme disease a year [1, 2]. Lyme borreliosis was first recognized in the United States in 1977, based on the investigation of an epidemic form of oligoarticular arthritis in the towns of Lyme, Old Lyme, and East Haddam in eastern Connecticut [3]. The epidemiology suggested transmission by ticks, as cases clustered geographically in heavily wooded areas, their occurrence peaked in summer months, and there was a lack of other common exposures. Moreover, in 25% of the patients, the arthritis was preceded by a characteristic skin lesion that fitted the description of erythema migrans, which was described in Europe and associated with the bite of *Ixodes ricinus* ticks. Additionally, a cluster of erythema migrans cases had recently been described in southeastern Connecticut [4], while a previous case was reported in Wisconsin [5]. The pathogen, *Borrelia burgdorferi,* was discovered in 1982 [6] and recognized as a new species of the genus *Borrelia* in 1984 [7]. Soon after, it was found that European strains were more heterogenous and could differ from American strains of *B. burgdorferi* [8, 9]. *B. burgdorferi* sensu lato was then classified into three main divisions or genospecies (I, II, and III), with genospecies I strains named *B. burgdorferi* sensu stricto (henceforward *B. burgdorferi*), since it contained the type strain for the species [10, 11]. Genospecies II was named *Borrelia garinii* sp. nov., while genospecies III was initially referred to as group VS461 and later named

A. R. Marques (✉)
Laboratory of Clinical Immunology and Microbiology, National Institute of Allergy and Infectious Diseases, National Institutes of Health, Bethesda, MD, USA
e-mail: amarques@niaid.nih.gov

G. P. Wormser
Division of Infectious Diseases, New York Medical College, Valhalla, NY, USA
e-mail: gwormser@nymc.edu

K.-P. Hunfeld, J. Gray (eds.), *Lyme Borreliosis*,
https://doi.org/10.1007/978-3-030-93680-8_5

Borrelia afzelii sp. nov. [12, 13]. There have been recent revisions to the taxonomy of the spirochetes that cause Lyme borreliosis from *Borrelia* to *Borreliella*, to differentiate them from the spirochetes that cause relapsing fever, which retain the genus name *Borrelia* [14]. This name change has been challenged and is controversial [15–17]. *B. burgdorferi* causes the vast majority of human infections in the United States, with *B. mayonii* causing a few cases of human illness in the upper Midwest [18, 19]. Other Lyme borrelia that are the leading causes of the disease in Europe (*B. afzelii* and *B. garinii*) are not found in the United States (Table 5.1).

Table 5.1 Lyme Borreliosis—United States versus Europe

Variable	United States	Europe
Tick vector	*Ixodes scapularis* *Ixodes pacificus*	*Ixodes ricinus* *Ixodes persulcatus*
Speed of tick transmission of Lyme borrelia	Rarely before 36 hours	*I. ricinus* may transmit *B. afzelii* within 24 hours
Lyme borrelia	Principally *B. burgdorferi*; but *B. mayonii* may occur in the upper midwestern United States	Principally *B. afzelii* and *B. garinii*, but several other species cause human disease including *B. bavariensis, B. spielmanii, B. bissetii*, plus others rarely
Clinical manifestations		
Asymptomatic infection	Approximately 10% of cases	Appears to be more frequent in Europe, although the exact frequency is unknown, as the data originate from serosurveys.
Lyme arthritis	More common in the United States	Occurs in Europe
Acrodermatitis chronica atrophicans	Does not occur in the United States	Occurs in Europe
Borrelia lymphocytoma	Does not occur in the United States	Occurs in Europe
Multiple EM skin lesions	More common in the United States	Occurs in Europe
Systemic symptoms in conjunction with EM	65% of cases	37% of cases
Lyme encephalopathy	Controversial in the United States	Not recognized to occur
Diffuse axonal peripheral neuropathy	Controversial in the United States	Occurs, but only in conjunction with ACA
Radicular pain from Lyme neuroborreliosis	Less in the United States	More common in Europe
EM mimics	STARI only occurs in the United States	STARI does not occur in Europe

Table 5.1 (continued)

Variable	United States	Europe
"Chronic Lyme disease"	More common in the United States	Less common in Europe
Gender	No female predominance for any manifestation	Female predominance for EM and ACA
Diagnosis	Serologic testing is principal laboratory test	Serologic testing is principal laboratory test. Interpretation is more complicated due to the greater number of Lyme borrelia species causing human disease
Coinfections	Anaplasmosis and babesiosis are the most common, with prevalence varying depending on the geographic areas and on the case definition	Tick-borne encephalitis virus is the most common in endemic areas. Anaplasmosis, rickettsiosis, and *B. miyamotoi* may also occur. Data are based on serosurveys and studies of the prevalence of pathogens in ticks. See Chap. 9
Treatment		
Oral penicillin	Usually not used	Oral penicillin is used in some European countries and is the preferred treatment for patients with EM in Norway
Pregnant women with Lyme borreliosis	Same as for nonpregnant patients, except that doxycycline is not usually used	Often IV ceftriaxone in Europe
Postexposure antibiotic prophylaxis after a tick bite	Commonly used in the United States	Not routinely used in Europe

EM erythema migrans, *ACA* acrodermatitis chronica atrophicans, *STARI* Southern tick-associated rash illness, *IV* intravenous

5.2 The Area of Risk for Lyme Borreliosis Is Expanding in the United States

Tickborne diseases, particularly Lyme borreliosis, are an increasing threat in the United States. As reported by the United States Centers for Disease Control and Prevention (CDC), the number of cases of tickborne diseases had gradually increased, doubling in the period from 2004 to 2016. Lyme borreliosis accounted for 82% of the cases of reportable tick-borne diseases [20]. Geographically, most cases of Lyme borreliosis occur in the mid-Atlantic, Northeast, and upper Midwest regions (Fig. 5.1), where the disease is transmitted by *Ixodes scapularis* (the blacklegged tick or deer tick), and over 20% of the ticks may be infected with *B. burgdorferi* [19]. Highly endemic areas include Maine, New Hampshire, Rhode Island, Pennsylvania, Vermont, Delaware, Connecticut, New Jersey, West Virginia, Wisconsin, Minnesota, Maryland, Massachusetts, New York, and Virginia. These 15 states accounted for

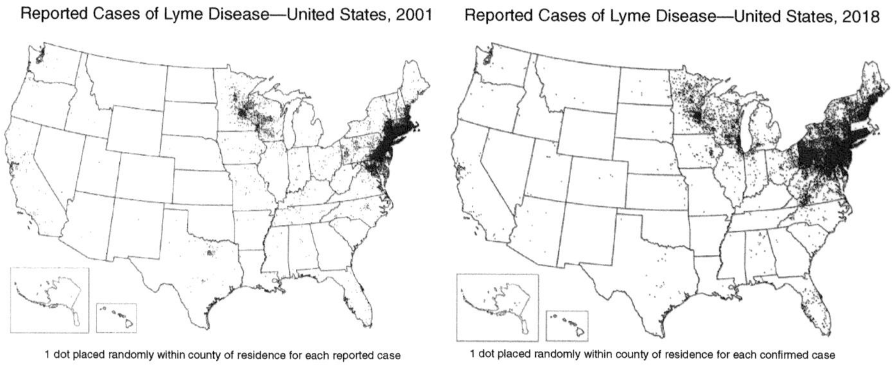

Fig. 5.1 Expansion of Lyme borreliosis—United States. Content source: Centers for Disease Control and Prevention (CDC), National Center for Emerging and Zoonotic Infectious Diseases (NCEZID), Division of Vector-Borne Diseases (DVBD)

more than 93% of reported US cases in 2018 [21]. The disease also occurs in areas of the Pacific Coast, where it is transmitted by *Ixodes pacificus*, the Western black-legged tick. Both the geographic locations and the number of infections in established Lyme borreliosis risk areas in the mid-Atlantic, Northeast, and Midwest regions have been steadily increasing [22–24], a change likely related to environmental factors such as climate changes, increasing forest fragmentation, and the resurgence and expansion of the white-tailed deer population, which is the key host for the adult stage of *I. scapularis* [25, 26]. These factors appear to have contributed to an increased density and range of host-seeking nymphal *I. scapularis* ticks, leading to more human encounters with infected ticks [27].

Interestingly, while *I. scapularis* is present throughout the Southern United States, these ticks are rarely infected with *B. burgdorferi*, and relatively few cases of Lyme borreliosis are reported from, or acquired in, the South [19]. Differences in questing behavior of immature forms of *I. scapularis*, as well as local ecological factors, and genetic factors of the tick, are believed to play a role in the low risk for human disease. In the South, *I. scapularis* larvae feed primarily on reservoir incompetent lizards, rather than reservoir-competent small mammals [28], and consequently nymphs are infrequently infected with *B. burgdorferi*. Additionally, nymphs can seldom be collected by standard tick collection methods of flagging and dragging [29], remaining under the leaf litter and consequently rarely bite humans. These behaviors are thought to be key factors contributing to the low incidence of Lyme borreliosis in the South [30, 31].

5.3 Differences in Lyme Borrelia Species between United States and Europe

In the United States, the only borrelial species recognized to cause Lyme borreliosis are *B. burgdorferi* and *B. mayonii*, whereas in Europe the majority of cases are caused by *B. afzelii* and *B. garinii*, with some cases caused by *B. burgdorferi*,

B. bavariensis, *B. spielmanii, and B. lusitaniae* [32] (Table 5.1). Differences in the species of Lyme borrelia between the United States and Europe have led to both subtle and substantive differences in the clinical features of this infection between the two geographic locations.

In addition, although the vast majority of United States cases of Lyme borreliosis are caused by *B. burgdorferi*, different strains within this species can be distinguished that impact pathogenicity and virulence in humans [27, 33, 34]. *B. burgdorferi* can be classified into subtypes based on genetic variations in the intergenic spacer regions of rRNA genes (RST), or in the outer surface protein (Osp) C gene, or on multilocus sequence typing. *B. burgdorferi* RST1 strains, which appear to account for approximately 40% of Lyme borreliosis cases in the northeastern United States, are more likely to disseminate hematogenously and are associated with a higher risk of post-infectious Lyme arthritis [35, 36]. Similarly, certain variations in OspC have been shown to be associated with disseminated infection in humans [34, 37].

5.4 Differences in Clinical Features between the United States and Europe

5.4.1 Erythema Migrans

Once *B. burgdorferi* is deposited in the human dermis by the feeding *Ixodes* ticks, it typically establishes a localized infection at that site and causes the characteristic skin lesion, erythema migrans (EM). EM is the most common manifestation of Lyme borreliosis in both the United States and Europe, occurring in about 80–90% of patients [38, 39], but there are some differences in presentation.

In the United States, EM lesions have a shorter incubation period and duration of the disease at presentation, and lesions expand faster. Patients with EM in the United States are more likely than patients in Europe to have concomitant systemic symptoms (65% vs. 37%), more likely to have multiple skin lesions (21% vs. 12%), and more likely to have regional lymphadenopathy (22% vs. 13%) [40]. In addition, the EM skin lesions in patients in the United States are less likely to manifest central clearing (19% vs. 79%), and patients in the United States are less likely to recall a tick bite at the site of the EM skin lesion (26% vs. 64%).

Multiple very small EM skin lesions in the United States have been observed in patients infected with *B. mayonii*. Similarly, differences in the infecting species of Lyme borrelia in Europe may also affect some of the clinical features of patients with EM in Europe (see Chap. 4 "The History, Epidemiology, Clinical Manifestations and Treatment of Lyme Borreliosis").

5.4.2 EM Versus STARI

One issue particular to the United States, which is becoming an increasingly significant problem, is distinguishing between EM and Southern tick-associated rash illness (STARI). A skin lesion very similar in appearance to EM occurs in STARI

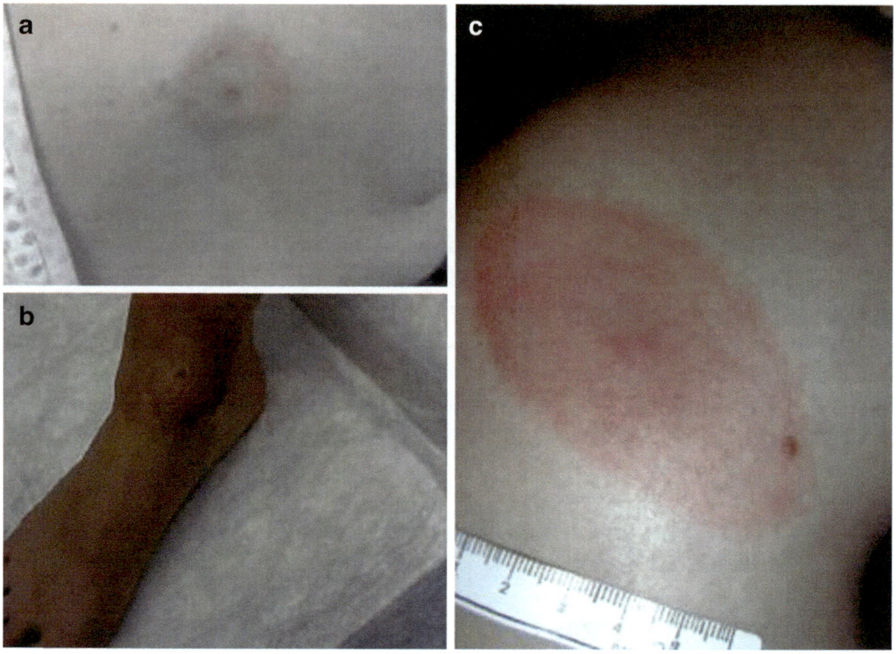

Fig. 5.2 Southern Tick-Associated Rash Illness (STARI) and Erythema Migrans (EM). STARI (Panel **a** and **b**) can be very similar in appearance to EM (Panel **c**). STARI follows the bite of the lone star tick, *Amblyomma americanum.* Neither the cause of STARI nor the natural history of the illness has been defined

(Fig. 5.2). Neither the cause of STARI nor the natural history of the illness has been defined. STARI follows the bite of the lone star tick, *Amblyomma americanum,* which is not a competent vector for Lyme borrelia [41]. *A. americanum* is the most abundant human-biting tick in the southeastern and southcentral United States, but its range has spread northwards along the eastern seaboard and overlaps areas where *I. scapularis* bites are common [42]. The potential for diagnostic confusion clearly exists in areas where both tick species coexist and this could impact Lyme borreliosis surveillance, characterization of laboratory tests for early Lyme borreliosis, and evaluation of future Lyme borreliosis vaccines. Experimentally, however, the two diseases could be distinguished based on different serum metabolic profiles [43].

5.4.3 "Summer Flu"

About 10–18% of patients in the United States diagnosed with Lyme borreliosis present with a nonspecific febrile illness in the summer (*a "summer flu"*). This is due in some cases to lack of recognition of an existing EM skin lesion, or alternatively the EM lesion may first appear after the start of systemic symptoms. Common symptoms include fatigue, malaise, myalgias, arthralgias, headache, and neck pain.

Respiratory symptoms and diarrhea would not be expected [39, 44, 45]. Moreover, it is possible that some of the summer flu cases attributed to Lyme borreliosis have been misdiagnosed and are actually due to other tickborne infections, particularly ones caused by *B. miyamotoi* [46–48] and *Anaplasma phagocytophilum*, since both of these infections can result in positive serologic tests for Lyme borreliosis [49], as can other infectious agents that may cause a febrile illness, including parvovirus B19 [50] and Epstein-Barr virus [51].

5.4.4 Lyme Neuroborreliosis

Patients with early Lyme neuroborreliosis typically present with cranial nerve palsy, particularly seventh nerve palsy, as well as lymphocytic meningitis and painful radiculitis. Facial palsy is the most common manifestation of early Lyme neuroborreliosis in the United States. Compared with Europe where most cases of early Lyme neuroborreliosis are caused by *B. garinii* and *B. bavariensis* [32, 52–54], patients in the United States seem to present less frequently with severe radicular pain. Levels of intrathecally produced specific antibodies to Lyme borrelia in the cerebrospinal fluid are lower in patients in the United States, both early and late in the course of the illness [55].

Late Lyme neuroborreliosis, i.e., progressive encephalitis, myelitis, or encephalomyelitis due to Lyme borrelia infection, which has been reported in Europe, is very rare in the United States [56]. On the other hand, there are two neurologic manifestations that seem particular to the United States and that have been immersed in controversy. The first is Lyme encephalopathy, a poorly defined entity, which was mostly described in studies published many years ago [57–59]. This is a subtle encephalopathic syndrome affecting memory and cognition, but without cerebrospinal fluid pleocytosis, intrathecal production of antiborrelia antibody, or molecular or culture evidence of *B. burgdorferi* infection in the central nervous system. Symptoms include headache, memory and concentration disturbances, anxiety, sleeping disorders, paresthesias, fatigue, arthralgias, and myalgias. The difference may be semantic, as some reports of late Lyme borreliosis in Europe seem to overlap with Lyme encephalopathy in the United States [60]. Another source of confusion is the addition of patients with posttreatment Lyme disease syndrome (PTLDS) showing abnormal neurocognitive test results to this category [61, 62], because criteria were not used in the early descriptions of Lyme encephalopathy to clearly distinguish between encephalopathy and PTLDS [63, 64]. Memory complaints are common in PTLDS [64–67]. Adding to the confusion is the question of what represents an abnormality in a single test or battery of neuropsychological tests and their clinical significance [68].

The second manifestation, which has become controversial, is a chronic, primarily axonal, distal sensory neuropathy. In Europe, distal axonal neuropathy in the context of Lyme borreliosis is exclusively associated with acrodermatitis chronica atrophicans (ACA), a manifestation of Lyme borreliosis principally associated with *B. afzelii* infection and therefore not seen in the United States. In patients with ACA, the neuropathy is predominantly sensory and more marked in the affected skin areas [69–71]. In the United States, a similar neuropathy, but without evidence of ACA, was described in early reports of small case series in adult patients [72–76]. The typical symptoms are paresthesias, which may be intermittent or radicular pain. Neurologic deficits are predominantly sensory and distal. The distribution is typically symmetric, but it can be asymmetric. Electrophysiologic studies indicated that the neuropathy is primarily axonal, and the pathogenesis is thought to be a mononeuropathy multiplex, which can be confluent [56]. These patients will usually have normal cerebrospinal fluid findings. More recently, there has been a discussion as to whether this entity has been appropriately validated as a manifestation of *B. burgdorferi* infection [61].

5.4.5 Lyme Arthritis

Lyme arthritis occurs in approximately 60% of patients with untreated EM in the United States [3, 77, 78] and comprises 28% of confirmed cases reported to the CDC with data on symptoms available [79]. Lyme arthritis appears to be less frequent in Europe [80–84], but some prospective studies found an incidence of Lyme arthritis of 6% or less in both children and adults in the United States [85, 86], rates that seem similar to Europe. Lyme arthritis is a migratory, asymmetric, oligoarticular arthritis of large joints, usually presenting with intermittent episodes of joint swelling and pain, especially involving the knee. Joint inflammation can last days to weeks or sometimes many months. While arthritis will resolve in the majority of patients after antibiotic therapy, some patients will have persistent arthritis (post-infectious Lyme arthritis) [87–90], which seems to be less common in Europe [91]. Moreover, pediatric Lyme arthritis in the United States can have an acute presentation that overlaps with septic arthritis [92–96]. Patients can present with fever and joint pain, along with large joint effusions, resulting in a limited range of motion. The peripheral white blood cell count and the inflammatory markers, erythrocyte sedimentation rate, and C-reactive protein may be elevated. The synovial fluid white cell count can exceed 80,000 cells/mm^3 with a percentage of polymorphonuclear cells greater than 75%. These findings can result in significant problems if children with Lyme arthritis are treated as acute septic arthritis, including the possibility of unnecessary surgical procedures, since the results of serologic testing for Lyme borreliosis are not immediately available. This acute presentation of pediatric Lyme arthritis does not appear to occur in Europe [97, 98].

5.4.6 Asymptomatic Infections

In the United States, *B. burgdorferi* is apparently associated with fewer asymptomatic infections than in Europe. According to data from the Lymerix vaccine study, asymptomatic infection may occur in approximately 10% of infected patients in the United States [99]. In comparison, serosurveys in Europe have provided indirect evidence of a much higher proportion of asymptomatic infections [100–105].

5.4.7 Other Clinical and/or Demographic Differences: United States Versus Europe

Differences between the most common clinical presentations of Lyme borreliosis in the United States versus Europe (Table 5.1) have been noted since the early years of the recognition of the disease and the discovery of *B. burgdorferi.* In the United States, untreated *B. burgdorferi* infection is particularly linked with arthritis [106, 107]. Borrelial lymphocytoma and ACA are not seen in the United States, presumably because these cutaneous manifestations of Lyme borreliosis are primarily caused by *B. afzelii,* a Lyme borrelia species not found in the United States [39]. Lyme borreliosis in the United States is associated with a male predominance, with males accounting for 56% of the reported cases from 2008 to 2018 [108]. In the United States, none of the clinical manifestations has been associated with a female predominance, whereas in Europe, the majority of cases of EM and ACA occur in women [109–113], with many studies (but not all) demonstrating a male predominance among cases of neuroborreliosis and arthritis [82, 114–116].

5.5 Laboratory Testing for Lyme Borreliosis in the United States

In both the United States and Europe, most laboratory tests performed to diagnose Lyme borreliosis are based on the detection of the antibody responses against Lyme borrelia in serum. Because Lyme borreliosis in the United States is mainly caused by *B. burgdorferi*, criteria for test interpretation were somewhat easier to standardize than in Europe. About 3.4 million Lyme serologic tests are done in the United States per year [117], likely being ordered in populations with a low probability of having Lyme borreliosis. Therefore, high specificity is an essential requirement of the testing. The two-tier approach has been recommended by the CDC since 1995 [118]. The first step uses a sensitive enzyme immunoassay (EIA) or rarely, an indirect immunofluorescence assay. If the test is negative, there is no further testing. If the test is borderline or positive, the sample is retested using separate IgM and IgG Western blots (WB) as the second step. The WB is interpreted using standardized criteria, requiring at least two of three signature bands for a positive IgM WB and five of ten signature bands for a positive IgG WB. The IgM WB results are used only for patients with an illness of less than or equal to 30 days duration. The IgM WB is also irrelevant for diagnosing Lyme arthritis, irrespective of the duration of symptoms, as this is a late manifestation of Lyme borreliosis and requires IgG seropositivity. While the current two-tier algorithm performs relatively well, there are areas in need of improvement. Problems include low sensitivity during early infection (due to the delay in the development of a reactive IgM WB), subjective interpretation of bands leading to inter- and intra-laboratory variability, high cost, long turnaround time, and confusion by health care providers and patients regarding how to the interpret the results. Use of a two-EIA approach as an alternative (or modified) two-tiered testing strategy (Fig. 5.3) has been shown to have higher sensitivity

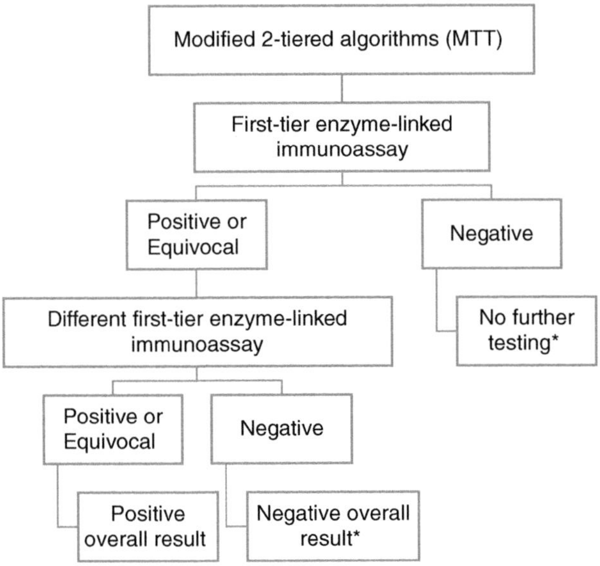

Fig. 5.3 Suggested modified two-tiered algorithms (MTT) for serodiagnosis of Lyme borreliosis. *Patients with erythema migrans (EM) should receive treatment on the basis of the clinical diagnosis. For patients with illnesses suspicious for early Lyme borreliosis, that do not present with EM, and have a disease duration of less or equal to 30 days, the provider may empirically treat the patient for Lyme borreliosis and follow up with serologic testing for antibodies to Lyme borrelia on a convalescent phase serum sample

in early disease, while maintaining similar specificity [119], when at least one of the EIA assays is based on the antibody response against VlsE (the variable surface antigen of *B. burgdorferi*) or the C6 peptide (derived from the invariable region 6 of VlsE). This strategy can be used in the United States, or in Europe, to diagnose Lyme borrelia infections acquired in either region. Hopefully, this will lead to new developments in the field, including a possible point-of-care test, which will be particularly useful for patients with manifestations of early disseminated Lyme borreliosis, like facial palsy or carditis, as well as for children with Lyme arthritis.

5.5.1 Intrathecal Production of Antibodies Against *B. burgdorferi*—Testing in the United States

Because direct tests for the presence of *B. burgdorferi* in cerebrospinal fluid have very low sensitivity, laboratory diagnosis relies on the detection of intrathecal production of anti-Lyme borrelia antibodies, referred to as the intrathecal antibody index. Detection of intrathecal production of anti-Lyme borrelia antibodies is recommended to diagnose Lyme neuroborreliosis with central nervous system involvement in both the United States and Europe [120–124]. The vast majority of studies on the value of the intrathecal antibody index for the diagnosis of Lyme neuroborreliosis, however, originate from Europe, where *B. garinii* and *B. bavariensis* are the species most often associated with neurologic disease. Studies have used different case definitions, different assays, and interpretative criteria, and there is little comparison among assays or among performing laboratories. In the United States, the situation is much worse, with no new research published on the value of tests for intrathecal antibody production to diagnose neuroborreliosis since the very early studies [52, 55, 57, 125]. While the available data are from very few studies, it appears that a positive intrathecal antibody index is less common in the United States [55, 126, 127]. To compound the issue, tests offered in the United States vary substantially in methods, assays, and interpretation [52, 128].

5.6 Some Differences in Treatment Recommendations between the United States and Europe

Recommendations for the treatment of Lyme borreliosis are very similar between the United States and European guidelines [129]. One difference is in the use of phenoxymethylpenicillin (penicillin V), which is recommended in some of the guidelines in Europe, but usually not prescribed in the United States [130, 131]. Phenoxymethylpenicillin is the most commonly used antibiotic to treat EM in Norway [132]. Another difference is the recommendation of intravenous ceftriaxone for treatment of EM, as well as other manifestations of Lyme borreliosis, in pregnant women by some authorities [130, 133]. The United States recommendations for antibiotic treatment of the different manifestations of Lyme borreliosis in pregnancy are the same as for nonpregnant patients, except that doxycycline is usually avoided in pregnancy [131].

5.6.1 Postexposure Chemoprophylaxis United States Versus Europe

Transmission of *B. burgdorferi* and *B. mayonii* by *I. scapularis* is very infrequent during the first 36 hours after tick attachment but steadily increases after 48 hours of attachment, with similar results with *I. pacificus*. While transmission of *B. afzelii* by *I. ricinus* may occur within 24 hours, the majority of transmission occurs after 48–72 hours [134–136]. Antibiotic prophylaxis with a single dose of doxycycline has been shown to reduce the risk of Lyme borreliosis after an *I. scapularis* bite [137, 138]. A recently published European trial showed that a single 200 mg dose doxycycline was successful for the prevention of Lyme disease after a tick bite [139], with efficacy of 67% by modified-intention-to-treat analysis and 77% in the per protocol analysis. We compared these results with the results from Nadelman et al. [138], using a Z-score of the log odds ratio from the studies and calculated a two-sided *p* value from the Normal distribution associated with the Z-score. We found no evidence of a significant difference in efficacy between the studies. For both studies, it was estimated that one case of Lyme borreliosis would be prevented for about 50 patients treated [138, 139]. Therefore, to limit the unnecessary use of doxycycline, in the United States, it is recommended that antibiotic prophylaxis be restricted to *I. scapularis* tick bites in geographic areas where *B. burgdorferi* infection rates in the ticks are at least 20%, the tick has been attached for at least 36 hours, and the prophylaxis can be given within 72 hours of tick removal [131]. In contrast, there are no official recommendations for chemoprophylaxis after an *I. ricinus* tick bite, and a watch-and-wait approach is the standard practice [130].

5.7 Coinfections United States Versus Europe

Ixodes ticks can carry multiple pathogens, and a single tick bite may result in the transmission of more than one infectious agent. Infectious agents transmitted by *I. scapularis* to humans include *B. burgdorferi, B. mayonii, B. miyamotoi, A. phagocytophilum, Babesia microti, Ehrlichia muris eauclairensis,* and the deer tick virus subtype of Powassan virus [140, 141]. The incidence of coinfections will depend on the prevalence of the infectious agents in ticks, which vary in different geographic areas [142–145]. The majority of recognized coinfections in the United States involve two of the three most common pathogens, *B. burgdorferi, A. phagocytophilum,* and *B. microti.* Ten states (Massachusetts, New York, Maine, Wisconsin, Minnesota, Vermont, New Hampshire, Rhode Island, New Jersey, and Connecticut) account for more than 93% of all reported cases of anaplasmosis and babesiosis [146]. All of these states also report a high incidence of Lyme borreliosis. Regarding how commonly coinfection occurs, most studies have examined patients using serological evidence of exposure, showing that a small proportion of patients with Lyme borreliosis are coinfected with *B. microti* or *A. phagocytophilum.* Patients with concurrent Lyme borreliosis and untreated babesiosis were more likely to be symptomatic for 3 months or longer in one study [147], but in another study, acute Lyme borreliosis was not more severe in patients with serological evidence of exposure to babesiosis [148]. Regarding anaplasmosis, coinfected patients seem to have more symptoms than patients with Lyme borreliosis alone (but this is very much dependent on the case definition of coinfection) [149], and children with recognized concurrent infections had higher rates of hospitalization [150].

About 11% of the patients with *B. miyamotoi* infection in the Northeastern United States also had concomitant Lyme borreliosis [151]. *B. miyamotoi* infection can cause a positive result on EIA used as first-tier tests for Lyme borreliosis, including the C6 peptide EIA [47]. Cases of encephalitis due to deer tick virus are relatively rare, but the number of cases is increasing, possibly due to better recognition of the disease and/or greater access to diagnostic tests, as well as to an increase in the number of cases [152–154]. The rate of infection of *I. scapularis* ticks in the Northeast and upper Midwest United States with deer tick virus is variable, with reports of up to 5% in certain regions [144, 155, 156]. There is no convincing evidence that *Bartonella spp.* is transmitted by *I. scapularis* ticks to humans or that coinfection with *B. burgdorferi* occurs.

In Europe, *I. ricinus* can transmit tick-borne encephalitis virus, *A. phagocytophilum*, species of the bacterial genus *Rickettsia*, *B. miyamotoi,* and *Babesia* protozoans (see Chap. 9 "Other Ixodes-Borne Diseases") Tick-borne encephalitis virus is well established as a cause of coinfection in patients with Lyme borreliosis [157–160]. More data on the frequency of coinfection with the other *I. ricinus*-transmitted pathogens are needed [159, 161–166].

5.8 Chronic Lyme Disease United States Versus Europe

A major controversial issue in the United States, which is also developing in Europe, is the diagnosis of "chronic Lyme disease" (CLD). CLD is a very confusing term, as it has been applied to vastly different patient populations. Initially used to describe patients with objective manifestations of late Lyme borreliosis, it has since been used to describe patients with PTLDS; however, in the majority of the cases, it is applied to patients suffering from medically unexplained nonspecific symptoms who received the CLD diagnosis based on unproven clinical criteria, with or without, the support of non-validated laboratory tests [167–174]. Almost any symptom has been attributed to CLD. Alternatively diagnosed chronic Lyme syndrome (ADCLS) has been suggested as a term to describe these patients [175, 176]. Moreover, CLD has grown into a disorder presumed to be caused by multiple coinfections; metabolic, hormonal, and immune imbalances; toxin damage; heavy metal toxicity; and other dysfunctions; all diagnosed by unconfirmed criteria. The diagnosis is based on clinical judgment, conventional laboratory tests are not diagnostic, and the disease will require prolonged treatment with antibiotics and supplements [177]. Treatments may also include a gamut of unorthodox, alternative therapies [177–181]. This view of CLD has been advocated by alternative treatment providers, activists, and support groups in the United States, with similar groups appearing in Europe in the last few years. While this has created much confusion [182–184], there has been little formal research performed on this heterogeneous patient population, and the underlying issues affecting these patients are poorly understood.

5.9 Conclusion

Tickborne infections, particularly Lyme borreliosis, are significant health problems in many areas of the United States, and the geographical range of the risk area is likely to continue to expand. Lyme borreliosis presents with a variety of manifestations, and variations within Lyme borrelia, together with differences in the host response, and time to antibiotic treatment, play a role in the diversity of disease manifestations and/or in their severity. In the United States, early Lyme borreliosis presenting with EM is associated with more symptomatic disease than in Europe. It will be important to delineate the specific virulence factors that contribute to more severe disease. There has been progress toward new approaches for the laboratory diagnosis of Lyme borreliosis, including simplification of the current algorithm for serologic testing, potentially opening the door for the development of point-of-care tests. More research in the United States on Lyme neuroborreliosis and its laboratory diagnosis is needed. The controversial issue of chronic Lyme disease is a growing problem. Creative, well-designed scientific approaches to investigate this heterogeneous group of patients are required to set up the groundwork for more effective treatment strategies for patients.Funding and DisclaimerFunding for this study was provided in part by the Division of Intramural Research, National Institute of Allergy and Infectious Diseases, National Institutes of Health. The content of this publication does not necessarily reflect the views or policies of the Department of Health and Human Services, nor does the mention of trade names, commercial products, or organizations imply endorsement by the United States Government.

References

1. Schwartz AM, Kugeler KJ, Nelson CA, Marx GE, Hinckley AF. Use of commercial claims data for evaluating trends in Lyme disease diagnoses, United States, 2010-2018. Emerg Infect Dis. 2021;27(2):499–507. https://doi.org/10.3201/eid2702.202728.
2. Kugeler KJ, Schwartz AM, Delorey MJ, Mead PS, Hinckley AF. Estimating the frequency of Lyme disease diagnoses, United States, 2010-2018. Emerg Infect Dis. 2021;27(2):616–9. https://doi.org/10.3201/eid2702.202731.
3. Steere AC, Malawista SE, Snydman DR, Shope RE, Andiman WA, Ross MR, et al. Lyme arthritis: an epidemic of oligoarticular arthritis in children and adults in three Connecticut communities. Arthritis Rheum. 1977;20(1):7–17. https://doi.org/10.1002/art.1780200102.
4. Mast WE, Burrows WM Jr. Erythema chronicum migrans in the United States. JAMA. 1976;236(7):859–60.
5. Scrimenti RJ. Erythema chronicum migrans. Arch Dermatol. 1970;102(1):104–5.
6. Burgdorfer W, Barbour AG, Hayes SF, Benach JL, Grunwaldt E, Davis JP. Lyme disease-a tick-borne spirochetosis? Science. 1982;216(4552):1317–9. https://doi.org/10.1126/science.7043737.
7. Johnson RC, Schmid GP, Hyde FW, Steigerwalt AG, Brenner DJ. *Borrelia burgdorferi* sp nov.: - etiologic agent of Lyme-disease. Int J Syst Bacteriol. 1984;34(4):496–7. https://doi.org/10.1099/00207713-34-4-496.
8. Wilske B, Preac-Mursic V, Schierz G. Antigenic heterogeneity of European *Borrelia burgdorferi* strains isolated from patients and ticks. Lancet. 1985;1(8437):1099. https://doi.org/10.1016/s0140-6736(85)92396-7.
9. Barbour AG, Heiland RA, Howe TR. Heterogeneity of major proteins in Lyme disease borreliae: a molecular analysis of North American and European isolates. J Infect Dis. 1985;152(3):478–84. https://doi.org/10.1093/infdis/152.3.478.
10. Boerlin P, Peter O, Bretz AG, Postic D, Baranton G, Piffaretti JC. Population genetic analysis of *Borrelia burgdorferi* isolates by multilocus enzyme electrophoresis. Infect Immun. 1992;60(4):1677–83. https://doi.org/10.1128/iai.60.4.1677-1683.1992.
11. Baranton G, Postic D, Saint Girons I, Boerlin P, Piffaretti JC, Assous M, et al. Delineation of *Borrelia burgdorferi* sensu stricto, *Borrelia garinii* sp. nov., and group VS461 associated with Lyme borreliosis. Int J Syst Bacteriol. 1992;42(3):378–83. https://doi.org/10.1099/00207713-42-3-378.
12. Canica MM, Nato F, du Merle L, Mazie JC, Baranton G, Postic D. Monoclonal antibodies for identification of *Borrelia afzelii* sp. nov. associated with late cutaneous manifestations of Lyme borreliosis. Scand J Infect Dis. 1993;25(4):441–8. https://doi.org/10.3109/00365549309008525.

13. Belfaiza J, Postic D, Bellenger E, Baranton G, Girons IS. Genomic fingerprinting of *Borrelia burgdorferi* sensu lato by pulsed-field gel electrophoresis. J Clin Microbiol. 1993;31(11):2873–7. https://doi.org/10.1128/jcm.31.11.2873-2877.1993.
14. Barbour AG, Adeolu M, Gupta RS. Division of the genus *Borrelia* into two genera (corresponding to Lyme disease and relapsing fever groups) reflects their genetic and phenotypic distinctiveness and will lead to a better understanding of these two groups of microbes (Margos et al. 2016) there is inadequate evidence to support the division of the genus *Borrelia*. Int J Syst Evol Microbiol. 2017;67(6):2058–67. https://doi.org/10.1099/ijsem.0.001815.
15. Stevenson B, Fingerle V, Wormser GP, Margos G. Public health and patient safety concerns merit retention of Lyme borreliosis-associated spirochetes within the genus *Borrelia*, and rejection of the genus novum *Borreliella*. Ticks Tick Borne Dis. 2019;10(1):1–4. https://doi.org/10.1016/j.ttbdis.2018.08.010.
16. Margos G, Marosevic D, Cutler S, Derdakova M, Diuk-Wasser M, Emler S, et al. There is inadequate evidence to support the division of the genus *Borrelia*. Int J Syst Evol Microbiol. 2017;67(4):1081–4. https://doi.org/10.1099/ijsem.0.001717.
17. Margos G, Castillo-Ramirez S, Cutler S, Dessau RB, Eikeland R, Estrada-Pena A, et al. Rejection of the name *Borreliella* and all proposed species comb. nov. placed therein. Int J Syst Evol Microbiol. 2020;70(5):3577–81. https://doi.org/10.1099/ijsem.0.004149.
18. Pritt BS, Mead PS, Johnson DKH, Neitzel DF, Respicio-Kingry LB, Davis JP, et al. Identification of a novel pathogenic *Borrelia* species causing Lyme borreliosis with unusually high spirochaetaemia: a descriptive study. Lancet Infect Dis. 2016;16(5):556–64. https://doi.org/10.1016/S1473-3099(15)00464-8.
19. Mead PS. Epidemiology of Lyme disease. Infect Dis Clin N Am. 2015;29(2):187–210. https://doi.org/10.1016/j.idc.2015.02.010.
20. Rosenberg R, Lindsey NP, Fischer M, Gregory CJ, Hinckley AF, Mead PS, et al. Vital signs: trends in reported vectorborne disease cases - United States and territories, 2004-2016. MMWR Morb Mortal Wkly Rep. 2018;67(17):496–501. https://doi.org/10.15585/mmwr.mm6717e1.
21. CDC: Lyme Disease Maps: Most Recent Year. 2019. https://www.cdc.gov/lyme/datasurveillance/maps-recent.html Accessed 05 Dec 2021.
22. Kugeler KJ, Farley GM, Forrester JD, Mead PS. Geographic distribution and expansion of human Lyme disease. United States Emerg Infect Dis. 2015;21(8):1455–7. https://doi.org/10.3201/eid2108.141878.
23. Lantos PM, Nigrovic LE, Auwaerter PG, Fowler VG Jr, Ruffin F, Brinkerhoff RJ, et al. Geographic expansion of Lyme disease in the Southeastern United States, 2000–2014. Open Forum Infect Dis. 2015;2(4):ofv143. https://doi.org/10.1093/ofid/ofv143.
24. Lantos PM, Tsao J, Nigrovic LE, Auwaerter PG, Fowler VG, Ruffin F, et al. Geographic expansion of Lyme disease in Michigan, 2000–2014. Open Forum Infect Dis. 2017;4(1):ofw269. https://doi.org/10.1093/ofid/ofw269.
25. Wood CL, Lafferty KD. Biodiversity and disease: a synthesis of ecological perspectives on Lyme disease transmission. Trends Ecol Evol. 2013;28(4):239–47. https://doi.org/10.1016/j.tree.2012.10.011.
26. Dumic I, Severnini E. "Ticking bomb": the impact of climate change on the incidence of Lyme disease. Can J Infect Dis Med Microbiol. 2018;2018:5719081. https://doi.org/10.1155/2018/5719081.
27. Pepin KM, Eisen RJ, Mead PS, Piesman J, Fish D, Hoen AG, et al. Geographic variation in the relationship between human Lyme disease incidence and density of infected host-seeking *Ixodes scapularis* nymphs in the Eastern United States. Am J Trop Med Hyg. 2012;86(6):1062–71. https://doi.org/10.4269/ajtmh.2012.11-0630.
28. Oliver JH Jr, Lin T, Gao L, Clark KL, Banks CW, Durden LA, et al. An enzootic transmission cycle of Lyme borreliosis spirochetes in the southeastern United States. Proc Natl Acad Sci U S A. 2003;100(20):11642–5. https://doi.org/10.1073/pnas.1434553100.
29. Diuk-Wasser MA, Gatewood AG, Cortinas MR, Yaremych-Hamer S, Tsao J, Kitron U, et al. Spatiotemporal patterns of host-seeking *Ixodes scapularis* nymphs (Acari: Ixodidae) in the

United States. J Med Entomol. 2006;43(2):166–76. https://doi.org/10.1603/0022-2585(2006)043[0166:spohis]2.0.co;2.
30. Ogden NH, Pang G, Ginsberg HS, Hickling GJ, Burke RL, Beati L, et al. Evidence for geographic variation in life-cycle processes affecting phenology of the Lyme disease vector *Ixodes scapularis* (Acari: Ixodidae) in the United States. J Med Entomol. 2018;55(6):1386–401. https://doi.org/10.1093/jme/tjy104.
31. Arsnoe I, Tsao JI, Hickling GJ. Nymphal *Ixodes scapularis* questing behavior explains geographic variation in Lyme borreliosis risk in the eastern United States. Ticks Tick Borne Dis. 2019;10(3):553–63. https://doi.org/10.1016/j.ttbdis.2019.01.001.
32. Coipan EC, Jahfari S, Fonville M, Oei GA, Spanjaard L, Takumi K, et al. Imbalanced presence of *Borrelia burgdorferi* s.l. multilocus sequence types in clinical manifestations of Lyme borreliosis. Infect Genet Evol. 2016;42:66–76. https://doi.org/10.1016/j.meegid.2016.04.019.
33. Wormser GP, Brisson D, Liveris D, Hanincova K, Sandigursky S, Nowakowski J, et al. *Borrelia burgdorferi* genotype predicts the capacity for hematogenous dissemination during early Lyme disease. J Infect Dis. 2008;198(9):1358–64. https://doi.org/10.1086/592279.
34. Hanincova K, Mukherjee P, Ogden NH, Margos G, Wormser GP, Reed KD, et al. Multilocus sequence typing of *Borrelia burgdorferi* suggests existence of lineages with differential pathogenic properties in humans. PLoS One. 2013;8(9):e73066. https://doi.org/10.1371/journal.pone.0073066.
35. Strle K, Jones KL, Drouin EE, Li X, Steere AC. *Borrelia burgdorferi* RST1 (OspC type A) genotype is associated with greater inflammation and more severe Lyme disease. Am J Pathol. 2011;178(6):2726–39. https://doi.org/10.1016/j.ajpath.2011.02.018.
36. Jones KL, McHugh GA, Glickstein LJ, Steere AC. Analysis of *Borrelia burgdorferi* genotypes in patients with Lyme arthritis: high frequency of ribosomal RNA intergenic spacer type 1 strains in antibiotic-refractory arthritis. Arthritis Rheum. 2009;60(7):2174–82. https://doi.org/10.1002/art.24812.
37. Seinost G, Dykhuizen DE, Dattwyler RJ, Golde WT, Dunn JJ, Wang IN, et al. Four clones of *Borrelia burgdorferi* sensu stricto cause invasive infection in humans. Infect Immun. 1999;67(7):3518–24. https://doi.org/10.1128/IAI.67.7.3518-3524.1999.
38. Shapiro ED, Wormser GP. Controversies about Lyme disease-reply. JAMA. 2018;320(23):2482–3. https://doi.org/10.1001/jama.2018.17207.
39. Steere AC, Strle F, Wormser GP, Hu LT, Branda JA, Hovius JW, et al. Lyme borreliosis. Nat Rev Dis Primers. 2016;2:16090. https://doi.org/10.1038/nrdp.2016.90.
40. Tibbles CD, Edlow JA. Does this patient have erythema migrans? JAMA. 2007;297(23):2617–27. https://doi.org/10.1001/jama.297.23.2617.
41. Wormser GP, Masters E, Nowakowski J, McKenna D, Holmgren D, Ma K, et al. Prospective clinical evaluation of patients from Missouri and New York with erythema migrans-like skin lesions. Clin Infect Dis. 2005;41(7):958–65. https://doi.org/10.1086/432935.
42. Raghavan RK, Peterson AT, Cobos ME, Ganta R, Foley D. Current and future distribution of the lone star tick, *Amblyomma americanum* (L.) (Acari: Ixodidae) in North America. PLoS One. 2019;14(1):e0209082. https://doi.org/10.1371/journal.pone.0209082.
43. Molins CR, Ashton LV, Wormser GP, Andre BG, Hess AM, Delorey MJ, et al. Metabolic differentiation of early Lyme disease from southern tick-associated rash illness (STARI). Sci Transl Med. 2017;9(403) https://doi.org/10.1126/scitranslmed.aal2717.
44. Steere AC, Dhar A, Hernandez J, Fischer PA, Sikand VK, Schoen RT, et al. Systemic symptoms without erythema migrans as the presenting picture of early Lyme disease. Am J Med. 2003;114(1):58–62. https://doi.org/10.1016/s0002-9343(02)01440-7.
45. Feder HM, Gerber MA, Krause PJ, Ryan R, Shapiro ED. Early Lyme-disease - a flu-like illness without erythema migrans. Pediatrics. 1993;91(2):456–9.
46. Wormser GP, Shapiro ED, Fish D. Borrelia miyamotoi: an emerging tick-borne pathogen. Am J Med. 2019;132(2):136–7. https://doi.org/10.1016/j.amjmed.2018.08.012.
47. Molloy PJ, Weeks KE, Todd B, Wormser GP. Seroreactivity to the C6 peptide in *Borrelia miyamotoi* infections occurring in the northeastern United States. Clin Infect Dis. 2018;66(9):1407–10. https://doi.org/10.1093/cid/cix1023.

48. Telford SR 3rd, Goethert HK, Molloy PJ, Berardi VP, Chowdri HR, Gugliotta JL, et al. *Borrelia miyamotoi* disease: neither Lyme disease nor relapsing fever. Clin Lab Med. 2015;35(4):867–82. https://doi.org/10.1016/j.cll.2015.08.002.
49. Wormser GP, Horowitz HW, Dumler JS, Schwartz I, Aguero-Rosenfeld M. False-positive Lyme disease serology in human granulocytic ehrlichiosis. Lancet. 1996;347(9006):981–2. https://doi.org/10.1016/s0140-6736(96)91475-0.
50. Tuuminen T, Hedman K, Soderlund-Venermo M, Seppala I. Acute parvovirus B19 infection causes nonspecificity frequently in *Borrelia* and less often in *Salmonella* and *Campylobacter* serology, posing a problem in diagnosis of infectious arthropathy. Clin Vaccine Immunol. 2011;18(1):167–72. https://doi.org/10.1128/CVI.00367-10.
51. Pavletic AJ, Marques AR. Early disseminated Lyme disease causing false-positive serology for primary Epstein-Barr virus infection: report of 2 cases. Clin Infect Dis. 2017;65(2):336–7. https://doi.org/10.1093/cid/cix298.
52. Marques AR. Lyme neuroborreliosis. Continuum (Minneap Minn). 2015;21(6 Neuroinfectious Disease):1729–44. https://doi.org/10.1212/CON.0000000000000252.
53. Ogrinc K, Lusa L, Lotric-Furlan S, Bogovic P, Stupica D, Cerar T, et al. Course and outcome of early European Lyme neuroborreliosis (Bannwarth syndrome): clinical and laboratory findings. Clin Infect Dis. 2016;63(3):346–53. https://doi.org/10.1093/cid/ciw299.
54. Barstad B, Quarsten H, Tveitnes D, Noraas S, Ask IS, Saeed M, et al. Direct molecular detection and genotyping of *Borrelia burgdorferi* sensu lato in cerebrospinal fluid of children with Lyme neuroborreliosis. J Clin Microbiol. 2018;56(5) https://doi.org/10.1128/JCM.01868-17.
55. Steere AC, Berardi VP, Weeks KE, Logigian EL, Ackermann R. Evaluation of the intrathecal antibody response to *Borrelia burgdorferi* as a diagnostic test for Lyme neuroborreliosis. J Infect Dis. 1990;161(6):1203–9. https://doi.org/10.1093/infdis/161.6.1203.
56. Halperin JJ. Diagnosis and management of Lyme neuroborreliosis. Expert Rev Anti-Infect Ther. 2018;16(1):5–11. https://doi.org/10.1080/14787210.2018.1417836.
57. Logigian EL, Kaplan RF, Steere AC. Chronic neurologic manifestations of Lyme disease. N Engl J Med. 1990;323(21):1438–44. https://doi.org/10.1056/NEJM199011223232102.
58. Kaplan RF, Meadows ME, Vincent LC, Logigian EL, Steere AC. Memory impairment and depression in patients with Lyme encephalopathy: comparison with fibromyalgia and non-psychotically depressed patients. Neurology. 1992;42(7):1263–7. https://doi.org/10.1212/wnl.42.7.1263.
59. Logigian EL, Kaplan RF, Steere AC. Successful treatment of Lyme encephalopathy with intravenous ceftriaxone. J Infect Dis. 1999;180(2):377–83. https://doi.org/10.1086/314860.
60. Ogrinc K, Logar M, Lotric-Furlan S, Cerar D, Ruzic-Sabljic E, Strle F. Doxycycline versus ceftriaxone for the treatment of patients with chronic Lyme borreliosis. Wien Klin Wochenschr. 2006;118(21–22):696–701. https://doi.org/10.1007/s00508-006-0698-7.
61. Wormser GP, Strle F, Shapiro ED, Dattwyler RJ, Auwaerter PG. A critical appraisal of the mild axonal peripheral neuropathy of late neurologic Lyme disease. Diagn Microbiol Infect Dis. 2017;87(2):163–7. https://doi.org/10.1016/j.diagmicrobio.2016.11.003.
62. Fallon BA, Keilp JG, Corbera KM, Petkova E, Britton CB, Dwyer E, et al. A randomized, placebo-controlled trial of repeated IV antibiotic therapy for Lyme encephalopathy. Neurology. 2008;70(13):992–1003. https://doi.org/10.1212/01.WNL.0000284604.61160.2d.
63. Klempner MS, Hu LT, Evans J, Schmid CH, Johnson GM, Trevino RP, et al. Two controlled trials of antibiotic treatment in patients with persistent symptoms and a history of Lyme disease. N Engl J Med. 2001;345(2):85–92. https://doi.org/10.1056/NEJM200107123450202.
64. Krupp LB, Hyman LG, Grimson R, Coyle PK, Melville P, Ahnn S, et al. Study and treatment of post Lyme disease (STOP-LD): a randomized double masked clinical trial. Neurology. 2003;60(12):1923–30. https://doi.org/10.1212/01.wnl.0000071227.23769.9e.
65. Kaplan RF, Trevino RP, Johnson GM, Levy L, Dornbush R, Hu LT, et al. Cognitive function in post-treatment Lyme disease: do additional antibiotics help? Neurology. 2003;60(12):1916–22. https://doi.org/10.1212/01.wnl.0000068030.26992.25.

66. Gaudino EA, Coyle PK, Krupp LB. Post-Lyme syndrome and chronic fatigue syndrome. Neuropsychiatric similarities and differences. Arch Neurol. 1997;54(11):1372–6. https://doi.org/10.1001/archneur.1997.00550230045015.
67. Shadick NA, Phillips CB, Logigian EL, Steere AC, Kaplan RF, Berardi VP, et al. The long-term clinical outcomes of Lyme disease. A population-based retrospective cohort study. Ann Intern Med. 1994;121(8):560–7. https://doi.org/10.7326/0003-4819-121-8-199410150-00002.
68. Binder LM, Iverson GL, Brooks BL. To err is human: "abnormal" neuropsychological scores and variability are common in healthy adults. Arch Clin Neuropsychol. 2009;24(1):31–46. https://doi.org/10.1093/arclin/acn001.
69. Kindstrand E, Nilsson BY, Hovmark A, Pirskanen R, Asbrink E. Peripheral neuropathy in acrodermatitis chronica atrophicans - a late *Borrelia* manifestation. Acta Neurol Scand. 1997;95(6):338–45. https://doi.org/10.1111/j.1600-0404.1997.tb00222.x.
70. Kristoferitsch W, Sluga E, Graf M, Partsch H, Neumann R, Stanek G, et al. Neuropathy associated with acrodermatitis chronica atrophicans. Clinical and morphological features. Ann N Y Acad Sci. 1988;539:35–45. https://doi.org/10.1111/j.1749-6632.1988.tb31836.x.
71. Hopf HC. Peripheral neuropathy in acrodermatitis chronica atrophicans (Herxheimer). J Neurol Neurosurg Psychiatry. 1975;38(5):452–8. https://doi.org/10.1136/jnnp.38.5.452.
72. Logigian EL, Steere AC. Clinical and electrophysiologic findings in chronic neuropathy of Lyme disease. Neurology. 1992;42(2):303–11. https://doi.org/10.1212/wnl.42.2.303.
73. Halperin JJ, Little BW, Coyle PK, Dattwyler RJ. Lyme disease: cause of a treatable peripheral neuropathy. Neurology. 1987;37(11):1700–6. https://doi.org/10.1212/wnl.37.11.1700.
74. Halperin JJ, Pass HL, Anand AK, Luft BJ, Volkman DJ, Dattwyler RJ. Nervous system abnormalities in Lyme disease. Ann N Y Acad Sci. 1988;539:24–34. https://doi.org/10.1111/j.1749-6632.1988.tb31835.x.
75. Halperin J, Luft BJ, Volkman DJ, Dattwyler RJ. Lyme neuroborreliosis. Peripheral nervous system manifestations. Brain. 1990;113(Pt 4):1207–21. https://doi.org/10.1093/brain/113.4.1207.
76. Halperin JJ, Krupp LB, Golightly MG, Volkman DJ. Lyme borreliosis-associated encephalopathy. Neurology. 1990;40(9):1340–3. https://doi.org/10.1212/wnl.40.9.1340.
77. Steere AC, Schoen RT, Taylor E. The clinical evolution of Lyme arthritis. Ann Intern Med. 1987;107(5):725–31. https://doi.org/10.7326/0003-4819-107-5-725.
78. Szer IS, Taylor E, Steere AC. The long-term course of Lyme arthritis in children. N Engl J Med. 1991;325(3):159–63. https://doi.org/10.1056/NEJM199107183250304.
79. CDC: Lyme disease—Relative frequency of clinical features among confirmed cases-United States, 2008–2018. 2019. https://www.cdc.gov/lyme/stats/graphs.html. Accessed 5 Dec 2021.
80. Enkelmann J, Bohmer M, Fingerle V, Siffczyk C, Werber D, Littmann M, et al. Incidence of notified Lyme borreliosis in Germany, 2013-2017. Sci Rep. 2018;8(1):14976. https://doi.org/10.1038/s41598-018-33136-0.
81. Vandenesch A, Turbelin C, Couturier E, Arena C, Jaulhac B, Ferquel E, et al. Incidence and hospitalisation rates of Lyme borreliosis, France, 2004 to 2012. Euro Surveill. 2014;19(34):20883. https://doi.org/10.2807/1560-7917.es2014.19.34.20883.
82. Strle F, Wormser GP, Mead P, Dhaduvai K, Longo MV, Adenikinju O, et al. Gender disparity between cutaneous and non-cutaneous manifestations of Lyme borreliosis. PLoS One. 2013;8(5):e64110. https://doi.org/10.1371/journal.pone.0064110.
83. Berglund J, Eitrem R, Ornstein K, Lindberg A, Ringer A, Elmrud H, et al. An epidemiologic study of Lyme disease in southern Sweden. N Engl J Med. 1995;333(20):1319–27. https://doi.org/10.1056/NEJM199511163332004.
84. Wilking H, Stark K. Trends in surveillance data of human Lyme borreliosis from six federal states in eastern Germany, 2009-2012. Ticks Tick Borne Dis. 2014;5(3):219–24. https://doi.org/10.1016/j.ttbdis.2013.10.010.
85. Gerber MA, Zemel LS, Shapiro ED. Lyme arthritis in children: clinical epidemiology and long-term outcomes. Pediatrics. 1998;102(4 Pt 1):905–8. https://doi.org/10.1542/peds.102.4.905.

86. Sigal LH, Zahradnik JM, Lavin P, Patella SJ, Bryant G, Haselby R, et al. A vaccine consisting of recombinant *Borrelia burgdorferi* outer-surface protein a to prevent Lyme disease. Recombinant outer-surface protein a Lyme disease vaccine study consortium. N Engl J Med. 1998;339(4):216–22. https://doi.org/10.1056/NEJM199807233390402.
87. Tory HO, Zurakowski D, Sundel RP. Outcomes of children treated for Lyme arthritis: results of a large pediatric cohort. J Rheumatol. 2010;37(5):1049–55. https://doi.org/10.3899/jrheum.090711.
88. Arvikar SL, Steere AC. Diagnosis and treatment of Lyme arthritis. Infect Dis Clin N Am. 2015;29(2):269–80. https://doi.org/10.1016/j.idc.2015.02.004.
89. Steere AC, Angelis SM. Therapy for Lyme arthritis: strategies for the treatment of antibiotic-refractory arthritis. Arthritis Rheum. 2006;54(10):3079–86. https://doi.org/10.1002/art.22131.
90. Brescia AC, Rose CD, Fawcett PT. Prolonged synovitis in pediatric Lyme arthritis cannot be predicted by clinical or laboratory parameters. Clin Rheumatol. 2009;28(5):591–3. https://doi.org/10.1007/s10067-009-1100-8.
91. Haugeberg G, Hansen IJ, Skarpaas T, Noraas S, Kjelland V. Lyme arthritis in Southern Norway—an endemic area for Lyme borreliosis. BMC Infect Dis. 2014;14:185. https://doi.org/10.1186/1471-2334-14-185.
92. Dart AH, Michelson KA, Aronson PL, Garro AC, Lee TJ, Glerum KM, et al. Hip synovial fluid cell counts in children from a Lyme disease endemic area. Pediatrics. 2018;141(5):e20173810. https://doi.org/10.1542/peds.2017-3810.
93. Cruz AI Jr, Anari JB, Ramirez JM, Sankar WN, Baldwin KD. Distinguishing pediatric Lyme arthritis of the hip from transient synovitis and acute bacterial septic arthritis: a systematic review and meta-analysis. Cureus. 2018;10(1):e2112. https://doi.org/10.7759/cureus.2112.
94. Deanehan JK, Nigrovic PA, Milewski MD, Tan Tanny SP, Kimia AA, Smith BG, et al. Synovial fluid findings in children with knee monoarthritis in Lyme disease endemic areas. Pediatr Emerg Care. 2014;30(1):16–9. https://doi.org/10.1097/PEC.0000000000000028.
95. Deanehan JK, Kimia AA, Tan Tanny SP, Milewski MD, Talusan PG, Smith BG, et al. Distinguishing Lyme from septic knee monoarthritis in Lyme disease-endemic areas. Pediatrics. 2013;131(3):e695–701. https://doi.org/10.1542/peds.2012-2531.
96. Bachman DT, Srivastava G. Emergency department presentations of Lyme disease in children. Pediatr Emerg Care. 1998;14(5):356–61.
97. Huppertz HI, Karch H, Suschke HJ, Doring E, Ganser G, Thon A, et al. Lyme arthritis in European children and adolescents. The pediatric rheumatology collaborative group. Arthritis Rheum. 1995;38(3):361–8. https://doi.org/10.1002/art.1780380310.
98. Moniuszko A, Popko J, Guszczyn T, Walinski T, Zukiewicz-Sobczak W, Pancewicz S. Lyme disease with effusion either in hip or knee in children from Podlaskie region treated in clinic in 2004-2010. Przegl Epidemiol. 2014;68(3):425–8, 535–7
99. Steere AC, Sikand VK, Schoen RT, Nowakowski J. Asymptomatic infection with *Borrelia burgdorferi*. Clin Infect Dis. 2003;37(4):528–32. https://doi.org/10.1086/376914.
100. Wilhelmsson P, Fryland L, Lindblom P, Sjowall J, Ahlm C, Berglund J, et al. A prospective study on the incidence of *Borrelia burgdorferi* sensu lato infection after a tick bite in Sweden and on the Aland Islands, Finland (2008-2009). Ticks Tick Borne Dis. 2016;7(1):71–9. https://doi.org/10.1016/j.ttbdis.2015.08.009.
101. Cetin E, Sotoudeh M, Auer H, Stanek G. Paradigm Burgenland: risk of *Borrelia burgdorferi* sensu lato infection indicated by variable seroprevalence rates in hunters. Wien Klin Wochenschr. 2006;118(21–22):677–81. https://doi.org/10.1007/s00508-006-0694-y.
102. Vos K, Van Dam AP, Kuiper H, Bruins H, Spanjaard L, Dankert J. Seroconversion for Lyme borreliosis among Dutch military. Scand J Infect Dis. 1994;26(4):427–34. https://doi.org/10.3109/00365549409008616.
103. Kuiper H, van Dam AP, Moll van Charante AW, Nauta NP, Dankert J. One year follow-up study to assess the prevalence and incidence of Lyme borreliosis among Dutch forestry workers. Eur J Clin Microbiol Infect Dis. 1993;12(6):413–8. https://doi.org/10.1007/BF01967434.

104. Carlsson H, Ekerfelt C, Henningsson AJ, Brudin L, Tjernberg I. Subclinical Lyme borreliosis is common in South-Eastern Sweden and may be distinguished from Lyme neuroborreliosis by sex, age and specific immune marker patterns. Ticks Tick Borne Dis. 2018;9(3):742–8. https://doi.org/10.1016/j.ttbdis.2018.02.011.
105. Rojko T, Ruzic-Sabljic E, Strle F, Lotric-Furlan S. Prevalence and incidence of Lyme borreliosis among Slovene forestry workers during the period of tick activity. Wien Klin Wochenschr. 2005;117(5–6):219–25. https://doi.org/10.1007/s00508-004-0306-7.
106. van Dam AP, Kuiper H, Vos K, Widjojokusumo A, de Jongh BM, Spanjaard L, et al. Different genospecies of *Borrelia burgdorferi* are associated with distinct clinical manifestations of Lyme borreliosis. Clin Infect Dis. 1993;17(4):708–17. https://doi.org/10.1093/clinids/17.4.708.
107. Stanek G, Wewalka G, Groh V, Neumann R, Kristoferitsch W. Differences between Lyme disease and European arthropod-borne *Borrelia* infections [letter]. Lancet. 1985;1(8425):401.
108. CDC: Lyme disease—Confirmed cases by age and sex—United States, 2008–2018. 2019. https://www.cdc.gov/lyme/stats/graphs.html. Accessed 5 Dec 2021.
109. Sajanti E, Virtanen M, Helve O, Kuusi M, Lyytikainen O, Hytonen J, et al. Lyme borreliosis in Finland, 1995-2014. Emerg Infect Dis. 2017;23(8):1282–8. https://doi.org/10.3201/eid2308.161273.
110. Strle F, Videcnik J, Zorman P, Cimperman J, Lotric-Furlan S, Maraspin V. Clinical and epidemiological findings for patients with erythema migrans. Comparison of cohorts from the years 1993 and 2000. Wien Klin Wochenschr. 2002;114(13–14):493–7.
111. Mehnert WH, Krause G. Surveillance of Lyme borreliosis in Germany, 2002 and 2003. Euro Surveill. 2005;10(4):83–5.
112. Bennet L, Stjernberg L, Berglund J. Effect of gender on clinical and epidemiologic features of Lyme borreliosis. Vector Borne Zoonotic Dis. 2007;7(1):34–41. https://doi.org/10.1089/vbz.2006.0533.
113. Stupica D, Maraspin V, Bogovic P, Ogrinc K, Blagus R, Cerar T, et al. Comparison of clinical course and treatment outcome for patients with early disseminated or early localized Lyme borreliosis. JAMA Dermatol. 2018;154(9):1050–6. https://doi.org/10.1001/jamadermatol.2018.2306.
114. Sodermark L, Sigurdsson V, Nas W, Wall P, Trollfors B. Neuroborreliosis in Swedish children: a population-based study on incidence and clinical characteristics. Pediatr Infect Dis J. 2017;36(11):1052–6. https://doi.org/10.1097/INF.0000000000001653.
115. Knudtzen FC, Andersen NS, Jensen TG, Skarphedinsson S. Characteristics and clinical outcome of Lyme neuroborreliosis in a high endemic area, 1995-2014: a retrospective cohort study in Denmark. Clin Infect Dis. 2017;65(9):1489–95. https://doi.org/10.1093/cid/cix568.
116. Rojko T, Bogovic P, Lotric-Furlan S, Ogrinc K, Cerar-Kisek T, Glinsek Biskup U, et al. *Borrelia burgdorferi* sensu lato infection in patients with peripheral facial palsy. Ticks Tick Borne Dis. 2019;10(2):398–406. https://doi.org/10.1016/j.ttbdis.2018.11.019.
117. Hinckley AF, Connally NP, Meek JI, Johnson BJ, Kemperman MM, Feldman KA, et al. Lyme disease testing by large commercial laboratories in the United States. Clin Infect Dis. 2014;59(5):676–81. https://doi.org/10.1093/cid/ciu397.
118. Centers for Disease C, Prevention. Recommendations for test performance and interpretation from the Second National Conference on Serologic Diagnosis of Lyme Disease. MMWR Morb Mortal Wkly Rep. 1995;44(31):590–1.
119. Marques AR. Revisiting the Lyme disease serodiagnostic algorithm: the momentum gathers. J Clin Microbiol. 2018;56(8) https://doi.org/10.1128/JCM.00749-18.
120. Dessau RB, van Dam AP, Fingerle V, Gray J, Hovius JW, Hunfeld KP, et al. To test or not to test? Laboratory support for the diagnosis of Lyme borreliosis: a position paper of ESGBOR, the ESCMID study group for Lyme borreliosis. Clin Microbiol Infect. 2018;24(2):118–24. https://doi.org/10.1016/j.cmi.2017.08.025.
121. Koedel U, Pfister HW. Lyme neuroborreliosis. Curr Opin Infect Dis. 2017;30(1):101–7. https://doi.org/10.1097/QCO.0000000000000332.

122. Rauer S, Kastenbauer S, Fingerle V, Hunfeld KP, Huppertz HI, Dersch R. Lyme neuroborreliosis. Dtsch Arztebl Int. 2018;115(45):751–6. https://doi.org/10.3238/arztebl.2018.0751.
123. Mygland A, Ljostad U, Fingerle V, Rupprecht T, Schmutzhard E, Steiner I. EFNS guidelines on the diagnosis and management of European Lyme neuroborreliosis. Eur J Neurol. 2010;17(1):8–16, e1–4. https://doi.org/10.1111/j.1468-1331.2009.02862.x.
124. Halperin JJ, Shapiro ED, Logigian E, Belman AL, Dotevall L, Wormser GP, et al. Practice parameter: treatment of nervous system Lyme disease (an evidence-based review): report of the Quality Standards Subcommittee of the American Academy of Neurology. Neurology. 2007;69(1):91–102. https://doi.org/10.1212/01.wnl.0000265517.66976.28.
125. Coyle PK, Schutzer SE, Deng Z, Krupp LB, Belman AL, Benach JL, et al. Detection of *Borrelia burgdorferi*-specific antigen in antibody-negative cerebrospinal fluid in neurologic Lyme disease. Neurology. 1995;45(11):2010–5. https://doi.org/10.1212/wnl.45.11.2010.
126. Smouha EE, Coyle PK, Shukri S. Facial nerve palsy in Lyme disease: evaluation of clinical diagnostic criteria. Am J Otol. 1997;18(2):257–61.
127. Halperin JJ, Golightly M. Lyme borreliosis in Bell's palsy. Long Island neuroborreliosis collaborative study group. Neurology. 1992;42(7):1268–70. https://doi.org/10.1212/wnl.42.7.1268.
128. Theel ES, Aguero-Rosenfeld ME, Pritt B, Adem PV, Wormser GP. Limitations and confusing aspects of diagnostic testing for neurologic Lyme disease in the United States. J Clin Microbiol. 2019;57(1) https://doi.org/10.1128/JCM.01406-18.
129. Wormser GP, O'Connell S. Treatment of infection caused by *Borrelia burgdorferi* sensu lato. Expert Rev Anti-Infect Ther. 2011;9(2):245–60. https://doi.org/10.1586/eri.10.174.
130. Stanek G, Strle F. Lyme borreliosis-from tick bite to diagnosis and treatment. FEMS Microbiol Rev. 2018;42(3):233–58. https://doi.org/10.1093/femsre/fux047.
131. Lantos PM, Rumbaugh J, Bockenstedt LK, Falck-Ytter YT, Aguero-Rosenfeld ME, Auwaerter PG, et al. Clinical practice guidelines by the Infectious Diseases Society of America (IDSA), American Academy of Neurology (AAN), and American College of Rheumatology (ACR): 2020 guidelines for the prevention, diagnosis and treatment of Lyme disease. Clin Infect Dis. 2021;72(1):1–8. https://doi.org/10.1093/cid/ciab049.
132. Eliassen KE, Berild D, Reiso H, Grude N, Christophersen KS, Finckenhagen C, et al. Incidence and antibiotic treatment of erythema migrans in Norway 2005-2009. Ticks Tick Borne Dis. 2017;8(1):1–8. https://doi.org/10.1016/j.ttbdis.2016.06.006.
133. Maraspin V, Strle F. How do I manage tick bites and Lyme borreliosis in pregnant women? Curr Probl Dermatol. 2009;37:183–90. https://doi.org/10.1159/000213076.
134. Strle F, Maraspin V, Furlan-Lotric S, Cimperman J. Epidemiological study of a cohort of adult patients with erythema migrans registered in Slovenia in 1993. Eur J Epidemiol. 1996;12(5):503–7. https://doi.org/10.1007/BF00144004.
135. Stanek G, Kahl O. Chemoprophylaxis for Lyme borreliosis? Zentralbl Bakteriol. 1999;289(5–7):655–65. https://doi.org/10.1016/s0934-8840(99)80025-5.
136. Eisen L. Pathogen transmission in relation to duration of attachment by *Ixodes scapularis* ticks. Ticks Tick Borne Dis. 2018;9(3):535–42. https://doi.org/10.1016/j.ttbdis.2018.01.002.
137. Warshafsky S, Lee DH, Francois LK, Nowakowski J, Nadelman RB, Wormser GP. Efficacy of antibiotic prophylaxis for the prevention of Lyme disease: an updated systematic review and meta-analysis. J Antimicrob Chemother. 2010;65(6):1137–44. https://doi.org/10.1093/jac/dkq097.
138. Nadelman RB, Nowakowski J, Fish D, Falco RC, Freeman K, McKenna D, et al. Prophylaxis with single-dose doxycycline for the prevention of Lyme disease after an *Ixodes scapularis* tick bite. N Engl J Med. 2001;345(2):79–84. https://doi.org/10.1056/NEJM200107123450201.
139. Harms MG, Hofhuis A, Sprong H, Bennema SC, Ferreira JA, Fonville M, et al. A single dose of doxycycline after an *Ixodes ricinus* tick bite to prevent Lyme borreliosis: an open-label randomized controlled trial. J Infect. 2021;82(1):98–104. https://doi.org/10.1016/j.jinf.2020.06.032.

140. Nelder MP, Russell CB, Sheehan NJ, Sander B, Moore S, Li Y, et al. Human pathogens associated with the blacklegged tick *Ixodes scapularis*: a systematic review. Parasit Vectors. 2016;9:265. https://doi.org/10.1186/s13071-016-1529-y.
141. Diuk-Wasser MA, Vannier E, Krause PJ. Coinfection by *Ixodes* tick-borne pathogens: ecological, epidemiological, and clinical consequences. Trends Parasitol. 2016;32(1):30–42. https://doi.org/10.1016/j.pt.2015.09.008.
142. Johnson TL, Graham CB, Maes SE, Hojgaard A, Fleshman A, Boegler KA, et al. Prevalence and distribution of seven human pathogens in host-seeking *Ixodes scapularis* (Acari: Ixodidae) nymphs in Minnesota, USA. Ticks Tick Borne Dis. 2018;9(6):1499–507. https://doi.org/10.1016/j.ttbdis.2018.07.009.
143. Johnson TL, Graham CB, Boegler KA, Cherry CC, Maes SE, Pilgard MA, et al. Prevalence and diversity of tick-borne pathogens in nymphal *Ixodes scapularis* (Acari: Ixodidae) in eastern National Parks. J Med Entomol. 2017;54(3):742–51. https://doi.org/10.1093/jme/tjw213.
144. Tokarz R, Tagliafierro T, Cucura DM, Rochlin I, Sameroff S, Lipkin WI. Detection of *Anaplasma phagocytophilum, Babesia microti, Borrelia burgdorferi, Borrelia miyamotoi*, and Powassan virus in ticks by a multiplex real-time reverse transcription-PCR assay. mSphere. 2017;2(2):e00151–17. https://doi.org/10.1128/mSphere.00151-17.
145. Stromdahl E, Hamer S, Jenkins S, Sloan L, Williamson P, Foster E, et al. Comparison of phenology and pathogen prevalence, including infection with the *Ehrlichia muris-like* (EML) agent, of *Ixodes scapularis* removed from soldiers in the midwestern and the northeastern United States over a 15 year period (1997-2012). Parasit Vectors. 2014;7:553. https://doi.org/10.1186/s13071-014-0553-z.
146. CDC: National Notifiable Infectious Diseases and Conditions: United States- 2018; 2018. https://wonder.cdc.gov/nndss/static/2018/annual/2018-table1.html, https://wonder.cdc.gov/nndss/static/2018/annual/2018-table2c.html, https://wonder.cdc.gov/nndss/static/2018/annual/2018-table2e.html. Accessed 05 Dec 2021.
147. Krause PJ, Telford SR 3rd, Spielman A, Sikand V, Ryan R, Christianson D, et al. Concurrent Lyme disease and babesiosis. Evidence for increased severity and duration of illness. JAMA. 1996;275(21):1657–60.
148. Wang TJ, Liang MH, Sangha O, Phillips CB, Lew RA, Wright EA, et al. Coexposure to *Borrelia burgdorferi* and *Babesia microti* does not worsen the long-term outcome of Lyme disease. Clin Infect Dis. 2000;31(5):1149–54. https://doi.org/10.1086/317465.
149. Horowitz HW, Aguero-Rosenfeld ME, Holmgren D, McKenna D, Schwartz I, Cox ME, et al. Lyme disease and human granulocytic anaplasmosis coinfection: impact of case definition on coinfection rates and illness severity. Clin Infect Dis. 2013;56(1):93–9. https://doi.org/10.1093/cid/cis852.
150. Schotthoefer AM, Hall MC, Vittala S, Bajwa R, Frost HM. Clinical presentation and outcomes of children with human granulocytic anaplasmosis. J Pediatric Infect Dis Soc. 2018;7(2):e9–e15. https://doi.org/10.1093/jpids/pix029.
151. Molloy PJ, Telford SR 3rd, Chowdri HR, Lepore TJ, Gugliotta JL, Weeks KE, et al. *Borrelia miyamotoi* disease in the northeastern United States: a case series. Ann Intern Med. 2015;163(2):91–8. https://doi.org/10.7326/M15-0333.
152. Piantadosi A, Rubin DB, McQuillen DP, Hsu L, Lederer PA, Ashbaugh CD, et al. Emerging cases of Powassan virus encephalitis in New England: clinical presentation, imaging, and review of the literature. Clin Infect Dis. 2016;62(6):707–13. https://doi.org/10.1093/cid/civ1005.
153. Krow-Lucal ER, Lindsey NP, Fischer M, Hills SL. Powassan virus disease in the United States, 2006-2016. Vector Borne Zoonotic Dis. 2018;18(6):286–90. https://doi.org/10.1089/vbz.2017.2239.
154. El Khoury MY, Camargo JF, White JL, Backenson BP, Dupuis AP 2nd, Escuyer KL, et al. Potential role of deer tick virus in Powassan encephalitis cases in Lyme disease-endemic areas of New York, USA. Emerg Infect Dis. 2013;19(12):1926–33. https://doi.org/10.3201/eid1912.130903.

155. Knox KK, Thomm AM, Harrington YA, Ketter E, Patitucci JM, Carrigan DR. Powassan/deer tick virus and *Borrelia burgdorferi* infection in Wisconsin tick populations. Vector Borne Zoonotic Dis. 2017;17(7):463–6. https://doi.org/10.1089/vbz.2016.2082.
156. Aliota MT, Dupuis AP 2nd, Wilczek MP, Peters RJ, Ostfeld RS, Kramer LD. The prevalence of zoonotic tick-borne pathogens in *Ixodes scapularis* collected in the Hudson Valley, New York State. Vector Borne Zoonotic Dis. 2014;14(4):245–50. https://doi.org/10.1089/vbz.2013.1475.
157. Veluscek M, Blagus R, Cerar Kisek T, Ruzic-Sabljic E, Avsic-Zupanc T, et al. Antibiotic use and long-term outcome in patients with tick-borne encephalitis and co-infection with *Borrelia burgdorferi* sensu lato in Central Europe. A retrospective cohort study. J Clin Med. 2019;8(10):1740. https://doi.org/10.3390/jcm8101740.
158. Moniuszko A, Dunaj J, Swiecicka I, Zambrowski G, Chmielewska-Badora J, Zukiewicz-Sobczak W, et al. Co-infections with *Borrelia* species, *Anaplasma phagocytophilum* and *Babesia* spp. in patients with tick-borne encephalitis. Eur J Clin Microbiol Infect Dis. 2014;33(10):1835–41. https://doi.org/10.1007/s10096-014-2134-7.
159. Lotric-Furlan S, Petrovec M, Avsic-Zupanc T, Nicholson WL, Sumner JW, Childs JE, et al. Prospective assessment of the etiology of acute febrile illness after a tick bite in Slovenia. Clin Infect Dis. 2001;33(4):503–10. https://doi.org/10.1086/322586.
160. Cimperman J, Maraspin V, Lotric-Furlan S, Ruzic-Sabljic E, Avsic-Zupanc T, Picken RN, et al. Concomitant infection with tick-borne encephalitis virus and *Borrelia burgdorferi* sensu lato in patients with acute meningitis or meningoencephalitis. Infection. 1998;26(3):160–4. https://doi.org/10.1007/BF02771842.
161. Koetsveld J, Tijsse-Klasen E, Herremans T, Hovius JW, Sprong H. Serological and molecular evidence for spotted fever group *rickettsia* and *Borrelia burgdorferi* sensu lato co-infections in the Netherlands. Ticks Tick Borne Dis. 2016;7(2):371–7. https://doi.org/10.1016/j.ttbdis.2015.12.010.
162. Honig V, Carolan HE, Vavruskova Z, Massire C, Mosel MR, Crowder CD, et al. Broad-range survey of vector-borne pathogens and tick host identification of *Ixodes ricinus* from Southern Czech Republic. FEMS Microbiol Ecol. 2017;93(11) https://doi.org/10.1093/femsec/fix129.
163. Blazejak K, Raulf MK, Janecek E, Jordan D, Fingerle V, Strube C. Shifts in *Borrelia burgdorferi* (s.l.) geno-species infections in *Ixodes ricinus* over a 10-year surveillance period in the city of Hanover (Germany) and *Borrelia miyamotoi*-specific reverse line blot detection. Parasit Vectors. 2018;11(1):304. https://doi.org/10.1186/s13071-018-2882-9.
164. Lotric-Furlan S, Rojko T, Jelovsek M, Petrovec M, Avsic-Zupanc T, Lusa L, et al. Comparison of clinical and laboratory characteristics of patients fulfilling criteria for proven and probable human granulocytic anaplasmosis. Microbes Infect. 2015;17(11–12):829–33. https://doi.org/10.1016/j.micinf.2015.09.017.
165. Jahfari S, Hofhuis A, Fonville M, van der Giessen J, van Pelt W, Sprong H. Molecular detection of tick-borne pathogens in humans with tick bites and erythema migrans, in the Netherlands. PLoS Negl Trop Dis. 2016;10(10):e0005042. https://doi.org/10.1371/journal.pntd.0005042.
166. Boyer PH, Koetsveld J, Zilliox L, Sprong H, Talagrand-Reboul E, Hansmann Y, et al. Assessment of *Borrelia miyamotoi* in febrile patients and ticks in Alsace, an endemic area for Lyme borreliosis in France. Parasit Vectors. 2020;13(1):199. https://doi.org/10.1186/s13071-020-04071-9.
167. Sigal LH. Summary of the first 100 patients seen at a Lyme disease referral center. Am J Med. 1990;88(6):577–81. https://doi.org/10.1016/0002-9343(90)90520-n.
168. Steere AC, Taylor E, McHugh GL, Logigian EL. The overdiagnosis of Lyme disease. JAMA. 1993;269(14):1812–6.
169. Rose CD, Fawcett PT, Gibney KM, Doughty RA. The overdiagnosis of Lyme disease in children residing in an endemic area. Clin Pediatr (Phila). 1994;33(11):663–8. https://doi.org/10.1177/000992289403301105.
170. Feder HM Jr, Hunt MS. Pitfalls in the diagnosis and treatment of Lyme disease in children. JAMA. 1995;274(1):66–8.

171. Reid MC, Schoen RT, Evans J, Rosenberg JC, Horwitz RI. The consequences of overdiagnosis and overtreatment of Lyme disease: an observational study. Ann Intern Med. 1998;128(5):354–62. https://doi.org/10.7326/0003-4819-128-5-199803010-00003.
172. Qureshi MZ, New D, Zulqarni NJ, Nachman S. Overdiagnosis and overtreatment of Lyme disease in children. Pediatr Infect Dis J. 2002;21(1):12–4. https://doi.org/10.1097/00006454-200201000-00003.
173. Aucott JN, Seifter A, Rebman AW. Probable late Lyme disease: a variant manifestation of untreated *Borrelia burgdorferi* infection. BMC Infect Dis. 2012;12:173. https://doi.org/10.1186/1471-2334-12-173.
174. Feder HM Jr, Johnson BJ, O'Connell S, Shapiro ED, Steere AC, Wormser GP, et al. A critical appraisal of "chronic Lyme disease". N Engl J Med. 2007;357(14):1422–30. https://doi.org/10.1056/NEJMra072023.
175. Patrick DM, Miller RR, Gardy JL, Parker SM, Morshed MG, Steiner TS, et al. Lyme disease diagnosed by alternative methods: a phenotype similar to that of chronic fatigue syndrome. Clin Infect Dis. 2015;61(7):1084–91. https://doi.org/10.1093/cid/civ470.
176. Bouquet J, Gardy JL, Brown S, Pfeil J, Miller RR, Morshed M, et al. RNA-seq analysis of gene expression, viral pathogen, and B-cell/T-cell receptor signatures in complex chronic disease. Clin Infect Dis. 2017;64(4):476–81. https://doi.org/10.1093/cid/ciw767.
177. Horowitz RI, Freeman PR. Precision medicine: the role of the MSIDS model in defining, diagnosing, and treating chronic Lyme disease/post treatment Lyme disease syndrome and other chronic illness: part 2. Healthcare (Basel). 2018;6(4) https://doi.org/10.3390/healthcare6040129.
178. Alexander W. Integrative healthcare symposium: cancer and chronic Lyme disease. P T. 2009;34(4):202–14.
179. Lantos PM, Shapiro ED, Auwaerter PG, Baker PJ, Halperin JJ, McSweegan E, et al. Unorthodox alternative therapies marketed to treat Lyme disease. Clin Infect Dis. 2015;60(12):1776–82. https://doi.org/10.1093/cid/civ186.
180. Lantos PM, Wormser GP. Chronic coinfections in patients diagnosed with chronic Lyme disease: a systematic review. Am J Med. 2014;127(11):1105–10. https://doi.org/10.1016/j.amjmed.2014.05.036.
181. Lantos PM, Auwaerter PG, Wormser GP. A systematic review of *Borrelia burgdorferi* morphologic variants does not support a role in chronic Lyme disease. Clin Infect Dis. 2014;58(5):663–71. https://doi.org/10.1093/cid/cit810.
182. Wormser GP. Should patients infected with *Borrelia burgdorferi* no longer be referred to as having Lyme disease? Am J Med. 2019;132(1):11–2. https://doi.org/10.1016/j.amjmed.2018.06.014.
183. Shapiro ED, Baker PJ, Wormser GP. False and misleading information about Lyme disease. Am J Med. 2017;130(7):771–2. https://doi.org/10.1016/j.amjmed.2017.01.030.
184. Auwaerter PG, Bakken JS, Dattwyler RJ, Dumler JS, Halperin JJ, McSweegan E, et al. Antiscience and ethical concerns associated with advocacy of Lyme disease. Lancet Infect Dis. 2011;11(9):713–9. https://doi.org/10.1016/S1473-3099(11)70034-2.

6 Laboratory Diagnosis of Lyme borreliosis

Benedikt Lohr, Volker Fingerle, and Klaus-Peter Hunfeld

6.1 Introduction

Lyme borreliosis (LB) is an infectious disease caused by tick-borne spirochetes of the *Borrelia (B.) burgdorferi* sensu lato (s.l.) complex. It is the most commonly reported vector-borne infection in the northern hemisphere [1–4]. In recent decades there has been tremendous scientific progress in understanding the clinical syndromes of LB and the pathophysiology of the infection as well as continuous improvement in laboratory testing and the establishment of well-recognized treatment options. Nevertheless, LB, like syphilis, remains a chameleon [5] for inexperienced clinicians, resulting in a range of problems. Therefore, clinical case definitions must be used in combination with the appropriate laboratory methods, especially when it comes to directly and indirectly detecting the pathogen and correctly interpreting the results in a clinical context (Table 6.1) [6]. We present here the current state of the art of laboratory diagnosis of LB, including a thorough discussion of the current pitfalls and limitations as well as future prospects in this challenging area of modern laboratory medicine.

B. Lohr · K.-P. Hunfeld (✉)
Institute for Laboratory Medicine, Microbiology, and Infection Control,
Northwest Medical Centre, Medical Faculty, Goethe University, Frankfurt/Main, Hessen, Germany
e-mail: K.hunfeld@em.uni-frankfurt.de

V. Fingerle
Bayerisches Landesamt für Gesundheit und Lebensmittelsicherheit (LGL),
Oberschleißheim, Germany
e-mail: Volker.fingerle@igl.bayern.de

K.-P. Hunfeld, J. Gray (eds.), *Lyme Borreliosis*,
https://doi.org/10.1007/978-3-030-93680-8_6

Table 6.1 Clinical case definitions and indications for medical laboratory testing, modified from Stanek et al. 2011 [44]

Symptom	Clinical case definition	Medical laboratory evidence necessary[b]	Supporting medical laboratory/clinical evidence
Erythema migrans (early localized infection)	Expanding red or bluish-red patch (>5 cm in diameter),[a] with or without central clearing. Advancing edge typically distinct, often intensely colored not markedly elevated.[a]	None for typical erythema	Detection of *B. burgdorferi* by culture and/or PCR in skin biopsy material
Borrelia lymphocytoma (localized infection)	Painless bluish-red nodule or plaque, usually on ear lobe, ear helix, nipple or scrotum. More frequent in children (especially on the ear) than in adults.	Seroconversion or positive serology	Skin biopsy in unclear cases; histology, detection of *B. burgdorferi* by culture and/or PCR; recent or concomitant EM
Lyme neuroborreliosis (early disseminated infection)	In adults mainly meningo-radiculitis (Bannwarth syndrome), meningitis; rarely encephalitis or myelitis; very rarely cerebral vasculitis; in children mainly symptom-poor meningitis and facial palsy.	Pleocytosis and demonstration of intrathecal specific antibody synthesis[c]	Detection of *B. burgdorferi* by culture and/or PCR in CSF. Intrathecal synthesis of total IgM, and/or IgG and/or IgA. Detection of borrelia-specific serum antibodies. Recent or concomitant EM.
Lyme carditis (rare) (early disseminated infection)	Acute onset of atrio-ventricular (I-III) conduction disturbances; rhythm disturbances, sometimes myocarditis or pancarditis. Alternative explanations must be ruled out.	Specific serum antibodies	Detection of *B. burgdorferi* by culture and/or PCR in endomyocardial biopsy material. Recent or concomitant erythema EM and/or typical neurological disorders.
Ocular manifestation (rare) (early disseminated infection)	Conjunctivitis, uveitis, papillitis, episcleritis, keratitis.	Specific serum antibodies	Recent or concomitant Lyme borreliosis manifestations. Detection of *B. burgdorferi* by culture and/or PCR in ocular fluid/biopsy.
Lyme arthritis (late manifestation)	Recurrent attacks or persisting objective joint swelling in one or a few large joints. Alternative explanations must be ruled out.	Specific serum IgG antibodies, usually in high concentrations	Synovial fluid analysis and detection of *B. burgdorferi* by PCR (and rarely culture) in synovial fluid and/or biopsy material.

Table 6.1 (continued)

Symptom	Clinical case definition	Medical laboratory evidence necessary[b]	Supporting medical laboratory/clinical evidence
Acrodermatitis chronica atrophicans (late manifestation)	Long-standing red or bluish-red lesions, usually on the extensor surfaces of extremities. Initial doughy swelling. Lesions eventually become atrophic. Possible skin indurations and fibroid nodules over bony prominences.	High level of specific serum IgG antibodies	Histology. Detection of *B. burgdorferi* by culture and/or PCR in skin biopsy.

[a]If <5 cm in diameter, a history of tick bite, a delay in appearance (after the tick bite) of at least 2 days and an expanding rash at the site of the tick bite is required. Can occur as single or, more rarely, as multiple erythema

[b]As a rule, initial and follow-up samples have to be tested in parallel in order to avoid changes due to inter-assay variation

[c]In early cases, specific intrathecally produced antibodies may still be absent

6.2 Direct Detection of *B. burgdorferi* s.l.

Direct detection of pathogens remains the gold standard for diagnosing infectious diseases [7–9] but suffers from clear limitations when it comes to the mainly paucibacillary disease manifestations of LB. There is a variety of ways to directly detect *B. burgdorferi* s.l. [2, 3, 10] or spirochete components (such as DNA or protein) in tick vectors, reservoir hosts, and patients [6].

Microbiological laboratories currently use five different methods of direct detection: i. culture ii. nucleic acid-based methods, iii. microscopic detection methods, iv. direct detection of *B. burgdorferi* s.l.-specific proteins, and v. xenodiagnoses. Of these, only culture and xenodiagnoses of *B. burgdorferi* s.l. detect viable organisms and represent the best way to confirm an active infection [2, 3]; however, neither of these methods are currently being used on a broader scale in routine diagnostic laboratories, mainly because they are costly, time-consuming, and not well standardized.

6.2.1 Direct Detection of Borrelia in Ticks

Various methods with partly unknown or highly variable sensitivity, specificity, and reliability have been used to detect the presence of LB agents in tick vectors [10, 11]. Such approaches include culture and multiple PCR formats (mostly nested PCR that targets different genomic loci), reverse-line blotting based on hybridization of amplified borrelia genes with specific probes, multilocus sequence analysis of amplified genetic fragments of borrelia, and microscopy of stained spirochetes in the tick midgut or salivary glands [2, 3, 12–14]. The most recently applied techniques also include next-generation sequencing (NGS), broad-range PCR combined with electrospray mass spectrometry (PCR/ESI MS), and proteomic approaches [6]. Alarmingly, there are even point-of-care-test kits (POCT) that can be used at home to test ticks for the presence of borrelia [11].

The reliability of such tests to directly detect borrelia in ticks is questionable as both false-negative and false-positive results occur even under routine conditions in certified microbiological laboratories. Moreover, such tests have not been standardized or evaluated by external quality control measures [11, 15], and there are few sound clinical application studies. Most importantly, the detection of a pathogen in the vector does not necessarily imply successful transmission to the host when feeding. This is why the use of such tests is of little value for routine diagnostic testing and should be limited to research or epidemiological studies [6, 11].

6.2.2 Xenodiagnostic Approaches

In a recent study, laboratory-reared larval *I. scapularis* ticks were placed on 36 subjects and allowed to feed to repletion [16]. Ticks were then tested for LB agents using a highly sensitive diagnostic approach that combined polymerase chain reaction (PCR), culture, and/or isothermal amplification followed by PCR and ESI MS. Attempts were also made to infect immunodeficient mice through tick bites or molted nymphal ticks or through inoculation with the tick content. In principle, xenodiagnosis was well tolerated, with the most common adverse events being a mild itching at the tick attachment site. However, further clinical evaluation is clearly needed to determine the sensitivity of xenodiagnosis in patients with LB, gauge the significance of a positive result, and address borrelial persistence post-treatment [17–19]. This is why xenodiagnostic methods are currently not recommended outside the experimental setting.

6.2.3 Direct Microscopy and Borrelia Antigen Detection from Clinical Samples

Direct microscopic detection of *B. burgdorferi* s.l. has limited clinical utility in laboratory confirmation of LB due to the sparseness of organisms in clinical samples [2, 3, 20–22]. This remains especially true for methods, such as the modified microscopy protocol (LM-method), which have recently received significant public attention. The LM-method claims to directly detect tick-borne pathogens in patient blood after a tick bite. In a recent clinical evaluation of the LM-method, structures interpreted as Borrelia and babesia could not be verified by PCR and the method was, thus, falsified [15]. Such clinical diagnostic studies underline the importance of doing proper test validation before new or modified assays are introduced [6, 15]. Antigen detection assays (aside from PCR) have the same limitations as microscopic detection. Although antigen capture tests have been used to detect *B. burgdorferi* s.l. antigens in CSF of patients with neuroborreliosis [2, 23, 24] and in urine samples from patients with suspected LB [25–27], such assays are not regarded as useful due to their insufficient diagnostic validity under routine laboratory conditions and many guidelines advise against their use [2, 3, 6, 28–30].

Recently a proposal was made to use a nano trap technique in combination with specific immunoassay technology for highly sensitive measurement of urinary excretion of the OspA carboxyl-terminus domain in early LB [31]. This interesting and novel approach cannot be regarded as an established diagnostic method without further evaluation and validation [32]. In summary, none of these procedures are recommended by current national and international guidelines for LB diagnostics [3, 28–30, 33–36].

6.2.4 Culture of *B. burgdorferi* s.l. Directly from Clinical Samples

Direct detection by culture with modified Kelly-Pettenkofer (MKP) and Barbour-Stoenner-Kelly-H (BSK-H) medium is considered to be the gold standard [6] and shows clear proof of infection with *B. burgdorferi* s.l. [2, 3, 11, 33]. Usually, the best borrelial growth is observed at 33 °C under microaerophilic conditions after 2–3 weeks, while no growth usually occurs at 4 °C. Although BSK-H medium supports better initial growth of borrelia, MKP is superior with regard to the isolation rate, morphology, and motility of cultured spirochetes [37]. Direct detection of spirochetes in LB skin manifestations by culture is frequently successful. The sensitivity of culture in European studies is between 40% and 90% for erythema migrans (EM) and between 20% and 60% for acrodermatitis chronica atrophicans (ACA) [10, 28–30, 33]. To a limited degree, detection by culture is also possible in CSF (10–26%), in very rare cases in synovial fluid, in synovial biopsies (anecdotal, <1%), and in blood culture (BC) (9% [Europe] to >40% [using larger volumes of blood from EM patients in the US]) [2, 3, 33]. Approximately 45% of untreated American patients with early EM-associated LB are known to have a positive BC based on microscopic detection of *B. burgdorferi* s.l. in BSK-H medium after 2–12 weeks of incubation [38]. Combing culture with real-time PCR can boost the detection of *B. burgdorferi* s.l. in BC to 70.8% and can also reduce the detection time to just 7 days of BC incubation, resulting in positive results for more than 90% of patients with EM and nearly 100% for patients with multiple EM [38]. This approach, however, is costly and not practical as larger amounts of blood must be taken from patients with EM who can usually be diagnosed and treated clinically. In addition, the positivity rate of BC is clearly much lower in late infections and with additional cutaneous disease manifestations [39]. *B. burgdorferi* s.l. has also been detected in other tissue samples, for example, heart muscle and iris biopsies [40, 41]; however, borrelia cultivation from patient samples generally remains laborious, costly, and usually takes more than 2 weeks to detect the growth of the spirochetes [2, 3, 28, 30, 33]. In addition, further molecular confirmation of positive culture results and the characterization of the isolate at the genospecies level is essential to guarantee the specificity of the results [28, 30]. In terms of the specificity of complex and accident-sensitive cultivation, it is important to note that contamination can occur. The authors of a recent study claimed they were able to cultivate *B. burgdorferi* s.l. from serum in 94% of 72 patients [42]; however, an assessment study showed that almost all of these isolates corresponded to one of the control strains [43]. Because of the invasiveness of sample acquisition, direct detection by culture should best be reserved for clear indications following case definitions such as those proposed by Stanek et al. [44], and the procedures should be explicitly undertaken by experienced reference centers and laboratories [6, 28, 30, 34–36].

6.2.5 Molecular Biological Detection Methods

For direct molecular detection of borrelia, the clinical presentation and stage of disease together with a clear-cut diagnostic indication dictate the type of specimen to use, such as skin biopsies for EM and ACA, CSF in suspected cases of neuroborreliosis, and synovial fluid or biopsies for Lyme arthritis (LA), as outlined by Stanek et al. [44]. Most European and American guidelines advise against using blood and urine specimens for molecular testing due to the low and mostly transient presence of spirochetes in such materials. This results in a highly variable testing performance, at least under routine diagnostic laboratory conditions [10, 28–30, 34–36, 45]. Although difficult to obtain clinically, the largest conceivable amount of any sample material (e.g. 2–3 mm biopsies, >1 mL of CSF or synovial fluid) should be collected due to the extremely variable borrelial load in most clinical materials (e.g. 10–11,000 spirochetes in 2 mm EM skin biopsies and 20-41,000 spirochetes per mL of synovial fluid as determined by quantitative real-time PCR) [2, 3, 46, 47]. These samples must be transported directly to the diagnostic laboratory as quickly as possible under optimal conditions (4–8 °C in under 2 h) [10]. Detection of specific DNA works better with fresh or fresh-frozen material compared to stored or fixed specimens [45, 48]. To circumvent the problems associated with a high ratio of human to bacterial DNA in most samples, modified manual and automated extraction methods have been developed based on specific lysis and degradation of the human tissue materials (cells and DNA), selective binding, separation and removal of human DNA, and CpG motive-based selection, with final enrichment of bacterial DNA. Some of these reagents are commercially available and extraction methods for PCR testing were extensively discussed in a recent review by Ružić-Sabljić and Cerar [10].

Conventional, isothermal, qualitative, and quantitative real-time PCR assays targeting the unique rRNA gene (16S rDNA, 23S rDNA, 5S–23S rDNA intergenic spacer) and a variety of other single-copy chromosomal targets (*fla*, *hbb*, *rrf-rrl*, *polC*, *SrRNK*, *p66*, *recA*, *bmpA*, *rpoB*, *rpoC*, and *gyr*), plasmid bound targets such as *dbpA*, *vlsE*, and outer surface proteins (*ospA*, *ospB*, *ospC*) have been developed and are, in part, commercially available [2, 3, 6, 10, 49]. An important drawback to a more standardized application of such assays is the fact that some molecular targets, especially the plasmid-encoded target genes (e.g. *ospA*, *ospB*, *ospC*), have high inter- and intra-strain variability, which can lead to amplification dropouts (false-negative results). Others (e.g. flagellin: *fla*) are unable to discriminate between the different *Borrelia* genospecies due to their more conserved genetic nature. An overview of correct indications and useful targets for the detection of borrelia in different clinical specimens is provided in Tables 6.1 and 6.2 [2, 3, 10, 50, 51]. Assays targeting plasmid-encoded genes (e.g., *osps*, *vlsE* etc.) are believed to be more sensitive than those targeting chromosomal ones (e.g., 16S rRNA-, flagellin (*fla*)-genes) [6]. Such analytical limitations and technical variabilities have led to the recommendation that molecular tests should employ at least two different DNA target sequences to increase diagnostic reliability [28, 30].

6.2.5.1 PCR Followed by Electrospray Ionization Mass Spectrometry (ESI MS)

A relatively recent molecular approach is broad-range PCR followed by electrospray ionization mass spectrometry (ESI MS). Briefly, this approach utilizes a conventional real-time PCR assay that uses broad-range primers targeting conserved sequences of eubacterial DNA. The resulting amplicons are subjected to ESI MS, which measures with sufficient accuracy the mass of the amplicons to determine the nucleic acid base composition [52, 53]. Unlike hybridization-based detection, ESI MS does not require prior knowledge of the target sequence but can identify without

Table 6.2 Sensitivity and specificity of molecular diagnostic detection methods for LB, modified from Ružić-Sabljić and Cerar (2017) [10]

Clinical specimen	No. of studies	No. of patients	Targets (genes)	Median sensitivity (range)	Specificity
Skin biopsy – EM	28	5–758	*p66, 23S rDNA, flagellin, rrf-rrl, ospA, recA, 16S rDNA, OspC*	68 (30–89)	98–100
Europe	19	5–758		70 (30–80)	
USA	9	23–139		59 (33–81)	
Skin biopsy – ACA	13	5–59	*p66, ospA, chromosomal DNA, 23S rDNA, rrf- rrl, flagellin*	75 (20–100)	100
CSF	22	8–190	*chromosomal DNA, ospA, flagellin, rrf-rrl, SrRNK, p66*	22.5 (5–100)	99–100
Europe	16	8–190		18 (9–100)	
USA	6	12–81		40.5 (5–93)	
Synovial fluid	12	4–124	*rrs-rrl, ospC, ospA, p66, flagellin*	77.5 (23–100)	100
Europe	7	4–20		72 (23–100)	
USA	5	7–124		85 (60–100)	
Blood, serum or plasma	11	7–557	*polC, ospA, 16S rDNA, rrf-rrl, rpoC*	18 (0–100)	95–100
Europe	5	10–557		16 (3.1–100)	
USA	6	7–76		29 (0–62)	

EM Erythema migrans, ACA acrodermatitis chronica atrophicans, CSF cerebrospinal fluid prejudice the composition of amplicons based on mass with reference to databases. PCR followed by ESI MS may be more useful for rapid borrelia detection but is currently not recommended for routine diagnostic testing because it needs more extensive clinical evaluation to demonstrate that it is not limited by the same general drawbacks in sensitivity in patients with late-stage disease as the other PCR-based detection methods [6]. In addition, costs are high for such a technically demanding diagnostic approach.

6.2.5.2 Sensitivity of Molecular Diagnostics

In general, the sensitivity of molecular test methods (mainly PCR-based) in detecting borrelia under routine laboratory conditions correlates with the known detection limits for culture [2, 3, 10, 28, 30, 50, 51]. In principle, the detection of borrelia from a skin biopsy from EM and ACA using nucleic acid amplification techniques (usually PCR) is very reliable (75%) and in the case of early manifestations may be even more sensitive (68%) than serological antibody detection (40–60%) [28, 30]. However, the question remains whether molecular testing and its related costs are necessary for most skin manifestations as the molecular test is clearly not warranted for a typical EM [44, 45, 52]. The diagnostic sensitivities of molecular diagnostics for clinical specimens other than skin biopsies based on a recent meta-analysis [10] are summarized in Table 6.2. These average 20% for CSF, approximately 77% for synovial fluid, and at best 18% for blood [10, 50, 54–58]. Patients with LA remain a diagnostic exception (Table 6.1) and molecular tests can achieve much higher sensitivities (77.5%; Table 6.2) than culture (<1%) with this form of manifestation [10, 28, 50, 56]. This is why a molecular investigation of synovial fluid or synovial biopsies is considered highly important in diagnosing LA [10, 28–30], whereas molecular testing of urine samples is generally not recommended due to its inadequate analytical specificity [59–61]. Positive results must be confirmed by amplicon sequencing and identification of the genospecies [28, 30]. After treatment, borrelia DNA can still be detected for weeks or even months in samples taken from previously affected areas of skin [62] and in treated LA [63, 64]. Since PCR does not discriminate between residual DNA and viable organisms, no conclusions should be drawn as to whether the therapy has failed, especially in patients without typical symptoms [62, 63]. Indeed, molecular detection of pathogens without the simultaneous presence of typical disease manifestations is of no clinical relevance [63, 65, 66].

6.2.5.3 Problems with Standardizing Molecular Testing

A significant drawback to molecular testing for LB has been the absence of standardized methods [10, 50, 67]. This relates to DNA isolation and selection of the clinical sample, as well as elution volumes, analytical conditions, and the selection of the molecular targets as outlined earlier. Studies on external quality control for these diagnostic techniques are currently too heterogeneous to recommend a particular method [50, 51, 68]. This supposition is further supported by evidence from INSTAND e.V.'s biannual external quality assessment scheme for molecular detection of *B. burgdorferi* s.l., which covers several major commercial manufacturers and many in-house assays. Between 2013 and 2015, the average pass rates for the 241 laboratories enrolled in this program were 86–97% for positive samples and 94–100% for negative samples [69], bringing to light the current situation surrounding molecular testing for LB.

Consequently, direct molecular (mostly PCR-based) detection methods should not be used as primary screening tools if LB is suspected. It is important to note that a negative PCR test result does not rule out LB. Positive results need to be confirmed with regard to specificity (e.g. probe hybridization and sequencing of the amplicon), and genospecies must be identified in the laboratory report. Direct molecular detection should be limited to defined skin and joint manifestations and performed exclusively by specialized reference laboratories [28–30, 33–36, 44, 51].

6.2.5.4 Genetic Typing Methods for Amplicons and Isolates

Genetic characterization of borrelia isolates is mainly relevant for epidemiological, clinical, and evolutionary studies [10, 14]. However, diagnostic laboratories also use the method to identify positive results of molecular and culture-based tests for LB [13]. A variety of molecular methods have been developed for these purposes, including large restriction fragment pattern (LRFP) analysis plus plasmid profiling, PCR-based typing techniques targeting single genes, PCR-based restriction fragment length polymorphism (RFLP) analysis of *rrs-rrlA* (16S–23S rDNA) and *rrfA-rrlB* (5S–23S rDNA) intergenic spacer, molecular *ospC*-analysis [13], flagellin typing, real-time PCR-based typing using melting temperature (TM) analysis, multilocus sequence typing (of mostly 8 housekeeping borrelia genes) [14], and whole-genome sequencing (WGS). While studies that use WGS and NGS from culture and field samples to diagnose LB are rare and the implementation of such techniques in the routine diagnostic laboratory is still under evaluation [10, 70–75], PCR-based RFLP analysis, restriction enzyme LFRP analysis in combination with pulsed-field gel electrophoresis (PFGE), and PCR-based flagellin typing have made their way into scientific and diagnostic laboratories with variable success [10]. In contrast, RT-PCR and melting temperature analysis can be automated and are much easier to use so that they are utilized by many laboratories for diagnostic and scientific purposes. Such assays, however, remain problematic if directly used with clinical samples [10]. PCR-based 5S–23S rDNA RFLP analysis using *Mse*I and *Dra*I enzymes [76] is a common method for confirming and characterizing borrelia isolates due to its relative ease of use, high discriminatory power, and excellent reproducibility [6].

6.3 Indirect Detection of the Pathogen (Serological Testing)

Because of its ease of use and substantial diagnostic value, indirect pathogen detection through serological testing is indicated in all cases where LB is clinically suspected (except with typical EM) to provide laboratory support in diagnosing the disease [28, 30, 34–36, 44, 77]. Case definitions for Europe, which should also work for most other parts of the northern hemisphere, contain descriptions of the various clinical manifestations of LB (Table 6.1). They provide guidance for clinical diagnosis and advice on the correct indication for diagnostic testing in cases of suspected LB [44]. Despite these definitions, laboratory testing for *B. burgdorferi* s.l.-specific antibodies continues to be frequently used in many clinical situations where testing is not recommended by current guidelines [28, 30, 34, 35, 77–80]. For example, in the Netherlands, only 9% of the patients tested had clinical symptoms outlined in the guidelines [80]. In Denmark, only 43% of samples from general practices originated from patients with suspected EM [79]. Unnecessary testing can delay proper diagnosis and treatment and increase healthcare costs. The annual cost of laboratory testing for LB in the outpatient sector in Germany alone was estimated to be €51 million, a substantial portion of which obviously resulted from overtesting [78].

6.3.1 Epidemiological Considerations for Adequate Serodiagnostics

It should be noted that the less specific the symptoms, the weaker the a priori probability of LB and the lower the predictive value of serological methods [2, 3, 33, 44, 77, 81]. Confirmed indications for serological testing in suspected LB are summarized in Table 6.1. The probability that a patient with a positive serological test actually has LB (positive predictive value) and the probability that a patient with a negative test does not have the disease (negative predictive value) depends on the performance characteristics of a given assay (sensitivity and specificity) and the prevalence of the disease in a given population and geographic region [44, 77, 82, 83]. The pretest probability of a patient having or not having LB determines the predictive value of a given test result. Therefore, the clinical significance of a test result for antibodies against *B. burgdorferi* s.l. must be interpreted with caution, especially outside endemic areas [82, 83]. Consequently, relevant clinical signs must be present before LB can be suspected [44, 77]. Serological testing is only indicated when such clinical symptoms are present [6] and a serological follow-up is only of use 2–3 weeks after a possible infection [28, 51].

6.3.2 Advantages and Limitations of Current Serological Test Strategies

Currently, many guidelines, including the US Centers for Disease Control and Prevention (CDC), recommend a two-tiered laboratory testing strategy that utilizes a screening test of high analytic sensitivity (e.g. enzyme-linked immunosorbent assay [ELISA]) with a highly specific confirmatory test (immunoblot) (Fig. 6.1) [28–30, 51, 84]. Recent attempts have been made to improve the current diagnostic testing strategies by integrating new antigen components, such as VlsE or closely related peptides (C6), into a new generation of immunoassays (IA) that could potentially replace the widely used two-step or two-tiered approach (e.g., confirmation of positive screening results by subsequent immunoblots) and that are more sensitive

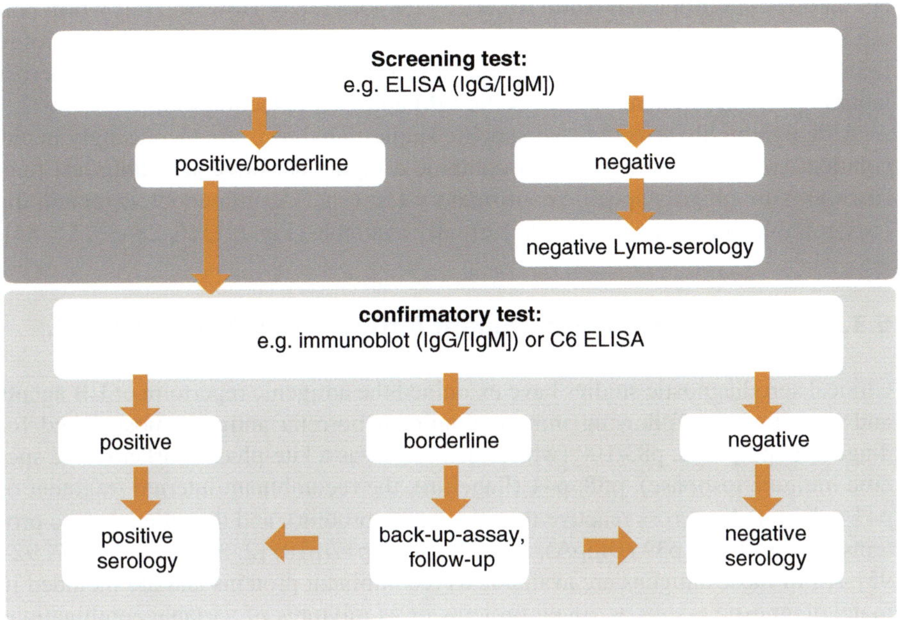

Fig. 6.1 Diagnostic algorithm for EIA and immunoblot-based two-tier testing, modified from Hunfeld et al. (2009) [112]

and specific than the tests currently being used in the United States [44]. In Europe, however, several investigations have raised doubts as to whether a single serological test is sensitive and specific enough to serve as a stand-alone test for diagnosing LB [44, 85–87]. *Borrelia* genospecies and strains have much higher biodiversity in Europe making it much more difficult to design an appropriate IA with a simple "one fits all" approach [51, 85, 87]. Therefore, this test strategy seems much more feasible in the United States due to the presence of fewer genospecies [6, 88]. This is underscored by a recent study, which confirmed that the standard two-tiered serological testing using assays developed for use in the United States performed more poorly than European assays in detecting LB acquired in Europe [89]. As outlined earlier, this result is not surprising as LB in North America is mainly caused by *B. burgdorferi* s.s. In Europe, an infection can be caused by *B. afzelii*, *B. garinii*, *B. bavariensis* , *B. burgdorferi* s.s., and less commonly, *B. spielmanii* [2, 3, 28, 30, 51]. Importantly, the specificity of stand-alone tests has been questioned by studies comparing the specificity of two-tiered (IA & C6 peptide ELISA) algorithms (99.5%) to the stand-alone C6 ELISA with a lower specificity of 98.4% [90]. Although this difference seems negligible, in the United States alone, where at least 3.4 million LB tests are performed annually [90], such a difference would lead to an additional 37,000 false-positive test results per year, more than the reported incidence of LB in the United States (>35,000 cases annually) [91]. The high specificity of the two-tiered approach (Fig. 6.3) is thus a critical advantage [88, 90] and therefore has prevailed as the gold standard for LB serology in most diagnostic laboratories in Europe and North America [28, 30, 51, 84]. However, it is worth noting that it is debatable as to whether the second tier needs to be an immunoblot in light of the limitations of immunoblot testing, with little standardization across laboratories and problems with specific IgM antibody detection [88].

Although highly sensitive and specific single-tiered tests are increasingly in circulation, two-tiered strategies that combine a highly sensitive screening test (e.g. ELISA) with a highly specific confirmatory test (e.g. IA, immunoblot) remain the most reliable diagnostic procedure currently available (Fig. 6.1) [6, 28–30, 51, 84].

6.3.3 Relevant Immunodominant Antigens of *B. burgdorferi* s.l.

Clinical serodiagnostic studies have examined the antigenic repertoire of LB agents and identified the following immunodominant borrelia antigens most suited for diagnostic purposes: p83/100 (which also serves as a late-phase marker of the specific immune response), p58, p41 (flagellin), the recombinant internal fragment of p41 (which is less cross reactive than the native protein), and the outer surface proteins OspA, OspC, p39 (BmpA), and DbpA (Osp17/p18) [2, 3, 28, 30, 51, 87, 92–95]. All of these antigens are available as recombinant proteins and are included in many diagnostic assays as single proteins or as mixtures of variable combinations and concentrations [6]. The known genospecies, and in part also strain-dependent variabilities of most borrelia antigens, can result in variable serodiagnostic sensitivities, especially within Europe but also between Europe and North America [28, 30, 51, 87, 89, 95, 96]. Such variability also significantly affects the proteins VlsE, OspA, OspC, and Osp17 with direct diagnostic impact because the resulting borrelial surface antigenic diversity impairs serodiagnostic performance, especially for methods such as the immunoblot [51, 88, 97]. For example, intraspecies differences in *B. garinii* detected using a panel of monoclonal antibodies have led to the recognition of at least 13 different OspC serotypes [98]. To a lesser extent, heterogeneity in the immunoreactivity to VlsE has been described in Europe [87]. As a result, European immunoassays are often prepared from mixtures of specific spirochetal lysates and/or purified antigens including fusion proteins, and then diagnostic criteria are adjusted to the diagnostic needs best suited for the local epidemiological situation [28, 30, 51, 99]. Due to strong cross-reactivity, the flagellin protein, a very sensitive but not very specific marker of early infection, should only be used as a recombinant truncated internal fragment (p41 int.) [93, 100]. A major improvement in serodiagnostics was the discovery and production of the recombinant VlsE protein and its conserved peptide region C6 [87, 101–105]. Interestingly, VlsE exhibits no recombination and a less intense expression in culture or ticks but considerable recombination and strong expression in the mammalian host [106]. Therefore, using recombinant VlsE as an important immunodominant antigen or the VlsE-derived C6 peptide for diagnostic purposes has dramatically improved the sensitivity and specificity of detecting IgG antibodies against *B. burgdorferi* by ELISA and immunoblot during the very early stages of infection and immune response [2, 3, 28, 30, 51, 87, 99].

6.3.4 Screening and Confirmatory Tests

Various IA modifications, such as ELISA, enzyme-linked fluorescence assays (ELFA), chemiluminescence-linked immunoassays (CLIA), and electrochemiluminescence immunoassays (ECLIA), are used as screening tests because they are well-suited for the polyvalent, selective, and quantitative determination of specific IgG and IgM antibodies [107]. Other serological tests, such as indirect hemagglutination assays, complement fixation, or indirect immunofluorescence, are no longer suitable [28, 30, 51]. In conventional whole-cell lysate assays, the patient's serum is absorbed by *Treponema phagedenis* to increase the specificity of the screening test. The serum must also be treated with a rheumatoid factor (RF) absorbent to selectively detect IgM antibodies and prevent false-positive results stemming from the possible presence of RF. Common causes of false-positive screening tests are summarized in Table 6.4 according to Branda and Steere [108]. Such pretreatment is normally not required for most recombinant test formats [30, 51]. The antigen fractions to specifically detect antibodies in ELISA and CLIA consist of ultrasonicate or borrelial whole-cell extract or purified recombinant proteins capable of stimulating a specific immune response in vivo; for example, Osp17/p18 (DbpA), flagellin (p41), p39, p58, OspC, VlsE (selective ELISA). Hybrid tests combining both cell-derived and recombinant antigens are also available, for example, enrichment of conventional antigen extracts with recombinant OspC or VlsE. CLIA and ELISA differ in the type of detection method and, to some extent, the antigen preparations they use. The specificity of advanced IAs is 80–90% [2, 3, 28, 30, 51]. Such assays are routine in serological laboratory testing for LB agents because they guarantee an automated reading, measurement accuracy, and ease of handling. These tools are also readily adapted for modern high-throughput laboratories using automated analytical chains [6, 51]. The results of the immunoassays can vary significantly depending on the specific antigen composition and the manufacturer of the test system [107]. Hence, the results of different tests and/or different laboratories are only comparable to a very limited extent [51, 78, 107, 109]. Standardization would require parallel testing across laboratories with archived control sera, but this is rarely carried out [28, 30, 51].

Traditional Western blots use ultrasonicated borrelia as an antigen source (Fig. 6.2). Thus, all borrelial antigens, that is, specific immunodominant and non-specific proteins, are involved in antibody detection. Optimal expression of the targeted immunodominant antigens of the *B. burgdorferi* strain is essential for the quality of such a blot [2, 3, 92]. Studies have shown that different strains of *B. burgdorferi* display pronounced variability in their immunodominant antigens. The *B. afzelii* strain PKo has proved to be particularly suitable for Europe [28, 95, 96, 110, 111]. Criteria have been compiled for interpreting, under standardized conditions, whole-cell antigen immunoblots that use the PKo strain [33, 95, 112] (Table 6.3). One disadvantage is that new immunodominant antigens such as VlsE are strongly expressed in vivo but show less intense expression in conventional culture [113]. Hence, many manufacturers of conventional lysate blots selectively add certain recombinantly produced proteins (VlsE, OspC) to create hybrid tests that

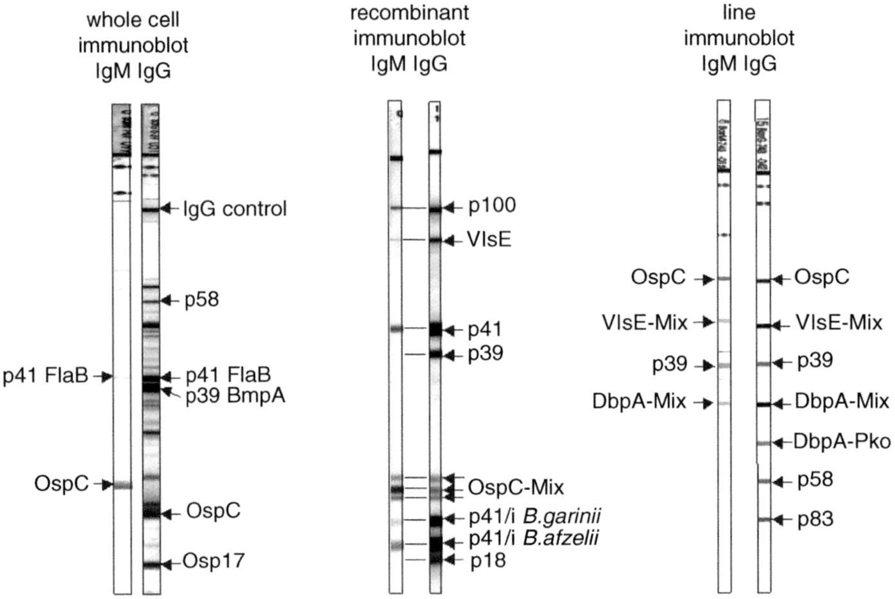

Fig. 6.2 Different formats of diagnostic immunoblots for the antigen and antibody class-specific detection of the anti-borrelia immune response, modified from Hunfeld et al. (2009) [112]

Table 6.3 Examples of established interpretative criteria for immunoblots, modified from *Hunfeld KP & Kraiczy P*, 2009 [112]

***B. afzelii* (strain PKo) whole cell antigen immunoblot evaluation criteria for Europe**	
IgG positive: ≥ 2 bands	IgM positive: ≥ 1 band
p100, p58, p43, p39, p30, OspC, p21, p17, p14	p41 (strongly positive), p39, OspC, p17
***B. burgdorferi* s.s. (strain G39/40) whole cell antigen immunoblot evaluation criteria (CDC recommendations for the USA only)**	
IgG positive: ≥ 5 bands	IgM positive: ≥ 2 bands
p83/100, p66, p58 (not GroEL), p45, p41, p39, p30, p28, OspC, or p18	p39, OspC, p41
Recombinant immunoblot evaluation criteria	
IgG positive: ≥ 2 bands	IgM positive: ≥ 2 bands
p100, p58, p39, VlsE, OspC, p41 internal fragment, p18/p17	p39, OspC, p41 internal fragment, p18/p17 or strong reaction only against OspC

close these diagnostic gaps [112]. The use by manufacturers of lot-specific evaluation templates and antigen localization verification with monoclonal antibodies in whole-cell lysate immunoblots is essential for diagnostic quality [6, 28, 33, 95, 112].

Highly specific "recombinant immunoblots" (selective blot) that employ antigen preparations from recombinant proteins to detect borrelia antibodies are used to an increasing extent [33, 112]. Some of the most common recombinant antigens for

Table 6.4 Infections and inflammatory conditions associated with falsely positive Lyme EIA results, modified from Branda and Steere (2021) [108]

Condition	Subcategory
Infection	Spirochetal infections: syphilis, yaws, pinta, leptospirosis, relapsing fever, *Borrelia miyamotoi* infection
	Tick-borne infections: anaplasmosis, RMSF
	Viral infections: Epstein-Barr virus, cytomegalovirus, varicella,
	parvovirus B19
	Bacterial endocarditis
Inflammatory disorders	Autoimmune: rheumatoid arthritis, systemic lupus erythematosus, multiple sclerosis
	Periodontitis or ulcerative gingivitis
Pain syndromes	Fibromyalgia
Vaccination	Lymerix (OspA)

these assays are Osp17/p18 (DbpA), VlsE, OspC, OspA, p39 (BmpA), p41/I (flagellin, internal fragment), p41 (flagellin), and p83/100 (Fig. 6.2). In addition, specific antigens of different genospecies can be used in the same test mixture to counter the immunological variability of the different *B. burgdorferi* species [6, 95]. The diagnostic sensitivity of the recombinant immunoblots depends on the type and amount of antigens used. The colored bands of the antigen pattern are more easily assigned to defined antigens in the recombinant immunoblot than the whole-cell lysate blot (Fig. 6.2). The recombinant immunoblot is, therefore, particularly recommended for laboratories with little experience in LB serodiagnostics [6, 112].

Line blots represent a modification of conventional recombinant immunoblots in terms of the production and processing of the antigens used. However, no electrophoretic separation step is necessary prior to the blotting procedure [112]. For such tests, the individual antigens are gently and selectively sprayed directly onto the carrier membrane without previous denaturation (Fig. 6.2). The line immunoblot achieves high levels of sensitivity and specificity in detecting borrelia-specific antibodies [112]. Moreover, the line immunoblot is able to resolve differences in the diagnostic reactivity of sera by combining or supplementing tests with highly specific immunodominant antigens (e.g. VlsE, OspC) from different genospecies and strains from different geographic origins [28, 87, 112]. These test systems provide information on the quality and duration of the immune response by taking into account the number and type of borrelia-specific bands, thus allowing the result to be classified more accurately in the clinical context [44, 51, 77]. Identifying blot bands via lot-specific evaluation templates that are appropriately weighted, as well as the parallel testing of positive controls and cutoff controls, is essential for avoiding false positives and antigen confusion [28, 112]. Given these technically demanding issues and the resulting difficulties in standardizing tests and test results, interlaboratory comparisons and round-robin trials reveal the obvious limitations of commercially manufactured conventional and recombinant immunoblots [6, 78, 107, 109].

6.3.5 Multiplex Fluorescence Immunoassays (MFI)

The introduction of novel multiple parameter test systems based on single-antigen Luminex technology allows a large number of analytes, such as antigens, to be simultaneously analyzed in the same microtiter well or by flow cytometry in a single process [51]. This test method is based on tiny, antigen-coated polystyrene beads that serve as the solid phase for a variety of detection reactions, similar to the Western blot and ELISA [114]. As with closely related single-antigen-based multiwell immunoassay systems, the resulting multi-analyte profiles combine the advantages of immunoblots with the analytic principles of quantifiable immunoassays. A study recently evaluated a multiplex bead-based assay for the detection of serum antibodies against *B. burgdorferi* s.l. [115]. The assay tested IgG and IgM responses to 13 different borrelia antigens in 49 Danish and 61 Swedish patients with Lyme neuroborreliosis (LNB), 139 Swedish non-LNB patients, and 218 Danish blood donor controls. The VlsE IgG and OspC IgM testing showed an area under the curve (AUC) of 96% and a receiver–operating characteristic curve of ~80%. All other antigens were found to be much less discriminatory in LNB compared to the controls. So, the practical advantages of such tests over classical diagnostics in LB remain at least questionable [6].

6.3.6 Interpretation of Serological Test Results

Antibodies against borrelia antigens usually form approximately 2–6 weeks after the onset of the borrelia infection. In most cases, the IgM antibody response precedes that of the IgG antibody response [28, 30, 116–118]. The absence of an IgM response has been reported in some cases [28]. An IgM response may also be absent during reinfections, as these are usually associated with a significant IgG response without major IgM production [117]. In the early phase of infection, the immune response of both immunoglobulin classes is first directed against a narrow range of borrelia antigens, especially flagellin (p41), VlsE, and OspC. Antibodies against VlsE and OspC are of special diagnostic significance because of their relatively high specificity [6]. The introduction of the VlsE antigen has provided better sensitivity in serodiagnostic testing for borrelia [87, 99, 105]. If used in the early stages of disease manifestation (e.g. EM, LNB), this antigen achieves significantly higher detection rates for borrelia-specific IgG antibodies. However, many patients (50 to 70%) still remain seronegative in the early stage of infection [28, 30].

The number of seropositive patients increases to nearly 100% in late disease as the spirochete infection progresses [28, 30, 44, 77]. In these cases, the immune response is directed toward a wide range of borrelia-specific antigens. Antibodies against specific antigens such as the p83/100 protein, p39 (BmpA), and Osp17/p18 (DbpA) have a particularly high diagnostic significance during the late stage of the immune response. In contrast, antibodies against OspA, which are also specific, are rare and are most often observed in patients with LA [28, 30, 51, 112].

As with other infectious diseases, immunocompromised patients may show a delayed or complete absence of an immune response. As a rule, seronegative LB is extremely rare in immunocompetent patients, except in the very early stage of the disease [6]. Direct detection of the pathogen should always be considered in patients who experience a short duration of the disease [28, 30, 44, 51, 77]. IgM antibodies against LB agents are relevant for detecting early infection but do not contribute to a serodiagnosis in late LB [6, 44]. As outlined earlier, the use of stand-alone IgG assays clearly suffers from limitations, at least in the non-American setting but may suffice if highly sensitive screening tests are conducted that use the VlsE protein or C6 peptide [28, 30, 51]. In this instance, additional IgM detection appears to have little significant advantage over IgG testing for early LB and may actually reduce the specificity of diagnostic testing in ambiguous clinical situations although this may depend on the antigen mix used in the assay [119, 120]. In patients with extended disease manifestations, such as chronic Lyme neuroborreliosis (LNB), ACA, or LA, only the detection of IgG antibodies against *Borrelia* should be considered to be of diagnostic significance [44]. This is because some individuals experience a persistent low-grade IgM antibody response for months or even years after treatment or past infection, although this phenomenon is not associated with a (persistent) infection with *B. burgdorferi* s.l. [121–124]. In contrast, in late LB manifestations, the presence of an IgG response is essential for the diagnosis of LB based on the current case definitions [44]. An isolated and persisting IgM response in such cases clearly argues against a long-lasting infection or late manifestation of LB [28, 30, 44, 51].

Changes in test results must always be verified by parallel testing with previously collected serum in the same assay [28, 30, 92, 118, 125]. Moreover, borderline titers and immunoblot interpretations as well as diagnostic sensitivity and specificity depend on the test and manufacturer. Specified borderline titers and cutoffs are only guidance values and should be critically verified for each test used in a laboratory through in-house performance reviews on positive reference samples and negative blood donor sera that reflect the local epidemiological situation [6, 92, 125, 126].

6.3.6.1 Interpreting Screening Test Results

No further investigations are needed for negative screening test results. However, a negative serological finding does not rule out LB. Patients in early disease stages often present with negative serological results. If the infection continues to be suspected, the serological diagnosis can be repeated after 2–6 weeks [6]. In individual cases, a measurable immune response may have been suppressed by early initiation of antibiotic treatment, inhibiting seroconversion for IgG and IgM (so-called "abrogative antibody response"; absence of IgG and/or IgM seroconversion) [28, 30, 44, 51, 77].

A borderline or positive test result must be interpreted with caution because false-positive findings do occur, for example, in the case of syphilis, other bacterial infections, and EBV infections, despite absorption of cross-reacting antibodies by *T. phagedenis* (Table 6.4) [127]. In the case of a borderline or positive LB screening test result, a test for syphilis should be performed (see above) to rule out present or resolved syphilis as a possible cause of false-positive borreliosis serology [6].

A positive test result is a strong indication of an active or possibly past borrelia infection. If this serological finding unambiguously coincides with the suspected clinical diagnosis (Table 6.1), further laboratory investigations are not required. In all other cases, a further confirmatory test must be performed [28, 30, 44, 51, 77].

6.3.6.2 Interpreting Confirmatory Test Results

A negative confirmatory test (immunoblot, or line blot) suggests that the screening test provided a false-positive result and borrelia serology is to be reported as negative. Further investigations are usually unnecessary although it must be kept in mind that early infection stages (EM, LNB) may produce false-negative findings [30, 112]. Borderline immunoblot values are particularly difficult to interpret because of the absence of the above-mentioned criteria for detecting a borrelia infection and diagnosing the disease [6]. There is no standard on how to define or interpret indeterminate results [77]. Repeating the test using the same method achieves little since the reproducibility of modern automated immune assays is quite high with only small random variations in measurement results [77]. Reproducibility of immunoblot pass rates for proficiency testing has been reported to have achieved the same intended result in 82% of the 239 participating laboratories [78]. In these cases, performing a backup test (e.g. verification of a whole-cell antigen blot result by recombinant immunoblot) can be helpful. If screening and backup tests produce divergent results in the presence of a borderline immunoblot result, this provides strong evidence for a false positive serodiagnosis [30, 51]. In the case of a positive or borderline backup test, the serological finding is consistent with an early-stage LB infection. However, such results rarely indicate an existing, persistent, or late manifestation of LB [28, 30, 44, 51, 77, 118]. Only if a recent infection is suspected, a borderline or negative serological test should be repeated after 2–6 weeks when there are clinical symptoms and an indication for testing (Table 6.1). If the finding remains unchanged, active LB is unlikely [6, 28, 30, 44, 51, 77, 118].

6.3.6.3 Interpreting Positive Confirmatory Immunoblot Results

As stated earlier, many guidelines, including the US CDC, recommend a two-tiered strategy that combines a highly sensitive screening test (e.g. ELISA) with a highly specific confirmatory test (immunoblot) (Fig. 6.1) [28–30, 51, 84]. In the case of a positive immunoblot, an analysis of the banding pattern should be performed. Data on the class of reactive antibodies (IgM and/or IgG), the intensity of the bands, and the number of bands (antigens) and their molecular weight, are required to interpret the test [28, 51]. In suspected early- or late-stage LB, the diagnostic findings must also match the clinical presentation and current case definitions (Table 6.1). An isolated detection of IgM antibodies against VlsE, p41, or OspC is an important marker of early LB. An isolated p41 band is not proof of LB because the antigen may cross-react to the flagellin proteins of other bacteria; however, its presence is consistent with the clinical diagnosis of early LB if additional clinical information is present [28, 30, 51]. Early LB is much more probable when antibodies against p41 or p41/I, the borrelia-specific internal fragment of flagellin, and VlsE or OspC are detected—as long as one of the bands is strongly present in the blot [28, 30, 51]. A clinical late-stage diagnosis is only supported by laboratory testing if several bands with an intensive signal are recognizable across a wide range of antigens [6]. The specificity of the p83/p100 and Osp17/p18 bands make them of particular diagnostic significance. In combination with a wide band pattern, they point to a late-phase immune response [28, 30, 51]. Detailed clinical information (Table 6.1) is essential when assessing an immunoblot result, as outlined above. Importantly, no conclusions can be drawn as to the need for treatment based only on a positive immunoblot or ELISA result because antibodies (including IgM) do not point to active disease *per se* and may persist for long periods (months to even years) after resolution of the infection and even after treatment [28, 30, 51]. Therefore, the detection of antibodies does not automatically confirm a clinical infection. Confirmation requires the serodiagnostic test result to be examined in conjunction with the clinical symptoms (Table 6.1), especially since a real activity marker of disease (such as the venereal disease laboratory test (VDRL) for syphilis) is currently not available [28, 30, 51]. Any reinfections can only be unambiguously diagnosed by verifying significant serology changes through parallel testing with a previously collected sample. It should again be emphasized that the isolated positive detection of IgM antibodies in this context is not an indication of. late LB [28, 30, 51].

6.3.7 Laboratory Diagnosis of Lyme Neuroborreliosis (LNB)

6.3.7.1 Serology

LNB is a disorder of the central nervous system that can manifest primarily or follow EM. Around 10% of LB patients exhibit LNB with typical clinical symptoms and syndromes (Table 6.1). Laboratory diagnosis should follow the proven diagnostic approaches outlined earlier. Except in very early LNB and in cases with polyneuropathy of the peripheral nerves, conventional laboratory investigation of the CSF shows signs of inflammation including lymphocytic pleocytosis, activated plasma cells, and a disturbance of the blood-brain barrier (i.e. elevated protein and albumin) [6, 128]. CSF cell counts can vary between 6/μL and 1100/μL with a mean of 170/μL [128, 129]. In addition, general intrathecal immunoglobulin production is present in 80–100% of cases for IgM and in 60% of cases for IgG in early LNB [128, 130]. High general intrathecal IgG and IgA production frequently occurs in late LNB [128, 131, 132]. Lactate determination does not play a significant role in the diagnosis of LNB [128]. Depending on the duration of the disease and the antigen preparation used for diagnostic testing (which should preferably contain VlsE or C6 peptide), specific intrathecal antibodies are detected in 60–100% of LNB cases depending on the duration of the infection. An isolated intrathecal antibody response without a specific antibody response in peripheral blood has rarely been observed—mainly in very early LNB in children [6]. Antibody production in the central nervous system is only detectable by parallel quantitative testing of CSF and serum for borrelia-specific antibodies. For this purpose, the serum and CSF IgG concentration or albumin concentration is interrelated with the concentration of the pathogen-specific antibodies (IgG, IgM) determined in serum and CSF taken at the same point in time [44, 77, 128, 133]. These data are used to determine the liquor-serum index (LSI) according to the following formula [128]:

$$\mathrm{LSI} = \frac{\mathrm{IgG\,or\,albumin\,conc.}(\mathrm{serum}) \times \mathrm{spec.antibody\,conc.}\left[\mathrm{ELISA}(\mathrm{U/mL})\right]\mathrm{in\,CSF}}{\mathrm{IgG\,or\,albumin\,conc.}(\mathrm{CSF}) \times \mathrm{spec.antibody\,conc.}\left[\mathrm{ELISA}(\mathrm{U/mL})\right]\mathrm{in\,serum}}$$

Depending on the test, LSI values >2 in ELISA indicate intrathecal antibody production due to LNB unless otherwise indicated. LSI values of 1.5–1.9 are considered to be borderline results [44, 77, 128, 133]. Advanced CSF analysis should employ IT-based evaluation programs coupled with medical laboratory protein analysis to assess the CSF flow (function of the blood-brain barrier) to take into account special analytical constellations of up-to-date diagnostic algorithms [28, 51]. This remains true especially in cases with local general intrathecal IgG, IgA, or IgM production when the calculation of the LSI for borrelia-specific local antibody production must be based on Q-Lim (which is the empirical cutoff for the IgG- [or IgA and IgM] fraction originating from peripheral blood in relation to albumin) to avoid false-negative LSI determination [6, 28, 51, 128]. In this case, the following formula must be applied:

$$\mathrm{LSI} = \frac{\mathrm{specific\,IgG\text{-}Ab\,in\,CSF}(\mathrm{U/mL}) : \mathrm{spec.\ IgG\text{-}AB\,serum}(\mathrm{U/mL})}{\mathrm{Q\text{-}Lim}}$$

High diagnostic accuracy is also achieved by immunoblot analysis of concurrently collected CSF and serum samples that have been adjusted to equal concentrations of class-specific immunoglobulin (crossmatch immunoblot). Additional bands in CSF or higher band intensity compared to the serum are evidence of immunoglobulin class-specific and antigen-specific autochthonous antibody production in CSF [51, 112].

The diagnostic conclusiveness of positive findings must always be assessed in the context of other protein analysis and CSF serology data (presence of blood-brain-barrier disorders, presence of lymphocytic pleocytosis). The absence of inflammation and a lack of an antibody response would indicate there is no LNB if the duration of the disease is longer than 4–6 weeks [51]. However, in very early LNB, there may be no systemic and/or intrathecal antibody response even though signs of inflammation are present, except in peripheral neuropathy. Most importantly, due to past infections and even after adequately treated LNB, specific autochthonous antibody formation in the CSF can persist for months or even years [128, 133]. It should be noted that not all serological test systems achieve the same detection sensitivity for *B. garinii,* the primary causative agent of LNB [6]. This especially applies to tests that do not include VlsE or C6 peptide and only use *B. afzelii* or *B. burgdorferi* s.l. as an antigen source [128, 133]. LNB can be ruled out, however, by adequate tests if, in the absence of pleocytosis and the presence of normal CSF protein concentrations, neurological symptoms have persisted for more than 2 months [128, 133].

6.3.7.2 CXCL13 as a Lyme Neuroborreliosis Marker

The chemokine CXCL13 may be a useful parameter in the early diagnosis of LNB [134]. Among other effects, this chemotactic cytokine (chemokine) attracts B-lymphocytes to the central nervous system [133, 135]. The presence of B-lymphocytes in CSF in the case of LB (as well as in neurosyphilis) is an established phenomenon. Recent studies have suggested that CXCL13 reliably increases in the CSF of patients with well-defined early LNB and can precede specific antibody formation in the CSF [133, 135]. Some studies have reported that CXCL13 shows high sensitivity in early LNB even when the borrelia-specific LSI in CSF remains negative [136]. Contemporary clinical evaluation studies have found the diagnostic sensitivity and specificity of CXCL13 to be 94–100% and 63–96%, respectively [135, 136]. Moreover, the CSF CXCL13 concentration decreases relatively rapidly in treated patients and could act as a potential biomarker for treatment response [136].

There remains a lack of information on the diagnostic specificity and discriminatory power for other infectious and inflammatory CNS disorders. Elevated CXCL13 concentrations have been reported to be detectable in infections with closely related pathogens (e.g. *T. pallidum*), but also in tuberculous meningitis and CNS-lymphoma [134, 136–139]. Most importantly, there is no consensus on the standardized performance of the assay and the best clinical cutoff value [6]. The CXCL13 test may be a useful parameter, especially in the early diagnosis of LNB and for monitoring treatment success, but is not yet established as a routine diagnostic tool and needs further clinical and scientific standardization and evaluation [44, 77, 128, 133].

6.4 Quality Assurance

Following the guidelines of many national medical associations, diagnostic laboratories must participate in infection-related serological round-robin tests several times a year [140]. This also applies to serological antibody detection and direct molecular biological detection of *B. burgdorferi* s.l. The molecular detection of LB agents is also an option offered as part of the interlaboratory proficiency testing scheme on bacterial genome detection. The results of the external quality assessment schemes (EQAS) that INSTAND e.V. has been carrying out for years, reveal extensive heterogeneity in the testing systems currently on the market (see above) [6]. The pass rates for the conventional serological and molecular test systems, collected from meta-analytical data, show that, despite relatively good analytical pass rates for immunoassays and molecular tests, clinical diagnostic interpretation of the results often proves difficult and can hamper medical treatment in daily clinical

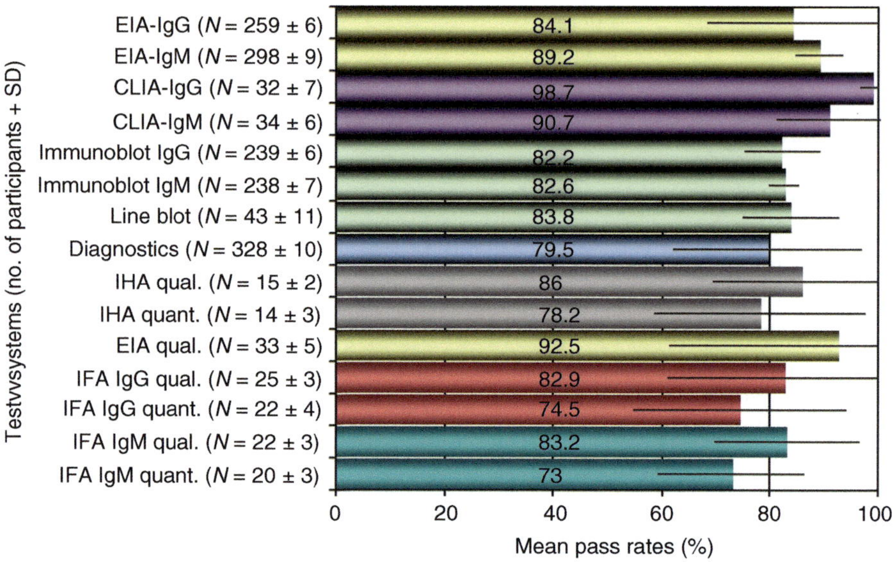

Fig. 6.3 Average number of participants and mean pass rates (%) with standard deviations (bars) for different assay systems observed between 2006 and 2008 as part of the German Lyme borreliosis proficiency testing program, modified from Müller et al. (2012) [78]

practice [69, 78, 112]. Figure 6.3 provides a summary of the pass rates for common test systems based on meta-analytical data in Germany from 2006 to 2008 [78]. Thus, when LB is suspected, infectious-disease testing should be conducted in laboratories that meet diagnostic standards in accordance with the guidelines of the expert medical societies [6, 30]. Physicians treating patients with LB should verify that these prerequisites are met in the laboratories charged with carrying out their diagnostic testing [30]. If questionable or implausible test results are produced, expert laboratories should be consulted.

6.5 Non-recommended Diagnostic Tests

In addition to the traditional diagnostic methods listed above, the literature describes a series of diagnostic techniques, some of which have been inconclusively evaluated [6]. This includes the immuno-histochemical detection of *B. burgdorferi* s.l. in biopsies and antigens in blood and urine as well as functional tests that test for cellular immunity (lymphocyte transformation tests [LTT] and cytokine detection) [141–144]. Currently, there is a paucity of scientific investigations that support the diagnostic benefit of such methods. In addition, LTT methods lack specificity and should not be used [142]. Immunohistochemical detection of borrelia in tissue is another method that is not recommended for use in diagnosing cutaneous manifestations of LB [30]. Similarly, the enzyme-linked immunospot assay (ELISPOT) [145] is not recommended. Detection of LB agents in engorged ticks through xenodiagnosis (see above) or molecular methods is similarly not recommended for disease diagnosis [16, 17]. The detection of cystic forms, L-forms or spheroplasts [146], CD57⁺/CD3-lymphocyte subpopulation tests [147], the detection of circulating immunocomplexes, and the visual contrast sensitivity test (VCS) [148] are neither helpful nor recommended. Also, point-of-care testing [149] is not recommended for diagnosing LB.

6.6 Conclusion

Over the last few decades, tremendous scientific progress has been achieved in improving laboratory diagnostic testing for LB; however, problems persist because of its variable clinical presentation and the lack of a sensitive and specific activity marker for the disease. As outlined earlier, direct detection methods, such as molecular testing and culture, currently have many limitations and cannot fulfill the expectations once raised when initially introduced on the diagnostic testing market. Although serology currently remains the gold standard for the laboratory diagnosis of LB, it also suffers from many drawbacks due to the obvious lack of standardized test systems and the given antigenic variability of the causative pathogens. Moreover, difficulties often arise concerning the correct interpretation of positive LB serology in a given clinical context as it can reflect a past or active infection depending on the constellation of test results and the patient's clinical symptoms [6]. Consequently, good knowledge of the currently established clinical case definitions (Table 6.1) and guidelines is necessary for making the right decisions at the right time to achieve the most effective, patient-oriented and stage-related application of up-to-date direct and indirect laboratory methods for detecting LB. This is also important for reducing over-testing which can mislead the attending clinician by providing a false diagnosis, thereby harming the patient by prolonging the time until a correct diagnosis can be made and treatment of the true underlying disease can be initiated. Such problems and ongoing limitations of LB diagnostic testing strongly underline the fact that research is urgently needed to establish better diagnostic options and new clinical markers to overcome the remaining diagnostic limitations of the many assays and test methods currently in use so that LB patient management can be optimized.

References

1. Berglund J, Eitrem R, Ornstein K, Lindberg A, Ringnér Å, Elmrud H, et al. An epidemiologic study of lyme disease in Southern Sweden. N Engl J Med. 1995;333(20):1319–24.
2. Aguero-Rosenfeld ME, Wang G, Schwartz I, Wormser GP. Diagnosis of Lyme borreliosis. Clin Microbiol Rev. 2005;18(3):484–509.
3. Aguero-Rosenfeld ME. Lyme disease: laboratory issues. Infect Dis Clin N Am. 2008;22(2):301–13. vii
4. Steere AC, Strle F, Wormser GP, Hu LT, Branda JA, Hovius JWR, et al. Lyme borreliosis. Nat Rev Dis Primers. 2016;2:16090.

5. Santino I, Comite P, Gandolfo GM. *Borrelia burgdorferi*, a great chameleon: know it to recognize it! Neurol Sci. 2010;31(2):193–6.
6. Lohr B, Fingerle V, Norris DE, Hunfeld K. Laboratory diagnosis of Lyme borreliosis: Current state of the art and future perspectives. Crit Rev Clin Lab Sci. 2018;55(4):219–45.
7. Koch R. Die Aetiologie der Tuberculose. Mitt Kaiser Gesundh. 1884;2:1–88.
8. Koch R. Ueber bakteriologische Forschung. Verh X Int Med Congr Berlin. 1890;1982:35.
9. Henle J. On Miasmata and Contagie. Baltimore: Johns Hopkins Press; 1938.
10. Ružić-Sabljić E, Cerar T. Progress in the molecular diagnosis of Lyme disease. Expert Rev Mol Diagn. 2016;17(1):19–30.
11. Cutler SJ, Rudenko N, Golovchenko M, Cramaro WJ, Kirpach J, Savic S, et al. Diagnosing Borreliosis. Vector-Borne and Zoonotic Dis. 2017;17(1):2–11.
12. Margos G, Vollmer SA, Ogden NH, Fish D. Population genetics, taxonomy, phylogeny and evolution of *Borrelia burgdorferi* sensu lato. Infect Genet Evol. 2011;11(7):1545–63.
13. Barbour AG, Cook VJ. Genotyping strains of lyme disease agents directly from ticks, blood, or tissue. Methods Mol Biol (Clifton, NJ). 2018;1690:1–11.
14. Margos G, Notter I, Fingerle V. Methods Mol Biol. 2018;1690(1):13–33.
15. Aase A, Hajdusek O, Øines Ø, Quarsten H, Wilhelmsson P, Herstad TK, et al. Validate or falsify: lessons learned from a microscopy method claimed to be useful for detecting *Borrelia* and *Babesia* organisms in human blood. Infect Dis. 2016;48(6):411–9.
16. Marques A, Telford SR, Turk S, Chung E, Williams C, Dardick K, et al. Xenodiagnosis to detect *Borrelia burgdorferi* infection: a first-in-human study. Clin Infect Dis. 2014;58(7):937–45.
17. Bockenstedt LK, Radolf JD. Editorial commentary: xenodiagnosis for posttreatment Lyme disease syndrome: resolving the conundrum or adding to it? Clin Infect Dis. 2014;58(7):946–8.
18. Telford SR, Hu LT, Marques A. Is there a place for xenodiagnosis in the clinic? Expert Rev Anti-Infect Ther. 2014;12(11):1307–10.
19. Turk S, Williams C, Marques A. Xenodiagnosis using *Ixodes scapularis* larval ticks in humans. Methods Mol Biol (Clifton, NJ). 2018;1690:337–46.
20. Berger BW, Clemmensen OJ, Ackerman AB. Lyme disease is a spirochetosis. A review of the disease and evidence for its cause. Am J Dermatopathol. 1983;5(2):111–24.
21. Bergler-Klein J, Sochor H, Stanek G, Globits S, Ullrich R, Glogar D. Indium 111-monoclonal antimyosin antibody and magnetic resonance imaging in the diagnosis of acute Lyme myopericarditis. Arch Intern Med. 1993;153(23):2696–700.
22. De Koning J, Bosma RB, Hoogkamp-Korstanje JAA. Demonstration of spirochaetes in patients with Lyme disease with a modified silver stain. J Med Microbiol. 1987;23(3):261–7.
23. Coyle PK, Deng Z, Schutzer SE, Belman AL, Benach J, Krupp LB, et al. Detection of *Borrelia burgdorferi* antigens in cerebrospinal fluid. Neurology. 1993;43(6):1093–8.
24. Coyle PK, Schutzer SE, Deng Z, Krupp LB, Belman AL, Benach JL, et al. Detection of *Borrelia burgdorferi*-specific antigen in antibody-negative cerebrospinal fluid in neurologic Lyme disease. Neurology. 1995;45(11):2010–5.
25. Dorward DW, Schwan TG, Garon CF. Immune capture and detection of *Borrelia burgdorferi* antigens in urine, blood, or tissues from infected ticks, mice, dogs, and humans. J Clin Microbiol. 1991;29(6):1162–70.
26. Hyde FW, Johnson RC, White TJ, Shelburne CE. Detection of antigens in urine of mice and humans infected with *Borrelia burgdorferi*, etiologic agent of Lyme disease. J Clin Microbiol. 1989;27(1):58–61.
27. Klempner MS, Schmid CH, Hu L, Steere AC, Johnson G, McCloud B, et al. Intralaboratory reliability of serologic and urine testing for Lyme disease. Am J Med. 2001;110(3):217–9.
28. Fingerle V, Eiffert H, Gesser A, Göbel UB, Hunfeld KP, Reischl U, et al. MiQ 12 Lyme-Borreliose. München: Elsevier Urban & Fischer Verlag; 2016.
29. Wormser GP, Dattwyler RJ, Shapiro ED, Halperin JJ, Steere AC, Klempner MS, et al. The clinical assessment, treatment, and prevention of Lyme disease, human granulocytic anaplasmosis, and babesiosis: clinical practice guidelines by the Infectious Diseases Society of America. Clin Infect Dis. 2006;43(9):1089–134.

30. Hofmann H, Fingerle V, Hunfeld K, Huppertz H, Krause A, Rauer S, et al. Cutaneous Lyme borreliosis: guideline of the German Dermatology Society. German Med Sci: GMS e-J. 2017;15. Doc14
31. Magni R, Espina BH, Shah K, Lepene B, Mayuga C, Douglas TA, et al. Application of nanotrap technology for high sensitivity measurement of urinary outer surface protein A carboxyl-terminus domain in early stage Lyme borreliosis. J Transl Med. 2015;13(1):311.
32. Magni R. Oral presentation. Vienna, Austria; 2017.
33. Wilske B, Fingerle V, Schulte-Spechtel U. Microbiological and serological diagnosis of Lyme borreliosis. FEMS Immunol Med Microbiol. 2007;49(1):13–21.
34. Dessau RB, Bangsborg J, Hansen K, Lebech A, Sellebjerg FT, Skarphédinson S, et al. Lyme Borreliose: Klinik, diagnostik og behandling i Danmark (2nd ed.) (Danish guideline) 2014. Available from: URL: www.dskm.dk.
35. Chidiac C, Bru JP, Choutet P, Decazes JM, Dubreuil L, Leport C, et al. 16e Conférence de consensus en thérapeutique anti-infectiese de la Spilf. Borréliose de Lyme: démarches diagnostiques, thérapeutiques et préventives. Texte long. Med Maladies Infect. 2007;37(Suppl. 3):S153–74.
36. Rijksinstituut voor Volksgezonheid en Milieu. LCI-richtlijn Lymeziekte; 2013 [cited 2017 Oct 23]. Available from: https://lci.rivm.nl/richtlijnen/lymeziekte.
37. Ružić-Sabljić E, Maraspin V, Cimperman J, Lotrič-Furlan S, Stupica D, Cerar T. Comparison of isolation rate of *Borrelia burgdorferi* sensu lato in two different culture media, MKP and BSK-H. Clin Microbiol Infect. 2014;20(7):636–41.
38. Liveris D, Schwartz I, Bittker S, Cooper D, Iyer R, Cox ME, et al. Improving the yield of blood cultures from patients with early Lyme disease. J Clin Microbiol. 2011;49(6):2166–8.
39. Nowakowski J, McKenna D, Nadelman RB, Bittker S, Cooper D, Pavia C, et al. Blood cultures for patients with extracutaneous manifestations of Lyme disease in the United States. Clin Infect Dis. 2009;49(11):1733–5.
40. Preac-Mursic V, Pfister HW, Spiegel H, Burk R, Wilske B, Reinhardt S, et al. First isolation of *Borrelia burgdorferi* from an iris biopsy. J Clin Neuroophthalmol. 1993;13(3):155–61. discussion 162
41. Stanek G, Klein J, Bittner R, Glogar D. Isolation of *Borrelia burgdorferi* from the myocardium of a patient with longstanding cardiomyopathy. N Engl J Med. 1990;322(4):249–52.
42. Sapi E, Pabbati N, Datar A, Davies EM, Rattelle A, Kuo BA. Improved culture conditions for the growth and detection of *Borrelia* from human serum. Int J Med Sci. 2013;10(4):362–76.
43. Johnson BJB, Pilgard MA, Russell TM. Assessment of new culture method for detection of *Borrelia* species from serum of Lyme disease patients. J Clin Microbiol. 2014;52(3):721–4.
44. Stanek G, Fingerle V, Hunfeld K, Jaulhac B, Kaiser R, Krause A, et al. Lyme borreliosis: clinical case definitions for diagnosis and management in Europe. Clin Microbiol Infect. 2011;17(1):69–79.
45. Alby K, Capraro GA. Alternatives to serologic testing for diagnosis of Lyme disease. Clin Lab Med. 2015;35(4):815–25.
46. Liveris D, Wang G, Girao G, Byrne DW, Nowakowski J, McKenna D, et al. Quantitative detection of *Borrelia burgdorferi* in 2-millimeter skin samples of erythema migrans lesions: correlation of results with clinical and laboratory findings. J Clin Microbiol. 2002;40(4):1249–53.
47. Schwaiger M, Péter O, Cassinotti P. Routine diagnosis of *Borrelia burgdorferi* (sensu lato) infections using a real-time PCR assay. Clin Microbiol Infect. 2001;7(9):461–9.
48. Schwartz I, Wormser GP, Schwartz JJ, Cooper D, Weissensee P, Gazumyan A, et al. Diagnosis of early Lyme disease by polymerase chain reaction amplification and culture of skin biopsies from erythema migrans lesions. J Clin Microbiol. 1992;30(12):3082–8.
49. Ojaimi C, Davidson BE, Girons IS, Old IG. Conservation of gene arrangement and an unusual organization of rRNA genes in the linear chromosomes of the Lyme disease spirochaetes *Borrelia burgdorferi*, *B. garinii* and *B. afzelii*. Microbiology. 1994;140(11):2931–40.
50. Schmidt BL. PCR in laboratory diagnosis of human *Borrelia burgdorferi* infections. Clin Microbiol Rev. 1997;10(1):185–201.

51. Hunfeld KP, Wichelhaus TA, Brade V Borreliosis TH-Books, English Edition. In: Clinical laboratory diagnostics. p. 1955–65.
52. Eshoo MW, Schutzer SE, Crowder CD, Carolan HE, Ecker DJ. Achieving molecular diagnostics for Lyme disease. Expert Rev Mol Diagn. 2014;13(8):875–83.
53. Ecker DJ, Sampath R, Li H, Massire C, Matthews HE, Toleno D, et al. New technology for rapid molecular diagnosis of bloodstream infections. Expert Rev Mol Diagn. 2014;10(4):399–415.
54. Roux F, Boyer E, Jaulhac B, Dernis E, Closs-Prophette F, Puéchal X. Lyme meningoradiculitis: prospective evaluation of biological diagnosis methods. Eur J Clin Microbiol Infect Dis. 2007;26(10):685–93.
55. Amouriaux P, Assous M, Margarita D, Baranton G, Saint GI. Polymerase chain reaction with the 30-kb circular plasmid of *Borrelia burgdorferi* B31 as a target for detection of the Lyme borreliosis agents in cerebrospinal fluid. Res Microbiol. 1993;144(3):211–9.
56. Priem S, Rittig MG, Kamradt T, Burmester GR, Krause A. An optimized PCR leads to rapid and highly sensitive detection of *Borrelia burgdorferi* in patients with Lyme borreliosis. J Clin Microbiol. 1997;35(3):685–90.
57. Gooskens J, Templeton K, Claas E, van Dam A. Evaluation of an internally controlled real-time PCR targeting the ospA gene for detection of *Borrelia burgdorferi* sensu lato DNA in cerebrospinal fluid. Clin Microbiol Infect. 2006;12(9):894–900.
58. Lebech AM, Hansen K. Detection of *Borrelia burgdorferi* DNA in urine samples and cerebrospinal fluid samples from patients with early and late Lyme neuroborreliosis by polymerase chain reaction. J Clin Microbiol. 1992;30(7):1646–53.
59. Brettschneider S, Bruckbauer H, Klugbauer N, Hofmann H. Diagnostic value of PCR for detection of Borrelia burgdorferi in skin biopsy and urine samples from patients with skin borreliosis. J Clin Microbiol. 1998;36(9):2658–65.
60. Aberer E, Bergmann AR, Derler AM, Schmidt B. Course of Borrelia burgdorferi DNA shedding in urine after treatment. Acta Derm Venereol. 2007;87(1):39–42.
61. Rauter C, Mueller M, Diterich I, Zeller S, Hassler D, Meergans T, et al. Critical evaluation of urine-based PCR assay for diagnosis of Lyme Borreliosis. Clin Vaccine Immunol. 2005;12(8):910–7.
62. Hunfeld K, Ruzic-Sabljic E, Norris DE, Kraiczy P, Strle F. In vitro susceptibility testing of *Borrelia burgdorferi* sensu lato isolates cultured from patients with erythema migrans before and after antimicrobial chemotherapy. Antimicrob Agents Chemother. 2005;49(4):1294–301.
63. Iyer R, Mukherjee P, Wang K, Simons J, Wormser GP, Schwartz I. Detection of *Borrelia burgdorferi* nucleic acids after antibiotic treatment does not confirm viability. J Clin Microbiol. 2013;51(3):857–62.
64. Gaubitz M, Dressler F, Huppertz HI, Krause A. Diagnostik und Therapie der Lyme-Arthritis. Empfehlungen der Kommission Pharmakotherapie der DGRh. Z Rheumatol. 2014;73(5):469–74.
65. Bockenstedt LK, Gonzalez DG, Haberman AM, Belperron AA. Spirochete antigens persist near cartilage after murine Lyme borreliosis therapy. J Clin Invest. 2012;122(7):2652–60.
66. Pícha D, Moravcová L, Vaňousová D, Hercogová J, Blechová Z. DNA persistence after treatment of Lyme borreliosis. Folia Microbiol. 2014;59(2):115–25.
67. van Dam AP. Molecular diagnosis of Borrelia bacteria for the diagnosis of Lyme disease. Expert Opin Med Diagn. 2011;5(2):135–49.
68. Reischl U, Schneider W, Maaß M, Straube E, Fingerle V, Bakteriengenom-Nachweis JE. PCR/NAT: Auswertung des Ringversuchs April 2010 von INSTAND e.V. zur externen Qualitätskontrolle molekularbiologischer Nachweisverfahren in der bakteriologischen Diagnostik. Der Mikrobiologe. 2010;(20):181–97.
69. Hunfeld KP, Reischl U. Oral presentation. Vienna, Austria: ICLB; 2015.
70. Wyres KL, Conway TC, Garg S, Queiroz C, Reumann M, Holt K, et al. WGS analysis and interpretation in clinical and public health microbiology laboratories: what are the requirements and how do existing tools compare? Pathogens (Basel, Switzerland). 2014;3(2):437–58.

71. Troy EB, Lin T, Gao L, Lazinski DW, Camilli A, Norris SJ, et al. Understanding Barriers to *Borrelia burgdorferi* dissemination during infection using massively parallel sequencing. Infect Immun. 2013;81(7):2347–57.
72. Leichty AR, Brisson D. Selective whole genome amplification for resequencing target microbial species from complex natural samples. Genetics. 2014;198(2):473–81.
73. Carpi G, Walter KS, Bent SJ, Hoen AG, Diuk-Wasser M, Caccone A. Whole genome capture of vector-borne pathogens from mixed DNA samples: a case study of *Borrelia burgdorferi*. BMC Genomics. 2015;16(1):469.
74. Margos G, Hepner S, Mang C, Sing A, Liebl B, Fingerle V. Completed genome sequences of *Borrelia burgdorferi* sensu stricto B31(NRZ) and closely related patient isolates from Europe. Genome Announc. 2017;5(28)
75. Margos G, Hepner S, Mang C, Marosevic D, Reynolds SE, Krebs S, et al. Lost in plasmids: next generation sequencing and the complex genome of the tick-borne pathogen *Borrelia burgdorferi*. BMC Genomics. 2017;18(1):422.
76. Postic D, Assous MV, Grimont PA, Baranton G. Diversity of *Borrelia burgdorferi* sensu lato evidenced by restriction fragment length polymorphism of rrf (5S)-rrl (23S) intergenic spacer amplicons. Int J Syst Bacteriol. 1994;44(4):743–52.
77. Dessau RB, van Dam AP, Fingerle V, Gray J, Hovius J, Hunfeld K, et al. To test or not to test? Laboratory support for the diagnosis of Lyme borreliosis. Clin Microbiol Infect. 2017;
78. Müller I, Freitag MH, Poggensee G, Scharnetzky E, Straube E, Schoerner C, et al. Evaluating frequency, diagnostic quality, and cost of Lyme borreliosis testing in Germany: a retrospective model analysis. Clin Dev Immunol. 2012;2012(2):1–13.
79. Dessau RB, Bangsborg JM, Ejlertsen T, Skarphedinsson S, Schønheyder HC. Utilization of serology for the diagnosis of suspected Lyme borreliosis in Denmark: survey of patients seen in general practice. BMC Infect Dis. 2010;10:317.
80. Coumou J, Hovius JWR, van Dam AP. *Borrelia burgdorferi* sensu lato serology in the Netherlands: guidelines versus daily practice. Eur J Clin Microbiol Infect Dis. 2014;33(10):1803–8.
81. Seltzer EG, Shapiro ED. Misdiagnosis of Lyme disease: when not to order serologic tests. Pediatr Infect Dis J. 1996;15(9):762–3.
82. Gordis L, editor. Assessing the validity and reliability of diagnostic and screening tests. 2nd ed. Philadelphia, London, New York: WB Saunders; 2000. (Epidemiology)
83. Rothman K, editor. Modern epidemiology. 2nd ed. Philadelphia, PA: Lippincott-Raven; 1998.
84. CDC. Recommendations for test performance and interpretation from the Second National Conference on Serologic Diagnosis of Lyme Disease. MMWR Morb Mortal Weekly Rep. 1995;44(31):590–1.
85. Sillanpää H, Lahdenne P, Sarvas H, Arnez M, Steere A, Peltomaa M, et al. Immune responses to borrelial VlsE IR6 peptide variants. Int J Med Microbiol. 2007;297(1):45–52.
86. Ang CW, Notermans DW, Hommes M, Simoons-Smit AM, Herremans T. Large differences between test strategies for the detection of anti-Borrelia antibodies are revealed by comparing eight ELISAs and five immunoblots. Eur J Clin Microbiol Infect Dis. 2011;30(8):1027–32.
87. Goettner G, Schulte-Spechtel U, Hillermann R, Liegl G, Wilske B, Fingerle V. Improvement of Lyme borreliosis serodiagnosis by a newly developed recombinant immunoglobulin G (IgG) and IgM line immunoblot assay and addition of VlsE and DbpA homologues. J Clin Microbiol. 2005;43(8):3602–9.
88. Schoen RT. Editorial commentary: better laboratory testing for Lyme disease: no more Western blot. Clin Infect Dis. 2013;57(3):341–3.
89. Branda JA, Strle F, Strle K, Sikand N, Ferraro MJ, Steere AC. Performance of United States serologic assays in the diagnosis of Lyme borreliosis acquired in Europe. Clin Infect Dis. 2013;57(3):333–40.
90. Branda JA, Linskey K, Kim YA, Steere AC, Ferraro MJ. Two-tiered antibody testing for Lyme disease with use of 2 enzyme immunoassays, a whole-cell sonicate enzyme immunoassay followed by a VlsE C6 peptide enzyme immunoassay. Clin Infect Dis. 2011;53(6):541–7.

91. CDC. Lyme disease--United States 2003–2005. MMWR Morb Mortal Weekly Rep. 2007;56(23):573–6.
92. Hamann-Brand A, Flondor M, Brade V. Evaluation of a passive hemagglutination assay as screening test and of a recombinant immunoblot as confirmatory test for serological diagnosis of Lyme disease. Eur J Clin Microbiol Infect Dis. 1994;13(7):572–5.
93. Hansen K, Asbrink E. Serodiagnosis of erythema migrans and acrodermatitis chronica atrophicans by the *Borrelia burgdorferi* flagellum enzyme-linked immunosorbent assay. J Clin Microbiol. 1989;27(3):545–51.
94. Jauris-Heipke S, Rössle B, Wanner G, Habermann C, Rössler D, Fingerle V, et al. Osp17, a novel immunodominant outer surface protein of *Borrelia afzelii*: recombinant expression in *Escherichia coli* and its use as a diagnostic antigen for serodiagnosis of Lyme borreliosis. Med Microbiol Immunol. 1999;187(4):213–9.
95. Hauser U, Lehnert G, Wilske B. Diagnostic value of proteins of three *Borrelia* species (*Borrelia burgdorferi* sensu lato) and implications for development and use of recombinant antigens for serodiagnosis of Lyme borreliosis in Europe. Clin Diagn Lab Immunol. 1998;5(4):456–62.
96. Hauser U, Krahl H, Peters H, Fingerle V, Wilske B. Impact of strain heterogeneity on Lyme disease serology in Europe: comparison of enzyme-linked immunosorbent assays using different species of *Borrelia burgdorferi* sensu lato. J Clin Microbiol. 1998;36(2):427–36.
97. Robertson J, Guy E, Andrews N, Wilske B, Anda P, Granström M, et al. A European multicenter study of immunoblotting in serodiagnosis of Lyme borreliosis. J Clin Microbiol. 2000;38(6):2097–102.
98. Wilske B, Jauris-Heipke S, Lobentanzer R, Pradel I, Preac-Mursic V, Rössler D, et al. Phenotypic analysis of outer surface protein C (OspC) of *Borrelia burgdorferi* sensu lato by monoclonal antibodies: relationship to genospecies and OspA serotype. J Clin Microbiol. 1995;33(1):103–9.
99. Hunfeld KP, Fingerle V, Stanek G, Dagnofer E, Brade V, Wilske B et al. European multicenter study for evaluation of a new enzyme immunoassay for detection of igg antibodies against *Borrelia burgdorferi* sensu lato [(unpublished poster presentation)]. Munich; 2005.
100. Wilske B, Fingerle V, Herzer P, Hofmann A, Lehnert G, Peters H, et al. Recombinant immunoblot in the serodiagnosis of Lyme borreliosis. Comparison with indirect immunofluorescence and enzyme-linked immunosorbent assay. Med Microbiol Immunol. 1993;182(5):255–70.
101. Liang FT, Jacobson RH, Straubinger RK, Grooters A, Philipp MT. Characterization of a *Borrelia burgdorferi* VlsE invariable region useful in canine Lyme disease serodiagnosis by enzyme-linked immunosorbent assay. J Clin Microbiol. 2000;38(11):4160–6.
102. Lawrenz MB, Hardham JM, Owens RT, Nowakowski J, Steere AC, Wormser GP, et al. Human antibody responses to VlsE antigenic variation protein of Borrelia burgdorferi. J Clin Microbiol. 1999;37(12):3997–4004.
103. Panelius J, Lahdenne P, Saxén H, Carlsson S, Heikkilä T, Peltomaa M, et al. Diagnosis of Lyme neuroborreliosis with antibodies to recombinant proteins DbpA, BBK32, and OspC, and VlsE IR6 peptide. J Neurol. 2003;250(11):1318–27.
104. Schulte-Spechtel U, Lehnert G, Liegl G, Fingerle V, Heimerl C, Johnson BJB, et al. Significant improvement of the recombinant *Borrelia*-specific immunoglobulin G immunoblot test by addition of VlsE and a DbpA homologue derived from *Borrelia garinii* for diagnosis of early neuroborreliosis. J Clin Microbiol. 2003;41(3):1299–303.
105. Eicken C, Sharma V, Klabunde T, Lawrenz MB, Hardham JM, Norris SJ, et al. Crystal structure of Lyme disease variable surface antigen VlsE of *Borrelia burgdorferi*. J Biol Chem. 2002;277(24):21691–6.
106. Indest KJ, Howell JK, Jacobs MB, Scholl-Meeker D, Norris SJ, Philipp MT. Analysis of Borrelia burgdorferi VlsE gene expression and recombination in the tick vector. Infect Immun. 2001;69(11):7083–90.
107. Leeflang MMG, Ang CW, Berkhout J, Bijlmer HA, van Bortel W, Brandenburg AH, et al. The diagnostic accuracy of serological tests for Lyme borreliosis in Europe: a systematic review and meta-analysis. BMC Infect Dis. 2016;16(1):31.

108. Branda JA, Steere AC. Laboratory diagnosis of Lyme Borreliosis. Clin Microbiol Rev. 2021;34(2):15.
109. Hunfeld K, Stanek G, Straube E, Hagedorn H, Schörner C, Mühlschlegel F, et al. Quality of Lyme disease serology. Lessons from the German proficiency testing program 1999–2001. A preliminary report. Wiener klinische Wochenschrift. 2002;114(13–14):591–600.
110. Hauser U, Lehnert G, Wilske B. Validity of interpretation criteria for standardized Western blots (immunoblots) for serodiagnosis of Lyme borreliosis based on sera collected throughout Europe. J Clin Microbiol. 1999;37(7):2241–7.
111. Norman GL, Antig JM, Bigaignon G, Hogrefe WR. Serodiagnosis of Lyme borreliosis by Borrelia burgdorferi sensu stricto, *B. garinii*, and *B. afzelii* Western blots (immunoblots). J Clin Microbiol. 1996;34(7):1732–8.
112. Hunfeld KP, Kraiczy P. When is the best time to order a Western blot and how should it be interpreted? Curr Probl Dermatol. 2009;37:167–77.
113. Bykowski T, Babb K, von Lackum K, Riley SP, Norris SJ, Stevenson B. Transcriptional regulation of the *Borrelia burgdorferi* antigenically variable VlsE surface protein. J Bacteriol. 2006;188(13):4879–89.
114. Porwancher RB, Hagerty CG, Fan J, Landsberg L, Johnson BJB, Kopnitsky M, et al. Multiplex immunoassay for Lyme disease using VlsE1-IgG and pepC10-IgM antibodies: improving test performance through bioinformatics. Clin Vaccine Immunol. 2011;18(5):851–9.
115. Dessau RB, Moller JK, Kolmos B, Henningsson AJ. Multiplex assay (Mikrogen recomBead) for detection of serum IgG and IgM antibodies to 13 recombinant antigens of *Borrelia burgdorferi* sensu lato in patients with neuroborreliosis: the more the better? J Med Microbiol. 2015;64(3):224–31.
116. Steere AC. Lyme disease. N Engl J Med. 1989;321(9):586–96.
117. Eiffert H, Hanefeld F, Thomssen R, Christen HJ. Reinfection in Lyme borreliosis. Infection. 1996;24(6):437–9.
118. Mauch H, Wellinghausen N, Abele-Horn M, Manthke OD. MiQ 35, Infektionsimmunologische Methoden Teil I. München: Urban & Fischer in Elsevier; 2017. p. 41–53.
119. Dessau RB. Diagnostic accuracy and comparison of two assays for *Borrelia*-specific IgG and IgM antibodies: proposals for statistical evaluation methods, cut-off values and standardization. J Med Microbiol. 2013;62(12):183–44.5.
120. Dessau R, Ejlertsen T, Hilden J. Simultaneous use of serum IgG and IgM for risk scoring of suspected early Lyme borreliosis: graphical and bivariate analyses. APMIS. 2010;118(4):313–23.
121. Glatz M, Golestani M, Kerl H, Müllegger RR. Clinical relevance of different IgG and IgM serum antibody responses to *Borrelia burgdorferi* after antibiotic therapy for erythema migrans. Arch Dermatol. 2006;142(7)
122. Goossens HA, van den Bogaard AE, Nohlmans MK. Reduced specificity of combined IgM and IgG enzyme immunoassay testing for Lyme borreliosis. Eur J Clin Microbiol Infect Dis. 2000;19(5):400–2.
123. Kalish RA, McHugh G, Granquist J, Shea B, Ruthazer R, Steere AC. Persistence of immunoglobulin M or immunoglobulin G antibody responses to *Borrelia burgdorferi* 10–20 years after active lyme disease. Clin Infect Dis. 2001;33(6):780–5.
124. Seriburi V, Ndukwe N, Chang Z, Cox M, Wormser G. High frequency of false positive IgM immunoblots for Borrelia burgdorferi in clinical practice. Clin Microbiol Infect. 2012;18(12):1236–40.
125. Mauch H, Wellinghausen N, Abele-Horn M, Manthke OD. MiQ 35, Infektionsimmunologische Methoden Teil I. München: Urban & Fischer in Elsevier; 2017. p. 12–20.
126. World Health Organization. Veterinary Public Health Unit: WHO Workshop on Lyme borreliosis diagnosis and surveillance. Document no. WHO/CDS/VPH/95.141. Geneva, Switzerland; 1995.
127. Bruckbauer HR, Preac-Mursic V, Fuchs R, Wilske B. Cross-reactive proteins of *Borrelia burgdorferi*. Eur J Clin Microbiol Infect Dis. 1992;11(3):224–32.
128. Rauer S, Kastenbauer S et al. S3-Leitlinie Neuroborreliose. 2017 [cited 2017 Oct 17]. Available from: http://www.awmf.org/leitlinien/detail/ll/030-071.html.

129. Oschmann P, Dorndorf W, Hornig C, Schäfer C, Wellensiek HJ, Pflughaupt KW. Stages and syndromes of neuroborreliosis. J Neurol. 1998;245(5):262–72.
130. Reiber H, Ressel CB, Spreer A. Diagnosis of neuroborreliosis—improved knowledge base for qualified antibody analysis and cerebrospinal fluid data pattern related interpretations. Neurol Psychiatry Brain Res. 2013;19(4):159–69.
131. Kaiser R. Variable CSF findings in early and late Lyme neuroborreliosis: a follow-up study in 47 patients. J Neurol. 1994;242(1):26–36.
132. Djukic M, Schmidt-Samoa C, Lange P, Spreer A, Neubieser K, Eiffert H, et al. Cerebrospinal fluid findings in adults with acute Lyme neuroborreliosis. J Neurol. 2012;259(4):630–6.
133. Mygland Å, Ljøstad U, Fingerle V, Rupprecht T, Schmutzhard E, Steiner I. EFNS guidelines on the diagnosis and management of European Lyme neuroborreliosis. Eur J Neurol. 2010;17(1):8–e4.
134. Rupprecht TA, Plate A, Adam M, Wick M, Kastenbauer S, Schmidt C, et al. The chemokine CXCL13 is a key regulator of B cell recruitment to the cerebrospinal fluid in acute Lyme neuroborreliosis. J Neuroinflammation. 2009;6:42.
135. Ljøstad U, Mygland Å. CSF B—lymphocyte chemoattractant (CXCL13) in the early diagnosis of acute Lyme neuroborreliosis. J Neurol. 2008;255(5):732–7.
136. Schmidt C, Plate A, Angele B, Pfister H, Wick M, Koedel U, et al. A prospective study on the role of CXCL13 in Lyme neuroborreliosis. Neurology. 2011;76(12):1051–8.
137. Dersch R, Hottenrott T, Senel M, Lehmensiek V, Tumani H, Rauer S, et al. The chemokine CXCL13 is elevated in the cerebrospinal fluid of patients with neurosyphilis. Fluids Barriers CNS. 2015;12:12.
138. Hytönen J, Kortela E, Waris M, Puustinen J, Salo J, Oksi J. CXCL13 and neopterin concentrations in cerebrospinal fluid of patients with Lyme neuroborreliosis and other diseases that cause neuroinflammation. J Neuroinflammation. 2014;11:103.
139. Rubenstein JL, Wong VS, Kadoch C, Gao H, Barajas R, Chen L, et al. CXCL13 plus interleukin 10 is highly specific for the diagnosis of CNS lymphoma. Blood. 2013;121(23):4740–8.
140. Richtlinie der Bundesärztekammer zur Qualitätssicherung laboratoriumsmedizinischer Untersuchungen; 2019.
141. Dattwyler RJ, Volkman DJ, Halperin JJ, Luft BJ, Thomas J, Golightly MG. Specific immune responses in Lyme borreliosis. Characterization of T cell and B cell responses to *Borrelia burgdorferi*. Ann N Y Acad Sci. 1988;539:93–102.
142. Dessau R, Fingerle V, Gray J, Hunfeld K, Jaulhac B, Kahl O, et al. The lymphocyte transformation test for the diagnosis of Lyme borreliosis has currently not been shown to be clinically useful. Clin Microbiol Infect. 2014;20(10):O786.
143. von Baehr V. The lymphocyte transformation test for *Borrelia* detects active Lyme borreliosis and verifies effective antibiotic treatment. Open Neurol J. 2012;6(1):104–12.
144. Valentine-Thon E, Ilsemann K, Sandkamp M. A novel lymphocyte transformation test (LTT-MELISA®) for Lyme borreliosis. Diagn Microbiol Infect Dis. 2007;57(1):27–34.
145. Nordberg M, Forsberg P, Nyman D, Skogman BH, Nyberg C, Ernerudh J, et al. Can ELISPOT be applied to a clinical setting as a diagnostic utility for neuroborreliosis? Cell. 2012;1(4):153–67.
146. Lantos PM, Auwaerter PG, Wormser GP. A systematic review of *Borrelia burgdorferi* morphologic variants does not support a role in chronic lyme disease. Clin Infect Dis. 2014;58(5):663–71.
147. Stricker RB, Winger EE. Decreased CD57 lymphocyte subset in patients with chronic Lyme disease. Immunol Lett. 2001;76(1):43–8.
148. Hartmann F, Mueller-Marienburg H. Indirekter Neurotoxinnachweis durch den "Visual Contrast Sensitivity"-Test bei Patienten mit einer chronischen Borreliose. Die Medizinische Welt. 2003;54:248–51.
149. Smit PW, Kurkela S, Kuusi M, Vapalahti O. Evaluation of two commercially available rapid diagnostic tests for Lyme borreliosis. Eur J Clin Microbiol Infect Dis. 2015;34(1):109–13.

Prophylactic Measures Against Lyme borreliosis Including Future Perspectives

7

Nathalie Boulanger

7.1 Introduction

Lyme borreliosis is the most prevalent tick-borne disease of the temperate northern hemisphere [1]. The twentieth century has seen an important geographic spread and impact of this human disease, associated with modifications in landscape patterns and socioeconomic changes but also with global warming [2, 3].

The rising incidence of Lyme borreliosis can be attributed to increased tick abundance (linked to the proliferation of the main hosts including deer and rodents), modifications of forestry culture and landscape use, changes in human behavior, and progress in clinical recognition and diagnosis [4]. The human disease is mainly caused by three *Borrelia* genospecies: *B. burgdorferi* sensu stricto (s.s.) in Eurasia and the United States, and *B. afzelii* and *B. garinii* in Eurasia [5]. There is a characteristic delay in *Borrelia* transmission after tick attachment to the vertebrate host. Indeed, in infected ticks, the bacteria are first located in the midgut. When blood enters the midgut, they modify their antigenic coat and migrate to the salivary glands where they are co-inoculated with tick saliva into the dermis [6]. Interestingly, delays of *Borrelia* transmission in Europe are usually shorter than in the United States where the tick vector and *Borrelia* species complex are different [7, 8].

Lyme *Borrelia* is transmitted by different *Ixodes* hard tick species in different regions: *I. ricinus* in Europe, *I. persulcatus* in East-Europe and Asia, *I. scapularis* in the Eastern part of the United States and *I. pacificus* in the western part of the United States [5]. *Ixodes* ticks can also transmit a large variety of other pathogens (see chapter "Other Ixodes-Borne Diseases"), the most common in humans being bacteria (*Borrelia, Anaplasma,* and *Rickettsia*), protozoan parasites (*Babesia*), and

N. Boulanger (✉)
UR 7290: Virulence bactérienne Précoce: Groupe Borrelia, Université de Strasbourg, Facultés de médecine et de pharmacie, Strasbourg, France

French Reference Center Borrelia, Centre Hospitalier Universitaire, Strasbourg, France
e-mail: nboulanger@unistra.fr

K.-P. Hunfeld, J. Gray (eds.), *Lyme Borreliosis*,
https://doi.org/10.1007/978-3-030-93680-8_7

viruses (tick-borne encephalitis virus in Europe and Powassan virus in the United States) [9]. Ticks are obligate blood-feeders that need a blood meal to molt from stage to stage: larvae, nymphs, and adults. In continental climate areas, they have two main periods of activity in spring and autumn [10]. The *Ixodes* complex feeds on a large variety of mammals, birds, and reptiles. They are equipped with sophisticated organs, such as Haller's Organs present on the first pair of legs, which enable them to find their host by detecting odors, carbon dioxide, or lactic acid released by the host. Once on the vertebrate host, the *Ixodes* tick secretes a complex panel of bioactive molecules targeting the pharmacology and the immunology of the host [6, 11].

Humans are accidental hosts, who normally encounter the tick in its typical biotope. In most cases, humans are bitten by the nymphal stage [12] and generally on the lower part of the body. Avoiding tick bites and rapid tick removal are the most effective measures to reduce the risk of contracting tick-borne diseases. There are mechanical or chemical tools available to prevent direct contacts between the tick and the host. Furthermore, collective interventions like modifications of the environment favorable to ticks can also be considered [13, 14]. Besides all these preventive strategies, an effective vaccine might constitute the future gold standard for protection against tick-borne diseases. Research is still in progress to identify protective antigens that might generate sufficient immunity against either *Borrelia* or the *Ixodes* vector [15, 16].

7.2 Tick Control in the Human Population

Although not discussed further in this chapter, education of people about tick biology and tick-borne diseases is one of the methods of choice to reduce the risk of tick bite and contracting tick-borne diseases, which is efficiently promoted in certain countries [17, 18].

In temperate zones, prevention relies on simple personal methods to avoid tick bites, such as mechanical protection or the use of skin repellents [19]. Furthermore, various collective measures to control ticks in their environment exist (Table 7.1).

7.2.1 Personal Protection

7.2.1.1 Mechanical Protection and Adequate Behavior

Although very simple, mechanical protection is the most reliable protection against ticks trying to climb up from the ground or low vegetation. Long trousers with light colors facilitate the detection of crawling ticks (Fig. 7.1). Further effective measures to avoid direct contact between the tick and human are to tuck the trousers into socks (rarely done), and to avoid open-toed shoes or sandals [20]. Gaiters (as shown in Fig. 7.1) can also be an efficient method to avoid tick bites. When hiking in tick-infested habitats, it is also essential to keep to the center of trails to reduce contact with ticks.

Table 7.1 Actual Management strategies and future development for Lyme borreliosis control

Usual methods to limit tick bite	
Personal protection	– Protective clothing (light colored cloth, gaiter) – Body examination and prompt tick removal – Use of skin repellents
Landscape management	– Mowing – Clearing leaves on the ground – Controlled burning of vegetation
Management of host abundance	– Use of fences to exclude deer – Deer reduction by hunting – Habitat control to reduce rodent reservoirs
Alternative methods to control tick population	
Acaricides	– Area spreading of acaricides – Host-targeted acaricides (rodents or deer)
Biological control	– Entomopathogenic fungi – Parasitoids/*Ixodiphagus hookeri* – Nematodes
Alternative methods to be developed	
Anti-*Borrelia* vaccine	– Identification of protective antigens – Clinical trials in progress with transmission blocking vaccine based on OspA antigen
Anti-tick vaccines	– Numerous tick proteins identified in *Ixodes* tick saliva
Transgenic ticks	– Modify tick genome to produce *Borrelia*-refractory ticks

Adapted from [4, 13, 54]

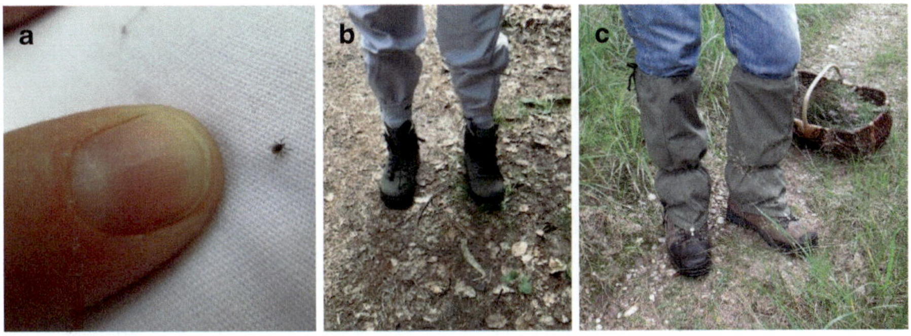

Fig. 7.1 Personal protective behavior: (**a**) Light-colored clothing for easier detection of *Ixodes* nymphs, (**b**) Pants tucked into socks, (**c**) Long pants and gaiters
Photos N Boulanger

Questing ticks are commonly found on the tips of the grass. Therefore, children aged 5–13 years are particularly at risk for tick bites. They are more likely to be bitten on the head because of their body size and their more careless behavior (e.g., rolling in the grass) [21]. The wearing of a hat or a cap and body checking after exposure (discussed later) can reduce tick bites at the level of the scalp. Unfortunately, most people do not observe these simple measures of tick bite prevention [4].

7.2.1.2 Repellents

Repellents are chemical substances that are applied topically and predominantly disturb the olfactory system of ticks, preventing them from detecting their host [22]. In principle, these molecules do not kill ticks. They must be applied carefully, depending on the age and activities of the subject (Table 7.2). Care must be taken to avoid contact with eyes or mucous membranes. The duration of repellent activity is

Table 7.2 Most important natural and synthetic repellents already marketed or in development

Molecules	Development	Concentration	Disadvantages	Advantages	Other specificity
Synthetic repellents registered in US, Canadian and European agencies					
DEET	1953	10–50%	Oily, plastics damage, eye irritation	Toxicology well-known Cheap Broad spectrum repellent	DEET 33%: slow release Polymer: Ultrathon® (3M)
Picaridin or KBR3023 (derived from piperidine)	1980s (BAYER)	20–30%	Possible skin irritation	Broad spectrum. Does not alter plastics. Low odor.	NA
IR3535 or EBAAP	1975 (MERCK)	20–35%	Eye irritation May damage plastic and clothing	Safe. Good record.	Low repellency at low concentrations.
Most important marketed plant-derived products					
P-menthane-3,8-diol (Quwenling)	NA	20–30%	Contains citral (skin irritating) eye irritating	NA	Eucalyptus: *Corymbia citriodora*
Permethrin (Pyrethrinoids)	1979	0.5%	Pesticide. Should not be applied to skin.	NA	Clothing repellent. Polymer-coating repellent
Most studied tick repellent compound derived from plants					
2-undecanone BioUD®	2007	7.75%	NA	NA	*Lycopersicon hirsutum*- wild tomato
Nootkatone	NA	0.0458 (wt/vol)	NA	NA	*Chamaecyparis nootkatensis*- Alaskan yellow cedar
Dodecanoic acid (DDA) Contrazeck®	NA	10%	NA	NA	Coconut and palm kernel oil

Adapted from [19, 22, 23]
NA Not applicable

variable and depends on the type of molecule, the formulation, and the concentration of the active compound. Special care is indicated with young children (under 2 years old), pregnant women, and allergic people [22–24].

Today, the most commonly used repellent is diethyltoluamide (DEET). In the United States, DEET has been used for several decennia and has proven to be efficient against ticks. The drawback is that it can damage synthetic fibers, plastics (glasses, watch-bracelets, etc.), and leather. It was first commercialized in 1956 with very few published side effects. Two more recently discovered molecules with repellent properties, IR35/35® (N-butyl, N-acétyl-3 éthylaminopropionate) and KBR 3023 or picaridin, also exhibit good activity against ticks [21]. Picaridin, which is the most used of the two against arthropods, has no odor, is not greasy, and does not damage plastics (Table 7.2). IR35/35 and picaridin have been the focus of several studies conducted by WHO (Pesticide Evaluation Scheme–WHOPES) [24].

Many essential oils and natural compounds are generally not recommended since they are too volatile and some of them cause skin irritation and induce allergies. However, oil of lemon eucalyptus (OLE) which is extracted from the eucalyptus *Corymbia citriodora* or P-menthane-3,8-diol (PMD), a synthesized version of OLE, is efficient and can be employed against ticks [19, 22]. Other natural molecules, including dodecanoic acid, 2-undecanone, and nootkatone, also have a potential to repel [19, 22, 23] (Table 7.2).

Permethrin, which was developed in the 1970s in the United States is toxic for reptiles and fish. Permethrin induces rapid immobilization and detachment of the tick when applied on fabric. The molecule is classified as a pesticide and must therefore not be applied directly to the skin. It should be used with caution; severe side effects are more and more documented [20, 23].

In summary, the use of tick repellents on skin can help to reduce tick bites and the incidence of Lyme borreliosis. The wearing of protective, light-colored clothes and long trousers has been reported as the most effective [25] as has bathing within 2 h of being exposed to ticks [26].

7.2.1.3 Body Checking

None of the above-mentioned techniques provide a 100% guarantee of protection [20]. Visual inspection of the entire body after activity in endemic areas for ticks is still the best prevention. Particular attention must be paid to the examination of moist areas of the body, such as the skin folds, navel, scalp, and ears. Tick bites are usually painless. In some individuals, a hypersensitive reaction to tick saliva may help to detect a tick. In the event of a bite, the best method is the mechanical removal of the tick with a specific tool such as thin-tipped tweezers or forceps so that the tick may be grasped as near to the skin as possible (Fig. 7.2). When the tick is pulled gently but firmly straight upward, the mouthparts can be removed intact. Should the mouthparts break off, a small nodule will persist in the skin for a few weeks and will finally be resorbed [27]. There are some commercial devices that work in certain circumstances but are generally less effective [20]. The application of chemicals to the tick such as petroleum, gasoline, fingernail polish, or 70% alcohol cannot be

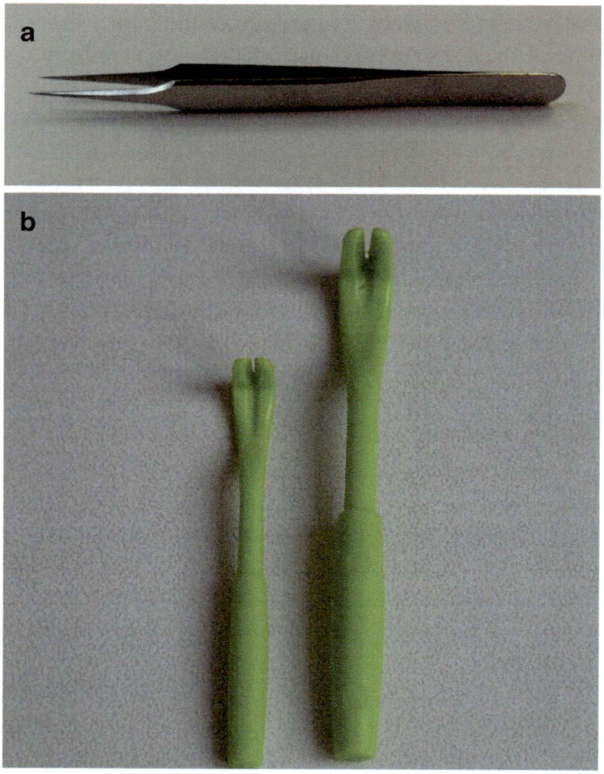

Fig. 7.2 Tools to remove ticks: (**a**) Fine tweezers, (**b**) commercial device to extract different sizes of *Ixodes* ticks
Photos N Boulanger

recommended. None of these products are really effective [28], and no study has conclusively proved that regurgitation of tick gut contents into the skin occurs after chemical application. Indeed, one laboratory study demonstrated that the method of tick removal has no impact on *Borrelia* transmission [28]. After removal, the tick bite site must be disinfected and hands should be washed. Topical antibiotics have not been shown to be effective in preventing the transmission of Lyme borreliosis [29]. It is recommended to note the site and date of the bite and watch for signs and symptoms (fever, flu-like symptoms, dizziness…). Erythema migrans, the only pathognomonic symptom of Lyme borreliosis, which occurs in a proportion of infected individuals, generally appear between 3 and 30 days after the infective tick bite [5] and should not be confused with a localized allergic reaction to the tick saliva, which can appear at the site of the bite and generally develops rapidly within 24–48 h [30].

7.2.2 Collective Measures: Management of Anthropogenic Environments

Ticks spend most of their time in their natural environment, dwelling primarily in forest leaf litter; the parasitic phase on the vertebrate host is very short, lasting just a few days during the time of the blood meal [13, 31]. Therefore, a suitable ecosystem, including the presence of its appropriate animal hosts, is essential for the tick to survive. Ticks quest for the vertebrate host and spend their time going up and down on the grass to rehydrate in the ground [31]. *Ixodes* ticks generally develop in shaded areas of mixed forest where the relative humidity is at least 80% [10]. All tick stages can regularly be encountered on woodland paths, adults especially like grass and bushes, even in urban and suburban areas [32].

Ecosystems typical for Lyme borreliosis are characterized by an environment that is favorable for tick development and survival as well as for rodents and deer (Fig. 7.3). Therefore, tick control relies on an integrated approach including simple methods such as leaf litter removal, controlled vegetation burning, management of invasive plant species, and lawn mowing around homes. Since deer play an essential role in proliferation of such tick populations, the installation of fences is very important to limit deer around housing [13, 14].

Forestry management is equally essential to control animal reservoirs for Lyme borreliosis, mainly rodents. Removal of deadwood on the ground and clearing of leaf litter makes an environment unattractive to rodents and also to the *Ixodes* tick population [14, 33]. The control of deer populations by regular hunting has been also proposed [34]. In certain areas, however, this intervention was not sufficiently successful to reduce the risk of Lyme borreliosis, as shown by a recent study performed in Scandinavia [35]. Opening up the land to direct solar exposure and lowering humidity on the ground contributes to the limitation of tick populations, and maintaining host diversity, thus promoting the dilution effect on *Borrelia* transmission, reduces the abundance of infected ticks [36, 37], although this does not apply everywhere [38].

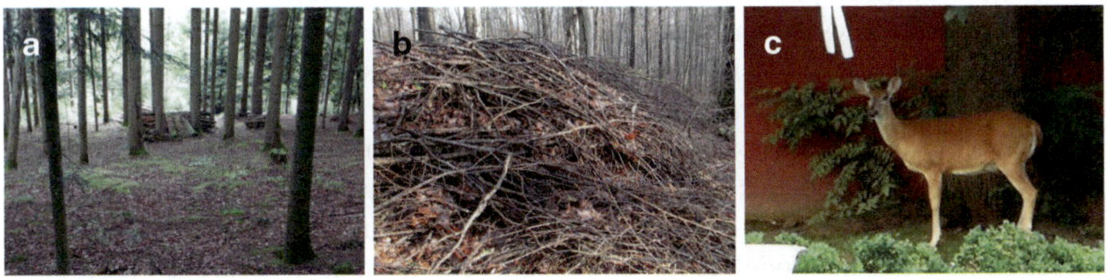

Fig. 7.3 Favorable environment for *Ixodes* ticks: (**a**) leaf litter, (**b**) branch bundles, (**c**) forested areas in American suburban area conducive for deer
Photos N Boulanger

7.3 Control of Ticks on Animals

7.3.1 Domestic Animals

Once a tick is attached and feeding, it will not detach to seek another animal or human host. Domestic animals such as dogs and cats can carry unattached ticks into the home. Therefore, living with pets increases the human risk of Lyme borreliosis due to their higher exposure to ticks crawling on dogs' and cats' coats [39]. Domestic animals can be bitten by *Ixodes* ticks and even be affected by Lyme borreliosis, but the risk seems to be associated with the genetic background of the animal. Clinical manifestations are rarely observed, although positive serology is found in a significant number of animals such as dogs, horses, and cats [40, 41]. It has therefore been proposed to use domestic animals as sentinels in Lyme borreliosis endemic areas. Some vaccines for dogs exist, but with variable efficacy [42].

Veterinarians promote various treatments to repel ticks on domestic animals, such as spot-on, sprays, collars, or powders. Active molecules include synthetic pyrethroids for dogs [43], but these molecules are toxic for cats.

7.3.2 Wild Animals

Lyme borreliosis is a zoonosis, and thus focusing on the reservoir hosts is an obvious approach to prevent the disease in humans [14]. A variety of small mammal and avian reservoirs exists in North America and Eurasia which serve as host for immature ticks. Deer are important hosts for adult *Ixodes*, known to contribute substantially to the maintenance of tick populations although they are not reservoirs as such for *Borrelia* [13]. Approaches to improve *Borrelia* control could be by treatment of animal reservoirs with antibiotics or insecticides, or the development of vaccines to block *Borrelia* acquisition.

7.3.2.1 Treatment of Hosts

Different treatment options are available for rodents and deer. Insecticides such as fipronil have been tested on rodent bait boxes to reduce larvae and nymphs on this primary reservoir [44]. A similar approach using 4-Poster bait boxes along with a barrier application of deltamethrin has also been tested for deer to reduce their tick burdens. This topical application of acaricide reduced the tick population efficiently [45]. An alternative approach is a doxycycline rodent-bait formulation. It was shown that an oral formulation of doxycycline was effective in preventing *B. burgdorferi* infection in a murine model. A major concern remains that widespread distribution of antibiotics used to treat animals could induce the development of resistance in target and non-target pathogens in humans [46].

7.3.2.2 Rodent Vaccination to Reduce Borrelia Infection

The principle of reservoir-targeted vaccines (RTV) is to reduce *B. burgdorferi* s.l. in reservoir hosts to reduce the abundance of infected ticks and thus decrease Lyme borreliosis incidence. For the development of RTV, it is essential to select the right antigen type, the appropriate route of delivery, and the optimal formulation. OspA is the major surface antigen on spirochetes during their development within the tick [47]. Vaccination of rodents with this antigen blocks the bacteria within the tick gut and inhibits their migration to the salivary glands from where bacteria would normally be inoculated into the host [48]. A baited oral vaccination strategy was very effective at selected pilot sites. Two main vaccination strategies were developed based on two different formulations: (1) oral vaccination based on *Escherichia coli* expressing recombinant OspA and (2) oral vaccination based on vaccinia virus (VV) expressing OspA. Both strategies were equally effective in producing protective levels of OspA-specific antibodies in laboratory mice and white-footed mice (*Peromyscus leucopus*) and in decreasing the prevalence of *B. burgdorferi* s.s. in infected ticks that had fed on vaccinated mice. In order to reduce the potential for human infection, another RTV was developed based on a VV encapsulated with pH-sensitive polymers (Eudragit) designed to prevent exposure to the virus until it is in contact with stomach fluids [49]. However, different technical problems need to be solved before extending this approach to natural conditions and increasing its scale [13].

7.3.2.3 Control of Deer Populations

Deer are the primary hosts of female *Ixodes,* and their populations have increased dramatically over the twentieth century [31]. Several studies have found a correlation between deer abundance and the incidence of Lyme borreliosis in humans [34, 50]. However, the culling programs that have been initiated to reduce deer populations as a means of controlling Lyme borreliosis have produced mixed results depending on the geographic areas studied and the numbers of shot animals [35, 51]. Alternatively, preventing deer from entering residential properties is possible by efficient fencing. This intervention reduces the introduction of immature tick stages and fed female ticks which can lay thousands of eggs [14]. It seems that targeting deer populations only is not sufficient to reduce the incidence of Lyme borreliosis and that an integrated approach would be more promising [13].

7.4 Control of *Ixodes* Ticks in the Environment

7.4.1 Biological Control of Ticks

Ticks have a variety of natural predators including ants, spiders, and birds, although most of them are generalists that only occasionally feed on ticks. Being non-specific predators for ticks, they do not contribute sufficiently to the reduction of tick populations [13]. Birds for example, such as guinea fowls and chicken, have been proposed to control tick populations. However, research indicates that their tick consumption is minimal and not effective enough to reduce local tick populations [52].

Other natural enemies of ticks have been studied in the laboratory; they include parasitoids, entomopathogenic fungi, and nematodes [13]. To be effective, these biological agents must be distributed over wide forest areas, and another limiting factor is the large quantities of these agents required for an effective application in nature.

7.4.1.1 Parasitoids

Some hymenoptera of the genus *Ixodiphagus* are known to be lethal for ticks. They lay their eggs in fed tick females. Their real utility for tick control is still controversial [13, 52].

7.4.1.2 Fungi

At least 20 fungi species can naturally infect ticks. For example, *Metarhizium anisopliae* and *Beauveria bassiana*, two entomopathogenic fungi, have been described as pathogens for ticks. They target the tick cuticle in specific environmental conditions and kill them [53].

7.4.1.3 Nematodes

Worms of the Steinernematidae and Heterorhabditidae families can infect ticks by entering via the genital pore. Here also, the conditions to use them effectively are very strict since a minimum temperature of 20 °C and the right soil are necessary to observe an effect. The effect of nematodes on ticks under natural conditions seems to be limited [13].

7.4.2 Chemical Control of *Ixodes* by Acaricides

The use of area-spread synthetic or natural product-based chemical acaricides to target host-seeking ticks is possible, and this approach is particularly developed in the United States [14]. Suitable molecules include three pyrethroid pesticides (bifenthrin, cyfluthrin, and deltamethrin), and one carbamate pesticide (carbaryl) [54]. They can be applied to the ground and to the vegetation as granules or as sprays, with specific regulations to protect the environment. On the east coast of the United States, the application of acaricides in residential landscapes has been shown to significantly reduce the number of host-seeking nymphs for at least 6 months. However, the acaricidal effect is not comprehensive since it is mainly the questing ticks that are targeted and not the ticks present in host microhabitats, in the soil, and in the leaf litter layer. The impact of weather conditions on the application and efficacy of various types of acaricides is still poorly understood. In Europe, synthetic acaricides are rarely spread because of concerns about the environment. Some products derived from plants have been tested as alternatives to synthetic chemical acaricides, such as pyrethrum derived from *Chrysanthemum* spp. or nootkatone derived from Alaska yellow cedar, many citrus products, and grapefruit [23]. As biopesticides, phytochemicals against ticks might offer promising alternatives to synthetic acaricides. However, additional assays are necessary to measure their toxicity and their impact on the environment [55].

7.5 Vaccination Against Lyme borreliosis: What Is the Future?

Vaccination could control the spread of tick-borne diseases, but the development of an effective human vaccine faces several important hurdles.

7.5.1 Human Vaccine Comprising *Borrelia* Outer Surface Protein Antigens

In Lyme borreliosis, the immunity to infection is strain-specific and not protective in the long term since it decreases within 1 year after the infection. Identifying suitable antigens for the induction of protective immunity is a great challenge. In 1998, Smith-Kline Beecham developed a vaccine with the trade name LYMErix, consisting of a recombinant OspA (Outer surface protein A). OspA is highly expressed in the gut of *Borrelia*-infected ticks and relatively well-conserved among different bacterial species [56]. This transmission-blocking vaccine contained lipidated OspA adsorbed onto aluminum hydroxide adjuvant in PBS. A portion of $OspA_{165\text{-}173}$ shared a very similar amino acid sequence with human protein LFA-1 (Lymphocyte Function Associated Antigen), and this cross-reactivity was potentially responsible for side effects such as autoimmunity. Marketed in 2002, LYMErix was withdrawn because of public perception of such potentially dangerous side-effects [57].

Lately, a new OspA vaccine has been successfully tested by BAXTER (Vienna, Austria) in a phase I/II trial. This new vaccine is a multivalent vaccine composed of 3 recombinant antigens from the three most pathogenic *Borrelia* species for humans. Three doses with or without aluminum hydroxide adjuvant were tested. It conferred protection against all *Borrelia* species in the United States and in Europe [58, 59]. The potential risk of antigen cross-reactivity was eliminated by the removal of the epitope responsible for autoimmunity. The vaccine proved itself to be safe with minimal adverse effects, well-tolerated, and immunogenic in healthy adults. The 30 μg adjuvanted dose was reported as the best formulation [25]. Meanwhile, another company, Valneva, has taken over this new vaccine, VLA15. This multivalent OspA vaccine targeting different pathogenic *Borrelia* species [16] is now being tested in various clinical trials to prove its efficacy in humans (source: Valneva website).

OspC, another outer surface protein, could in theory represent an interesting alternative to OspA antigen, since it is upregulated during tick feeding and expressed during spirochete transmission from tick to mammal and during the first weeks of mammalian infection [60]. However, OspC has been shown to be highly variable amongst *Borrelia* species. Therefore, vaccination with recombinant OspC might be protective only against those spirochetes bearing identical or very similar OspC. Eventually, OspC alone was considered as not being a reliable vaccine candidate [15].

Other *Borrelia* vaccine candidates have been tested such as BBK32, a 47 kDa protein [61] or RevA, a surface-exposed 17 kDa outer membrane protein [62], both fibronectin-binding proteins. DpbA (Decorin binding protein A), another *Borrelia* protein interacting with the extracellular matrix, has been identified as a further candidate. However, results were disappointing since immunization of mice with this protein protected animals only when they were challenged by syringe-inoculated *Borrelia* and not when spirochetes were transmitted by infected nymphs [63]. Alternative approaches using proteomics and RT-PCR on mouse skin have allowed the identification of additional *Borrelia* candidates [64], but up to now, none of these antigens have been used to develop a human vaccine [15].

7.5.2 Anti-tick Vaccine

Instead of targeting pathogen proteins, another approach could be to use a tick protein for a vaccine. Observations on the effects of sequential exposure of experimental animals to feeding ticks have shown the existence of acquired immunity to repeated tick bites. Very early studies performed by Trager in 1939 on rabbits infested with the hard tick *Dermacentor variabilis* showed that the animals develop an immune response against tick components resulting in rapid tick rejection after successive blood meals (for a review see [65]). It must be noted that successful tick vaccination experiments have mostly utilized abnormal hosts and in an attempt to evade the effects of the tick's immunomodulatory salivary proteins 'novel' antigens such as Bm86 were targeted. By using the midgut antigen, Bm86, derived from *Rhipicephalus* (*Boophilus*) *microplus* to immunize cattle [66], it was shown that Bm86-based vaccine reduced the number, weight, and reproductive capacity of fed females. However, its efficacy is limited to certain geographic areas because of variation between different tick strains [67].

Since hard ticks inject a large number of different tick saliva molecules into the host skin during its long-lasting blood meal, these molecules may constitute potential vaccine candidates, despite the existence of immunomodulatory saliva components [68]. They target different pharmacological processes in the host, such as the coagulation cascade and protease inhibitors, or host immune mechanisms such as innate and acquired immunity. Different antigens have already been tested in several vaccine assays (for a review see [69, 70]. The European project ANTIDotE consisted of a network of laboratories that attempted to identify and evaluate potential anti-tick vaccines [71]. Unfortunately, all attempts to identify such tick vaccine candidates have failed (*Final Report Summary - ANTIDOTE (Anti-tick Vaccines to Prevent Tick-borne Diseases in Europe)* | *FP7* | *CORDIS* | *European Commission* (*europa.eu*).

7.6 Conclusions

The prevention of Lyme borreliosis in humans can only be successful with an integrated strategy embracing different measures. They should include education campaigns leading to better information and awareness about ticks and TBDs, personal protection including appropriate clothing when walking in tick-infested areas, collective measures to limit tick populations in the environment, and the enhancement of research to find and develop efficient vaccines [25]. Lyme borreliosis is rapidly expanding into new geographical areas. This indicates that the natural control mechanisms within the enzootic cycle are becoming deregulated. Although humans are only accidental hosts, their vaccination alone, even if successful, will not confine *B. burgdorferi* s.l. to its natural cycle. Only multidisciplinary approaches, built upon effective methods to better control the dynamics in the enzootic cycle, together with successful vaccination of humans will lead to a synergistic effect in public health. Presently, increasing awareness about personal protection and seeking medical help are essential to limit the impact of tick-borne diseases in humans.

References

1. Mead P. Epidemiology of Lyme disease. Infect Dis Clin North Am. 2015;29(2):187–210.
2. Kilpatrick A, Randolph S. Drivers, dynamics, and control of emerging vector-borne zoonotic diseases. Lancet. 2012;380(9857):1946–55.
3. Medlock JM, Hansford KM, Bormane A, Derdakova M, Estrada-Peña A, George J-C, et al. Driving forces for changes in geographical distribution of *Ixodes ricinus* ticks in Europe. Parasit Vectors [Internet]. 2013;6:1. Jan [cited 2014 Mar 21]. Available from: http://www.pubmedcentral.nih.gov/articlerender.fcgi?artid=3549795&tool=pmcentrez&rendertype=abstract
4. Stafford K. Tick management handbook. Revised ed. The Connecticut Agricultural Experiment Station. The Connecticut General Assembly.; 2007. 77 p.
5. Stanek G, Wormser G, Gray J, Strle F. Lyme borreliosis. Lancet. 2012;379(9814):461–73. [cited 2014 Feb 21]. Available from: http://www.ncbi.nlm.nih.gov/pubmed/21903253
6. Bonnet S, Boulanger N. Ixodes Tick Saliva: a potent controller at the skin Interface of early *Borrelia burgdorferi* sensu lato transmission. In: Wikel S, Aksoy S, Dimopoulos G, editors. Arthropod vector: controller of disease transmission, vol. 2. London: Academic Press Ltd.-Elsevier Science Ltd.; 2017. p. 231–48.
7. Crippa M, Rais O, Gern L. Investigations on the mode and dynamics of transmission and infectivity of *Borrelia burgdorferi* sensu stricto and Borrelia afzelii in *Ixodes ricinus* ticks. Vector Borne Zoonotic Dis. 2002;2(1):3–9.
8. Piesman J, Eisen L. Prevention of tick-borne diseases. Annu Rev Entomol. 2008;53:323–43.
9. de la Fuente J, Antunes S, Bonnet S, Cabezas-Cruz A, Domingos A, Estrada-Peña A, et al. Tick-pathogen interactions and vector competence: identification of molecular drivers for tick-borne diseases. Front Cell Infect. 2017;7:114.
10. Humair P, Gern L. The wild hidden face of Lyme borreliosis in Europe. Microbes Infect. 2000;2(8):915–22.
11. Wikel S. Ticks and tick-borne infections: complex ecology, agents, and host interactions. Vet Sci. 2018;5(2):E60.
12. Barbour A, Fish D. The biological and social phenomenon of Lyme disease. Science. 1993;260(5114):1610–6.
13. Ginsberg H. Tick control. In: Sonenshine D, Roe RM, editors. Biol ticks; 2014. p. 409–44.
14. Eisen L. Control of ixodid ticks and prevention of tick-borne diseases in the United States: the prospect of a new Lyme disease vaccine and the continuing problem with tick exposure on residential properties. Ticks Tick-Borne Dis. 2021;12(3):101649. Elsevier GmbH; [cited 2021 May 29]. Available from: https://pubmed.ncbi.nlm.nih.gov/33549976/
15. Embers M, Narasimhan. Vaccination against Lyme disease: past, present, and future. Front Cell Infect Microbiol. 2013;3:6.

16. Nayak A, Schüler W, Seidel S, Gomez I, Meinke A, Comstedt P, et al. Broadly protective multivalent OspA vaccine against Lyme borreliosis, developed based on surface shaping of the C-terminal fragment. Infect Immun. 2020;88(4):e00917–9. Apr 1 [cited 2021 Jun 11]. Available from: https://pubmed.ncbi.nlm.nih.gov/31932330/
17. Kilpatrick A, Dobson A, Levi T, Salkeld D, Swei A, Ginsberg H, et al. Lyme disease ecology in a changing world: consensus, uncertainty and critical gaps for improving control. Philos Trans R Soc L B Biol Sci. 2017;372(1722):1722.
18. de Groot CG. Personal protection for people with occupational risk in the Netherlands. In: Braks MAH, van Wieren SE, Takken WSH, editors. Ecology and prevention of Lyme borreliosis. Wageningen Academic Publishers; 2016. p. 389–407.
19. Pages F, Dautel H, Duvallet G, Kahl O, de Gentile L, Boulanger N. Tick repellents for human use: prevention of tick bites and tick-borne diseases. Vector Borne Zoonotic Dis. 2014;14(2):85–93. [cited 2014 Mar 31]. Available from: http://www.ncbi.nlm.nih.gov/pubmed/24410143
20. Due C, Fox W, Medlock J, Pietzsch M, Logan J. Tick bite prevention and tick removal. BMJ. 2013;347:f7123.
21. Robertson J, Gray J, Stewart P. Tick bite and Lyme borreliosis risk at a recreational site in England. Eur J Epidemiol. 2000;16(7):647–52.
22. Debboun M, Frances SP, Strickman DA. In: Debboun M, Frances SP, Strickman DA, editors. Insect repellents handbook. 2nd ed. London, New York: CRC Press; 2015. p. 383.
23. Bissinger BW, Roe RM. Tick repellents: past, present, and future. Pestic Biochem Physiol. 2010;96(2):63–79. [cited 2014 Mar 25]. Available from: http://linkinghub.elsevier.com/retrieve/pii/S0048357509001412
24. Debboun M, Strickman D. Insect repellents and associated personal protection for a reduction in human disease. Med Vet Entomol. 2013;27(1):1–9. [cited 2014 Mar 31].Available from: http://www.ncbi.nlm.nih.gov/pubmed/22624654
25. Richardson M, Khouja C, Sutcliffe K. Interventions to prevent Lyme disease in humans: a systematic review. Prev Med Rep. 2018;13:16–22.
26. Connally N, Durante A, Yousey-Hindes K, Meek J, Nelson R, Heimer R. Peridomestic Lyme disease prevention: results of a population-based case-control study. Am J Prev Med. 2009;37(3):201–6.
27. Elston DM. Tick bites and skin rashes. Curr Opin Infect Dis. 2010;23(2):132–8. [cited 2014 Mar 10]. Available from: http://www.ncbi.nlm.nih.gov/pubmed/20071986
28. Kahl O, Janetzki-Mittmann C, Gray J, Jonas R, Stein J, de Boer R. Risk of infection with *Borrelia burgdorferi* sensu lato for a host in relation to the duration of nymphal *Ixodes ricinus* feeding and the method of tick removal. Zentralbl Bakteriol. 1998;287(1–2):41–52.
29. Wormser G, Daniels T, Bittker S, Cooper D, Wang G, Pavia C. Failure of topical antibiotics to prevent disseminated *Borrelia burgdorferi* infection following a tick bite in C3H/HeJ mice. J Infect Dis. 2012;205(6):991–4.
30. Aberer E. What should one do in case of a tick bite? Curr Probl Dermatol. 2009;37:155–66.
31. Földvári G. Life cycle and ecology of *Ixodes ricinus*: the roots of public health importance. In: Braks MAH, Van Wieren SE, Takken WSE, editors. Ecology and prevention of Lyme borreliosis. 1st ed. Wageningen Academic Publishers; 2016. p. 462.
32. Gassner F, Hansford K, Medlock J. Greener cities, a wild card for ticks ? In: Braks MAH, Van Wieren SE, Takken WSH, editors. Ecology and prevention of Lyme borreliosis. Ecology and control of vector-borne diseases. Wageningen Academic Publishers; 2016. p. 187–203.
33. Hubálek Z, Halouzka J, Juricová Z, Sikutová S, Rudolf I. Effect of forest clearing on the abundance of *Ixodes ricinus* ticks and the prevalence of *Borrelia burgdorferi* s.l. Med Vet Entomol. 2006;20(2):166–72. [cited 2014 Mar 25]; Available from http://www.ncbi.nlm.nih.gov/pubmed/16796612
34. Kilpatrick HJ, LaBonte AM, Stafford KC. The relationship between deer density, tick abundance, and human cases of Lyme disease in a residential community. J Med Entomol. 2014;51(4):777–84.

35. Mysterud A, Easterday W, Stigum V, Aas A, Meisingset E, Viljugrein H. Contrasting emergence of Lyme disease across ecosystems. Nat Commun. 2016;7:11882.
36. LoGiudice K, Ostfeld RS, Schmidt KA, Keesing F. The ecology of infectious disease: effects of host diversity and community composition on Lyme disease risk. Proc Natl Acad Sci U S A. 2003;100(2):567–71. Available from: http://www.pubmedcentral.nih.gov/articlerender.fcgi?artid=141036&tool=pmcentrez&rendertype=abstract
37. Ogden NH, Tsao JI. Biodiversity and Lyme disease: dilution or amplification? Epidemics. 2009;1(3):196–206. [cited 2014 Mar 19]. Available from: http://www.ncbi.nlm.nih.gov/pubmed/21352766
38. Randolph S, Dobson A. Pangloss revisited: a critique of the dilution effect and the biodiversity-buffers-disease paradigm. Parasitology. 2012;139(7):847–63.
39. Jones E, Hinckley A, Hook S, Meek J, Backenson B, Kugeler K, et al. Pet ownership increases human risk of encountering ticks. Zoonoses Public Heal. 2018;65(1):74–9.
40. Krupka I, Straubinger R. Lyme borreliosis in dogs and cats: background, diagnosis, treatment and prevention of infections with Borrelia burgdorferi sensu stricto. Vet Clin North Am Small Anim Pract. 2010;40(6):1103–19.
41. Wagner B, Erb H. Dogs and horses with antibodies to outer-surface protein C as on-time sentinels for ticks infected with *Borrelia burgdorferi* in New York State in 2011. Prev Vet Med. 2012;107(3–4):275–9.
42. Straubinger RK, Dharma Rao T, Davidson E, Summers BA, Jacobson RH, Frey AB. Protection against tick-transmitted Lyme disease in dogs vaccinated with a multiantigenic vaccine. Vaccine. 2001;20(1–2):181–93.
43. Emil Hovius K. The protection of European dogs againts infection with Lyme disease spirochaetes. In: Braks MAH, van Wieren SE, Takken W, Sprong H, editors. Ecology and prevention of Lyme borreliosis. Wageningen Academic Publishers; 2016. p. 409–26.
44. Piesman J. Strategies for reducing the risk of Lyme borreliosis in North America. Int J Med Microbiol. 2006;296(Suppl):17–22.
45. Grear JS, Koethe R, Hoskins B, Hillger R, Dapsis L, Pongsiri M. The effectiveness of permethrin-treated deer stations for control of the Lyme disease vector *Ixodes scapularis* on Cape Cod and the islands: a five-year experiment. Parasit Vectors. 2014;7:292. Available from: https://pubmed.ncbi.nlm.nih.gov/24965139
46. Dolan M, Zeidner N, Gabitzsch E, Dietrich G, Borchert J, Poché R, et al. A doxycycline hyclate rodent bait formulation for prophylaxis and treatment of tick-transmitted *Borrelia burgdorferi*. Am J Trop Med Hyg. 2008;(5):803–5.
47. Schuijt TJ, Hovius JW, van der Poll T, van Dam AP, Fikrig E. Lyme borreliosis vaccination: the facts, the challenge, the future. Trends Parasitol. 2011;27(1):40–7. [cited 2014 Mar 28]. Available from: http://www.ncbi.nlm.nih.gov/pubmed/20594913
48. Tsao JI, Wootton JT, Bunikis J, Luna MG, Fish D, Barbour AG. Elimination of *Borrelia burgdorferi* from vector ticks feeding on OspA-immunized mice. PNAS. 2004;89(12):5418–21. 28 [cited 2019 Nov 26]
49. Kern A, Zhou C, Jia F, Xu Q, Hu L. Live-vaccinia virus encapsulation in pH-sensitive polymer increases safety of a reservoir-targeted Lyme disease vaccine by targeting gastrointestinal release. Vaccine. 2016;34(38):4507–13.
50. Ostfeld R, Canham C, Oggenfuss K, Winchcombe R, Keesing F. Climate, deer, rodents, and acorns as determinants of variation in Lyme-disease risk. PLoS Biol. 2006;4(6):e145.
51. Kugeler K, Jordan R, Schulze T, Griffith K, Mead P. Will culling white-tailed deer prevent Lyme disease? Zoonoses Public Heal. 2016;63(5):337–45.
52. Ostfeld RS, Price A, Hornbostel VL, Benjamin MA, Keesing F. Controlling ticks and tick-borne zoonoses with biological and chemical agents. Bioscience. 2006;56(5):383–94. 1 [cited 2020 Jun 2]. Available from: https://academic.oup.com/bioscience/article/56/5/383/234709#.XtZMg5lFCRY.mendeley

53. Stafford KC, Allan SA. Field applications of entomopathogenic fungi *Beauveria bassiana* and *Metarhizium anisopliae* f52 (hypocreales: clavicipitaceae) for the control of *Ixodes scapularis* (Acari: Ixodidae). J Med Entomol. 2010;47(6):1107–15. 1 [cited 2020 Jun 2]. Available from: https://academic.oup.com/jme/article-lookup/doi/10.1603/ME10019
54. Eisen L, Dolan M. Evidence for personal protective measures to reduce human contact with Blacklegged Ticks and for environmentally based control methods to suppress host-seeking Blacklegged Ticks and reduce infection with lyme disease spirochetes in Tick vectors and rodent. J Med Entomol. 2016;53(5):1063–92.
55. Bharadwaj A, Stafford KC III, Behle RW. Efficacy and environmental persistence of Nootkatone for the control of the Blacklegged Tick (Acari: Ixodidae) in residential landscapes. J Med Entomol. 2012;49(5):1035–44. 1 [cited 2020 Jun 2]. Available from: https://academic.oup.com/jme/article-lookup/doi/10.1603/ME11251
56. Ohnishi J, Piesman J, de Silva A. Antigenic and genetic heterogeneity of *Borrelia burgdorferi* populations transmitted by ticks. PNAS. 2001;98(2):670–5. Available from: http://www.pubmedcentral.nih.gov/articlerender.fcgi?artid=14646&tool=pmcentrez&rendertype=abstract
57. Abbott A. Lyme disease: Uphill struggle. Nature. 2006;439:524–5.
58. Wressnigg N, Pöllabauer E, Aichinger G, Portsmouth D, Löw-Baselli A, Fritsch S, et al. Safety and immunogenicity of a novel multivalent OspA vaccine against Lyme borreliosis in healthy adults: a double-blind, randomised, dose-escalation phase 1/2 trial. Lancet Infect Dis. 2013;13(8):680–9.
59. Wressnigg N, Barrett P, Pöllabauer E, O'Rourke M, Portsmouth D, Schwendinger M, et al. A Novel multivalent OspA vaccine against Lyme borreliosis is safe and immunogenic in an adult population previously infected with *Borrelia burgdorferi* sensu lato. Clin Vaccine Immunol. 2014;21(11):1490–9.
60. Tilly K, Bestor A, Jewett MW, Rosa P. Rapid clearance of Lyme disease spirochetes lacking OspC from skin. Infect Immun. 2007;75(3):1517–9.
61. Seshu J, Esteve-Gassent MD, Labandeira-Rey M, Kim JH, Trzeciakowski JP, Höök M, et al. Inactivation of the fibronectin-binding adhesin gene bbk32 significantly attenuates the infectivity potential of *Borrelia burgdorferi*. Mol Microbiol. 2006;59(5):1591–601.
62. Brissette CA, Rossmann E, Bowman A, Cooley AE, Riley SP, Hunfeld K-P, et al. The borrelial fibronectin-binding protein RevA is an early antigen of human Lyme disease. Clin Vaccine Immunol. 2010;17(2):274–80. Feb [cited 2014 Mar 28]. Available from: http://www.pubmedcentral.nih.gov/articlerender.fcgi?artid=2815533&tool=pmcentrez&rendertype=abstract
63. Hagman K, Yang X, Wikel S, Schoeler G, Caimano M, Radolf J, et al. Decorin-binding protein A (DbpA) of *Borrelia burgdorferi* is not protective when immunized mice are challenged via tick infestation and correlates with the lack of DbpA expression by B. burgdorferi in ticks. Infect Immun. 2000;68(8):4759–64.
64. Schnell G, Boeuf A, Jaulhac B, Boulanger N, Collin E, Barthel C, et al. Proteomic analysis of three *Borrelia burgdorferi* sensu lato native species and disseminating clones: relevance for Lyme vaccine design. Proteomics. 2014; https://doi.org/10.1002/pmic.201400177.
65. Wikel SK. Ticks and tick-borne pathogens at the cutaneous interface: host defenses, tick countermeasures, and a suitable environment for pathogen establishment. Front Microbiol. 2013;4:337. Jan [cited 2014 Feb 8]. Available from: http://www.pubmedcentral.nih.gov/articlerender.fcgi?artid=3833115&tool=pmcentrez&rendertype=abstract
66. de la Fuente J, Rodriguez M, Montero C, Redondo M, Garcia-Garcia JC, Mendez L, et al. Vaccination against ticks (*Boophilus* spp.): the experience with the Bm86-based vaccine Gavac. Genet Anal. 1999;15:143–8. Available from: http://www.ncbi.nlm.nih.gov/pubmed/10596754
67. de la Fuente J, Kocan K. Development of vaccines for control of tick infestations and interruption of pathogen transmission. In: Sonenshine DRR, editor. Biology of ticks. 2nd ed. Oxford University Press; 2014. p. 333–52.

68. Šimo L, Kazimirova M, Richardson J, Bonnet S. The essential role of tick salivary glands and saliva in tick feeding and pathogen transmission. Front Cell Infect Microbiol. 2017;7:281.
69. Kotal J, Langhansova H, Lieskovska J, Andersen JF, Francischetti IM, Chavakis T, et al. Modulation of host immunity by tick saliva. J Proteomics. 2015;128:58–68. Available from: http://www.ncbi.nlm.nih.gov/pubmed/26189360
70. Nuttall P. Wonders of tick saliva. Ticks Tick Borne Dis. 2019;10(2):470–81. pii: S1877-959X(18)30255-3
71. Sprong H, Trentelman J, Seemann I, Grubhoffer L, Rego R, Hajdušek O, Kopáček P, et al. ANTIDotE: anti-tick vaccines to prevent tick-borne diseases in Europe. Parasit Vectors. 2014;7:77.

Public Health Aspects of Lyme Borreliosis: The German Experience

8

Hendrik Wilking and Klaus Stark

8.1 Introduction

Public health is the organized effort for promoting human health on a population level. Avoiding exposures and identifying and treating infection is, for most infectious diseases, the best way to decrease morbidity and mortality. For most infectious diseases several good starting points to interrupt transmission of most infections have been detailed [1]. For some robust surveillance leads to early detection and targeted countermeasures. Vaccines potentially decrease population susceptibility, and in other diseases, health promotion leads to less risky behavior. Lyme borreliosis is, for various reasons, difficult to combat and a challenge for public health. This problem is rooted in the fact that a clear stand-alone meaningful laboratory diagnostic test is not available. Furthermore, clinical manifestations are diverse and also vary in frequency and severity. These factors contribute to difficulties in surveillance. A vaccine is currently not marketed. The avoidance of tick bites seems to be a straightforward if not trivial idea but it is difficult to decrease the frequency of bites in the population by organized and targeted efforts.

8.2 Surveillance of Lyme Borreliosis, Incidence Estimates, and Disease Burden

Public health surveillance is the continuous, systematic collection, analysis, and interpretation of health-related data needed for the planning, implementation, and evaluation of public health practice [2]. In several European countries, there are notification systems for Lyme borreliosis in place. Either clinical cases or

H. Wilking (✉) · K. Stark
Department Infectious Disease Epidemiology, Robert Koch Institute, Unit Gastrointestinal Infections, Zoonoses and Tropical Infections, Berlin, Germany
e-mail: Wilkingh@rki.de; Starkk@rki.de

K.-P. Hunfeld, J. Gray (eds.), *Lyme Borreliosis*,
https://doi.org/10.1007/978-3-030-93680-8_8

laboratory diagnoses (or a combination of both) are reported to the public health offices or registries [3, 4]. The typical seasonal accumulation of cases between June and September is similar in different countries in Europe [5–7] and the United States [3]. The collection and analysis of these notifications allow detection of the onset and end of an infection season and they help in the assessment of the infection intensity of the season (Fig. 8.1). Moreover, the geographic distribution, especially the spread to new regions, can be assessed in a timely manner.

In Germany, there is currently mandatory notification for Lyme borreliosis in 9 federal states, while in five of nine states Lyme borreliosis has been notifiable since the 1990s without significant changes. Epidemiological data obtained refers only to the diagnosable manifestations of erythema migrans, acute neuroborreliosis, and acute Lyme arthritis. The onset of the Lyme borreliosis season is in April and May. The peak in most years is in August. Seasonal variations are minor and seasons of Lyme borreliosis are stable recurring processes. The intensity varies from year-to-year, but extremely atypical seasons do not occur.

In addition to the monitoring of the seasonality, notification systems provide valuable insights into trends. But the interpretation of year-to-year-differences, and especially geographical variation, is hampered by varying awareness of the need for notification among physicians and the predictable effects of underreporting and diagnostic inaccuracy [5, 8] (Fig. 8.2).

In these federal states of Germany, Lyme borreliosis has been continuously notifiable since the 1990s and in this overall awareness can be assumed to be stable for laboratories as well as for physicians.

The number of cases ranged from the lowest in 2002 (2,959) to the highest in 2006 (6,069). After several years of increasing trends up to 2006, lower case numbers followed for several years. Relatively high incidences were observed in the years 2016 to 2020.

Lyme borreliosis notification systems currently (status 2020) cover parts of Europe, and the status of notifiability of Lyme borreliosis remains a matter of controversy in Europe [4].

Supporters of notification claim that the obligation to notify is justified because of the medical importance and severity of the disease. Critics reply that to qualify

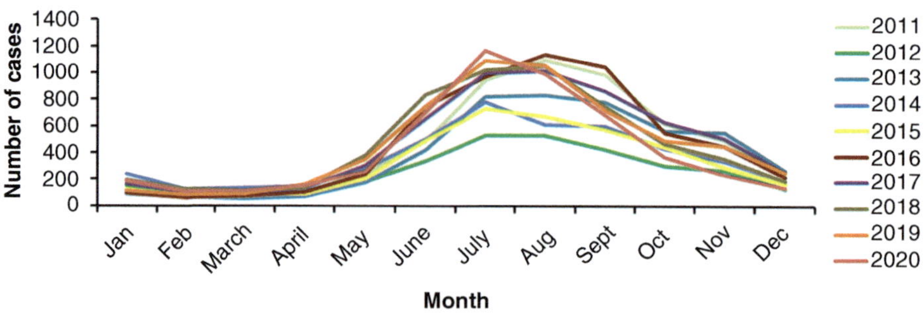

Fig. 8.1 Distribution of notified cases of Lyme borreliosis by month in 5 German federal state (Brandenburg, Mecklenburg-Vorpommern, Saxony-Anhalt, Saxony, Thuringia)

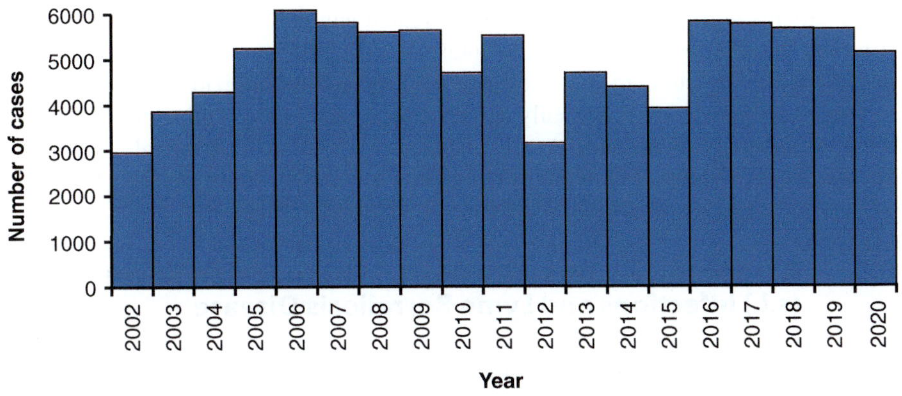

Fig. 8.2 Number of notified cases from 2002 to 2020 by year of notification in 5 German states (Brandenburg, Mecklenburg-Vorpommern, Saxony-Anhalt, Saxony, Thuringia)

for notification the infectious disease or pathogen should require action by the health authorities in relation to patients or disease outbreaks to prevent disease transmission. However, Lyme borreliosis is not contagious and cannot be transmitted from person to person. Furthermore, notification data are most meaningful when detailed information on individual patients and their clinical courses are available. But this creates a considerable administrative workload for the medical profession, for example, general practitioners, hospital doctors, and public health professionals, which in the view of the critics are not generally related to the scientific insights obtainable from analysis of notification data. In notification systems for Lyme borreliosis, it is important that clear-cut and comparable case definitions are used [9].

Information on the incidence of different Lyme borreliosis manifestations is best retrieved from epidemiological studies focusing on population incidence. These are difficult to setup and have rarely been conducted in Europe. A population-based study in southern Sweden in the 1990s showed an incidence of 69/100,000 inhabitants [10]. The most frequent clinical manifestation was erythema migrans (77%), 16% showed neuroborreliosis, and 7% Lyme arthritis. Another prospective, population-based study, in a south German city identified 313 cases of Lyme borreliosis over 12 months, corresponding to an incidence of 111 cases/100,000 inhabitants [11]. Altogether 89% of the patients showed classic erythema migrans, 3% an atypical disseminated erythema migrans, 2% a lymphocytoma, 3% early neuroborreliosis, and less than 1% Lyme carditis. Patients with late manifestations occurred in 5% (Lyme arthritis) and 1% (acrodermatitis chronica atrophicans). Patients with other manifestations were not found.

Secondary data analysis of health insurance data based on the International Classification of Diseases (ICD 10) coding and billings of doctors and hospitals leads to significantly higher case numbers in comparison to notification data. In a study in Germany, 214,000 billed case patients were estimated annually in Germany [12]. But the authors mention that this number might be overestimated due to clinical misdiagnosis or incorrect coding during the calculation. Another study estimated

7500 patients with Lyme borreliosis were treated annually in hospitals in Germany [6]. The same study calculated the total societal cost produced by hospitalized patients including direct medical cost and indirect medical cost (loss of productivity) as around 30 million euros annually in Germany. A study in the United States showed that the medical costs of Lyme borreliosis patients recorded in a medical claims database expenses averages nearly 3000 US dollars for each patient annually [13].

8.3 Associated Factors with Borrelia burgdorferi sensu lato (s.l.) Infections and Lyme Borreliosis Disease

The disease burden resulting from infections with *B. burgdorferi* s.l. varies strongly among population groups and geographical regions. Differences in incidence are the result of differences in the distribution of *Ixodes* ticks, the proportion of infected ticks, and the probability of human exposure to these infected ticks.

Data on the population distribution of the infection determined by serosurveys can be used as a surrogate for surveillance and provides population-representative estimates, not only for prevalence but also for factors associated with *B. burgdorferi* s.l. infections, although it always has to be kept in mind that infection (measured by antibodies) is not a disease, and manifestation-probability indices might differ between population groups. In this way, serosurveys were conducted in Germany in population-representative samples of children and adolescents as well as in adults (Fig. 8.3) [14, 15]. Especially high increases of seroprevalence by age can be shown in children and senior citizens (Fig. 8.4). Several studies, based on antibody prevalence, notification data, and health insurance data show that boys and men are much more affected by infection and Lyme borreliosis than girls and women [6, 8, 14]. Prevalence in the 14- to 17-year age group was already at 7%. In adults, the prevalence of *Borrelia* antibodies continues to rise. In the 70- to 79-year age group, 16.4% of adult women and 24.5% of adult men were seropositive. A similar distribution was found in other European countries such as Belgium [16], Sweden [17], Norway, [18], and Finland, [19].

It should be noted that IgG antibodies persist for more than 10 years. Therefore, the exact age at the time of infection cannot be determined by such an investigation, and the different seroprevalence rates in the age groups must be interpreted as a cumulative prevalence with an ascending curve as risk increases and a flat curve indicating a low risk. From Wilking et. al. [15, 20].

The increase in seroprevalence in the age-groups between 20 and 50 years is relatively low. This argues against Lyme borreliosis as a particular occupational medical problem, although studies focusing on occupational groups with obvious increased risk of exposure to ticks, such as forestry workers or farmers, have been reported to be at higher risks of infection [21].

People who reside in rural or small-town areas have a higher risk for *B. burgdorferi*-infections and for Lyme borreliosis, and residences in densely forested areas have previously been identified as a risk factor in the United States and Europe [14, 15,

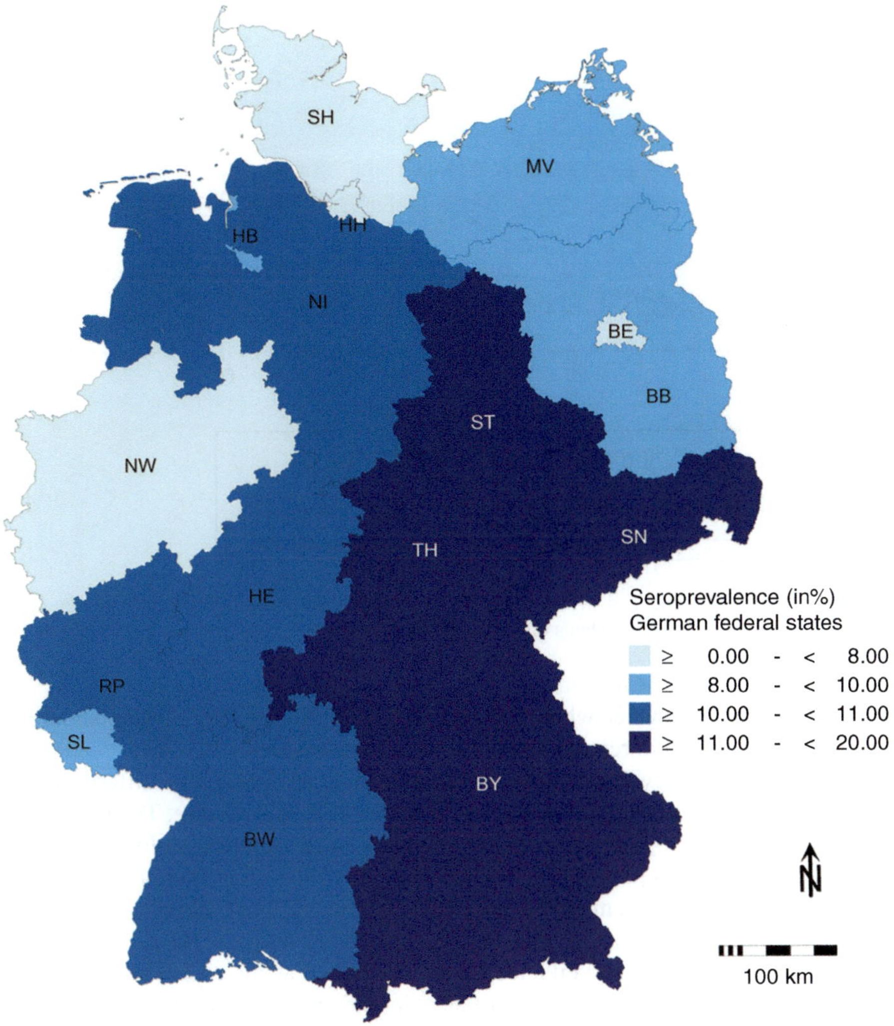

Fig. 8.3 Geographic distribution of representative seroprevalence estimates in adults (18–79 years) from 16 federal states of Germany

22–24]. In contrast, Lyme borreliosis risk is not absent in urban environments because *Borrelia*-infected ticks can be found in urban parks and private gardens in Europe [25–27]. In addition, rats (*Rattus norvegicus* and *Rattus rattus*) can function as reservoir hosts in urban areas. Studies in Sweden and France showed that the incidence of Lyme borreliosis can be significant in urban surroundings [10, 28].

Pet owners have long been regarded as a risk group and the focus has been mostly on dog walkers. However, data show that keeping cats is also a risk factor [14]. It is hypothesized that these animals become infested by ticks during the day, which then

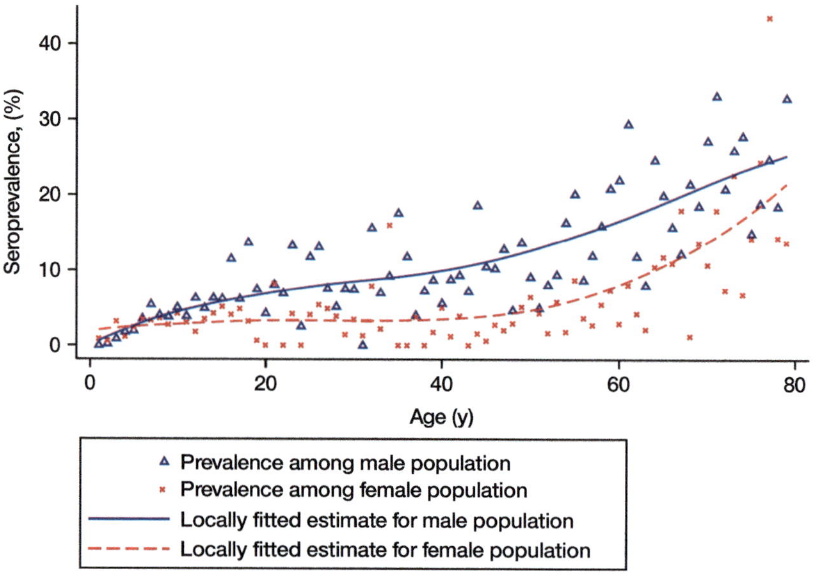

Fig. 8.4 Age and gender distribution of representative seroprevalance estimates in adults (18–79 years) from 16 federal states of Germany

transfers to the cat owner when the cat reenters the house. Pet owners should be specifically included in recommended prevention measures.

The analysis of surveillance data is ideal for illustration of spatial differences and geographic factors associated with the occurrence of Lyme disease. The local transmission of *B. burgdorferi* has been established in such disparate ecological areas as Dutch coastal regions [29, 30], forested highlands in Bavaria [5], and mountainous terrain (subalpine) with a mainly continental climate, such as Slovenia [31]. Despite this wide range, there is a characteristic heterogeneity between the regions and the districts in Europe and surveillance data can show that the risk is not uniformly distributed [5]. There is a large variance in the incidence of Lyme borreliosis between the European countries and regions [32, 33]. The highest reported incidence for Lyme borreliosis in Europe has been reported from Sweden with 464 erythema migrans patients per 100,000 inhabitants [34].

Schleswig-Holstein SH),Hamburg (HH), Lower Saxony (NI), Bremen (HB), North Rhine-Westphalia (NW), Hesse (HE), Rhineland-Palatinate (RP), Baden-Wurttemberg (BW), Bavaria (BY), Saarland (SL), Berlin (BE), Brandenburg (BB, Mecklenburg-Vorpommern (MV), Saxonia (SN), Saxonia-Anhalt (ST), Thuringia (TH).

Although epidemiological studies (including serosurveys) show heterogeneous risks of Lyme borreliosis in different geographic areas, it is undisputed that it is a widespread disease in many countries, and medical awareness and prevention measures must be taken seriously. Public health efforts in the fight against Lyme borreliosis are not necessarily in proportion to the exact number of disease cases each year. The infection may cause severe disease in some patients; however, the vast majority of cases present as erythema migrans and comparatively mild illnesses, which are easily treatable with antibiotics. A fatal outcome is very rare and only seen in Lyme carditis.

8.4 Disease Prevention Through Promotion of Tick-Bite Avoidance, Early Removal, and Awareness of Disease Symptoms

As far as is known all infections with *B. burgdorferi* s.l. are tick-borne. There are no well-documented medical reports of person-to-person transmission or blood-borne infections. Based on the biology it is conceivable that the pathogens are transmissible by blood transfusion, therefore Lyme borreliosis patients should not donate during the disease. Public health promotion should focus on tick-borne infections and aim to communicate these three items of information: (i) the ways to avoid tick bites, (ii) do's and don'ts in the removal of ticks, and (iii) knowledge of relevant symptoms of Lyme borreliosis and that the patient should seek medical care if symptoms consistent with the disease are observed.

The best personal action against Lyme borreliosis is avoidance of tick bites by preventing ticks from gaining access to the skin and by avoiding highly infested areas. Reducing exposure to ticks is one of the key public health intervention options promoted by public health agencies. Communicating that ticks are dangerous and may transmit serious infections is important, but overstatements and exaggeration should be avoided. Triggering fear in the general public might lead to irrational beliefs and behaviors of the population groups. For example, it is essential to communicate the likelihood of developing Lyme borreliosis following a tick bite, which, depending on the study and the geographical region, ranges from 0.3 to 1.4% [35–37].

The European Centre for Disease Prevention and Control (ECDC) recommendations include the wearing of long trousers and long-sleeved shirts as protective clothing [38]. Some institutions recommend tucking the socks into the trousers. The body should be checked periodically for ticks after being outdoors. Ticks prefer protected body sites such as the back of the knees or the armpits. Furthermore, they assemble on and around the scalp. The Centers for Disease Control and Prevention (CDC) recommends the application of a repellent from a specific list of active agents published on their website [39], among others permethrin on clothes and DEET on the body. It is important to communicate the limited period of protection and that products have to be chosen with a protection time that fits the duration of outdoor activity. Furthermore, it can be useful to recommend taking showers within 2 h after being outdoors. The water helps to wash off the ticks and washing is also a good opportunity to check for ticks.

Although documentaries and magazines dealing with outdoor activities promote these prevention measures, adherence to the recommendations by the public is rare. Presumably, people do not like to be reminded of such things during their leisure time or holidays. For reasons of convenience and personal style, people don't like to wear long trousers when it is hot outside. Daily evening showers and scanning for ticks are often omitted and during camping and long hiking tours is often not possible. Unfortunately, there is substantial evidence that even in high endemic regions and after years of promotion, compliance is poor [40, 41].

If a tick bite is experienced, the tick must be removed as quickly as possible. This timeliness is crucial and must be emphasized in the communication. The tick must feed for more than 12 h before the pathogen is transmitted and the risk of infection increases, depending on the study, after 12–36 h and become highest in 48–72 h after the bite [42, 43]. This "window of opportunity" for infectious disease control should be the keystone in any communication. But the time of onset of bite often cannot be determined by the bitten person or is even estimated to be shorter than it really is. Ticks should be removed with tweezers or fine-pointed forceps, grasping the tick close to the skin, pulling gently but straightforwardly upwards [44]. All manipulation of the tick beforehand (e.g. squeezing, suffocation with nail polish or glue) should be avoided [45]. The risk of infection with *B. burgdorferi* s.l. is not increased if tick mouthparts are left behind. A skin disinfectant can be applied after tick removal to prevent localized bacterial infection.

The results of tick testing for *B. burgdorferi* s.l. should not be used for decisions on treatment because positive results do not necessarily mean that the bitten persons are diseased or even infected. Negative results can lead to false assurance. Public health agencies do not recommend antimicrobial prophylaxis for the prevention of Lyme borreliosis after a recognized tick bite, as side effects are outweighed by the benefits in all but a very few instances [41, 46]. In some regions of the United States with extreme disease risk, single courses of doxycycline can have a positive risk–benefit ratio for some adult patients.

Good health-education material related to Lyme borreliosis is essential. In addition, for the control of Lyme borreliosis, local community-based approaches might be productive in raising education about disease symptoms and decreasing disease burden. There are often knowledge gaps in vulnerable and hard-to-reach groups that can be addressed by local stakeholders. For example, a Dutch study found that local scout groups are often not aware of infectious risks from ticks and do not regularly monitor young scouts [47]. A short training by stakeholders in environmental services (e.g. forest service) or the health sector (e.g. community healthcare workers) could readily fill these gaps. Special targeted communication for other vulnerable groups, for example, beekeepers or the geocaching community, are conceivable.

All in all, the fastest possible detection and removal of an attached tick is of great importance in the prevention of Lyme borreliosis. On the one hand, recommendations should result in a significant public health impact on the population in the reduction of infection exposure and disease. They should be strong enough that people see the relevance of the ticks for their health, and people should become confident to manage this risk by prompt tick removal. On the other hand, exaggerated messages might result in opposite effects. People lose confidence, become anxious, postpone tick removal before seeing a doctor or wait to purchase instruments until the next drugstore opening time.

8.5 Disease Prevention by Vaccination

A vaccine was marketed in the United States from 1998 to 2002. After three doses it was shown to be highly effective with only moderate side effects in the vaccinated persons [48–49]. It was removed from the market because of low acceptance in the US population and among doctors. Additionally, some groups suspected the vaccine to be associated with autoimmune reactions [50, 51]. In Europe, no licensed vaccine has ever reached the market. Because of the heterogeneity of *Borrelia* strains, it is more difficult to develop an effective vaccine for Europe [52–54]. However, new vaccine candidates are under development in both Europe [55, 56] and the United States [57].

8.6 Lyme Controversy, Evidence-Based Approaches to Both Public Health and the Practice of Medicine

In the current medical and societal contexts, Lyme borreliosis is not only a medical issue but also a societal problem and a subject of public controversy. Over the last 20 years, a considerable controversy has developed about Lyme borreliosis among medical societies, the medical scientific community, and evidence-based medicine on the one hand and some Lyme borreliosis activist groups and associations of physicians who claim to be experts in the diagnosis and treatment of patients (so-called "Lyme literate medical doctors" (LLMDs) on the other hand [58]. Among the latter groups some believe, unsupported by scientific evidence, that infections with *B. burgdorferi* s.l. can cause symptoms even in the absence of objective signs of Lyme borreliosis [59]. Furthermore, they allege that treatment with antibiotics and other therapeutics is efficient only if prescribed for months or years to suppress the symptoms of Lyme borreliosis. Diagnostic tests are often claimed to be falsely negative. People who experience suffering because of their symptoms are hastily assigned the diagnosis of Lyme disease and are thus prevented from receiving their actual correct diagnosis which is also a public health problem. Lyme borreliosis activist groups believe that due to the abovementioned circumstances the incidence of Lyme borreliosis is heavily underestimated by surveillance systems and is in reality a real plague for the masses. They have developed a significant international movement, and maintain a high level of pressure on health authorities, policymakers, and the medical scientific community. The dispute between the two groups is bitter and far from being resolved.

In several countries, such as the Netherlands, France, the United Kingdom, Belgium, and Germany, systematic reviews of the literature have been carried out. This research should be further developed into comprehensive, up-to-date information in centers of peer-reviewed information on Lyme borreliosis. The provision of public education in trustable access points related to Lyme borreliosis and the strong connection to medical scientific research might help to improve knowledge about this disease in the population. Additionally, health professionals have to be educated on the latest Lyme borreliosis research and resulting treatment options. The development of safe and effective vaccines against Lyme borreliosis and their roll out must be preceded by preparation of the public in order to increase the acceptance of a vaccine. Overall this might result in less disease burden and fewer misdiagnoses and misclassifications of the disease.

References

1. Nelson KE, Williams CM. Infectious disease epidemiology : theory and practice. 3rd ed. Burlington, Mass.: Jones & Bartlett Learning; 2014. xviii, 963 p. p.
2. CDC. Centers for Disease Control and Prevention (CDC): Public health surveillance. Available: https://www.cdc.gov/training/publichealth101/surveillance.html. Last access: June 6, 2021. 2018.
3. CDC. Centers for Disease Prevention and Control (CDC). Summary of notifiable infectious diseases and conditions-United States. Morb Mortal Weekly Report (MMWR). 2014;63(54):1–152.
4. Rizzoli A, Hauffe HC, Carpi G, Vourc'h GI, Neteler M, Rosà R. Lyme borreliosis in Europe. Euro Surveill. 2011, 2011;16(27) pii=19906
5. Enkelmann J, Böhmer M, Fingerle V, Siffczyk C, Werber D, Littmann M, et al. Incidence of notified Lyme borreliosis in Germany, 2013–2017. Sci Rep. 2018;8(1):14976.
6. Lohr B, Müller I, Norris DE, Schöffski O, Hunfeld K-P. Epidemiology and cost of hospital care for Lyme borreliosis in Germany: lessons from a health care utilization database analysis. Ticks Tick-Borne Dis. 2015;6:56–62.
7. Vandenesch A, Turbelin C, Couturier E, Arena C, Jaulhac B, Ferquel E, et al. Incidence and hospitalisation rates of Lyme borreliosis, France, 2004 to 2012. Euro Surveill. 2014;19(34) pii=20883
8. Wilking H, Stark K. Trends in surveillance data on human Lyme borreliosis from six federal states in eastern Germany, 2009-2012. Ticks Tick-Borne Dis. 2014;5:219–24.
9. Stanek G, Fingerle V, Hunfeld KP, Jaulhac B, Kaiser R, Krause A, et al. Lyme borreliosis: clinical case definitions for diagnosis and management in Europe. Clin Microbiol Infect. 2011;17(1):69–79.
10. Berglund J, Eitrem R, Ornstein K, al e. An epidemiological study of Lyme disease in southern Sweden. N Engl J Med. 1995;1995(333):1319–27.
11. Huppertz H, Böhme M, Standaert S, Karch H, Plotkin S. Incidence of Lyme borreliosis in the Würzburg region of Germany. Eur J Clin Microbiol Infect Dis. 1999;18:697–703.
12. Müller I, Freitag MH, Poggensee G, Scharnetzky E, Straube E, Schoerner C, et al. Evaluating frequency, diagnostic quality and cost of Lyme borreliosis testing in Germany: a retrospective model analysis. Clin Dev Immunol. 2012:595427. https://doi.org/10.1155/2012/595427.
13. Adrion ER, Aucott J, Lemke KW, Weiner JP. Health care costs, utilization and patterns of care following Lyme disease. PLoS One. 2015;10(2):e0116767.
14. Dehnert M, Fingerle V, Klier C, Talaska T, Schlaud M, Krause G, et al. Seropositivity of Lyme borreliosis and associated risk factors: a population-based study in children and adolescents in Germany (KIGSS). PLoS One. 2012;7(8):e41321. https://doi.org/10.1371/journalpone0041321.
15. Wilking H, Fingerle V, Klier C, Thamm M, Stark K. Antibodies against *Borrelia burgdorferi* sensu lato among adults, Germany, 2008–2011. Emerg Infect Dis. 2015;21(1):107–10.
16. De Keukeleire M, Vanwambeke SO, Cochez C, Heyman P, Fretin D, Deneys V, et al. Seroprevalence of *Borrelia burgdorferi*, *Anaplasma phagocytophilum*, and *Francisella tularensis* infections in Belgium: results of three population-based samples. Vector Borne Zoonotic Dis (Larchmont, NY). 2017;17(2):108–15.

17. Johansson M, Manfredsson L, Wistedt A, Serrander L, Tjernberg I. Significant variations in the seroprevalence of C6 ELISA antibodies in a highly endemic area for Lyme borreliosis: evaluation of age, sex and seasonal differences. APMIS. 2017;125(5):476–81.
18. Vestrheim DF, White RA, Aaberge IS, Aase A. Geographical differences in seroprevalence of *Borrelia burgdorferi* antibodies in Norway, 2011–2013. Ticks Tick-Borne Dis. 2016;7(5):698–702.
19. van Beek J, Sajanti E, Helve O, Ollgren J, Virtanen MJ, Rissanen H, et al. Population-based *Borrelia burgdorferi* sensu lato seroprevalence and associated risk factors in Finland. Ticks Tick-Borne Dis. 2018;9(2):275–80.
20. Wilking H, Dehnert M, Fingerle V, Klier C, Talaska T, Schlaud M, et al. Seroprävalenz der Lyme-Borreliose bei Kindern und Jugendlichen in Deutschland. Epidemiol Bull Nr 14, 10 April 2012. 2012.
21. Jurke A, Bannert N, Brehm K, Fingerle V, Kempf VA, Kompf D, et al. Serological survey of *Bartonella* spp., *Borrelia burgdorferi*, *Brucella* spp., *Coxiella burnetii*, *Francisella tularensis*, *Leptospira* spp., *Echinococcus*, Hanta-, TBE- and XMR-virus infection in employees of two forestry enterprises in North Rhine-Westphalia, Germany, 2011–2013. Int J Med Microbiol. 2015;305(7):652–62.
22. Glass GE, Schwartz BS, Morgan JM 3rd, Johnson DT, Noy PM, Israel E. Environmental risk factors for Lyme disease identified with geographic information systems. Am J Public Health. 1995;85(7):944–8.
23. Linard C, Lamarque P, Heyman P, Ducoffre G, Luyasu V, Tersago K, et al. Determinants of the geographic distribution of Puumala virus and Lyme borreliosis infections in Belgium. Int J Health Geogr. 2007;6:15.
24. Woudenberg T, Bohm S, Bohmer M, Katz K, Willrich N, Stark K, et al. Dynamics of *Borrelia burgdorferi*-specific antibodies: seroconversion and seroreversion between two population-based, cross-sectional surveys among adults in Germany. Microorganisms. 2020;8(12)
25. Guy EC, Farquhar RG. *Borrelia burgdorferi* in urban parks. Lancet (London, England). 1991;338(8761):253.
26. Junttila J, Peltomaa M, Soini H, Marjamaki M, Viljanen MK. Prevalence of *Borrelia burgdorferi* in *Ixodes ricinus* ticks in urban recreational areas of Helsinki. J Clin Microbiol. 1999;37(5):1361–5.
27. Maetzel D, Maier WA, Kampen H. *Borrelia burgdorferi* infection prevalences in questing *Ixodes ricinus* ticks (Acari: Ixodidae) in urban and suburban Bonn, western Germany. Parasitol Res. 2005;95(1):5–12.
28. Letrilliart L, Ragon B, Hanslik T, Flahault A. Lyme disease in France: a primary care-based prospective study. Epidemiol Infect. 2005;133(5):935–42.
29. Hofhuis A, Bennema S, Harms M, van Vliet AJH, Takken W, van den Wijngaard CC, et al. Decrease in tick bite consultations and stabilization of early Lyme borreliosis in the Netherlands in 2014 after 15 years of continuous increase. BMC Public Health. 2016;16(425):2016.
30. Hofhuis A, Harms M, van Wijngaard C, Sprong H, van Pelt W. Continuing increase of tick bites of Lyme disease between 1994 and 2009. Ticks Tick-Borne Dis. 2015;6(2015):69–74.
31. Strle F. Lyme borreliosis in Slovenia. Zentralblatt fur Bakteriologie: Int J Med Microbiol. 1999;289(5–7):643–52.
32. de Mik E, van Pelt W, Docters-van Leeuwen B, van der Veen A, Schellekens JFP, Borgdorff MW. The geographical distribution of tick bites and erythema migrans in general practice in the Netherlands. Int J Epidemiol. 1997;26(2):451–7.
33. Sykes RA, Makiello P. An estimate of Lyme borreliosis incidence in Western Europe. J Public Health. 2016:1–8. https://doi.org/10.1093/pubmed/fdw017.
34. Bennet L, Halling A, Berglund J. Increased incidence of Lyme borreliosis in southern Sweden following mild winters and during warm, humid summers. Eur J Clin Microbiol Infect Dis. 2006;25(7):426–32.
35. Heininger U, Zimmermann T, Schoerner C, Brade V, Stehr K. Tick bite and Lyme borreliosis. An epidemiologic study in the Erlangen area. Monatsschr Kinderheilkd. 1993;141(11):874–7.

36. Maiwald M, Oehme R, March O, Petney TN, Kimmig P, Naser K, et al. Transmission risk of *Borrelia burgdorferi* sensu lato from *Ixodes ricinus* ticks to humans in southwest Germany. Epidemiol Infect. 1998;121(1):103–8.
37. Nahimana I, Gern L, Blanc DS, Praz G, Francioli P, Peter O. Risk of *Borrelia burgdorferi* infection in western Switzerland following a tick bite. Eur J Clin Microbiol Infect Dis. 2004;23(8):603–8.
38. ECDC. European Centre for Disease Prevention and Control (ECDC). Factsheet on Lyme borreliosis, for healthcare professionals. Available from: https://ecdc.europa.eu/en/publications-data/factsheet-lyme-borreliosis-healthcare-professionals. Last access: June 6, 2021. 2015.
39. CDC. Centers for Disease Prevention and Control (CDC). Preventing tick bites 2018. Available from: https://www.cdc.gov/ticks/avoid/on_people.html. Last access: June 6, 2021. 2020;63(54):152.
40. Gould LH, Nelson RS, Griffith KS, Hayes EB, Piesman J, Mead PS, et al. Knowledge, attitudes, and behaviors regarding Lyme disease prevention among Connecticut residents, 1999–2004. Vector Borne and Zoonotic Dis(Larchmont, NY). 2008;8(6):769–76.
41. Hayes EB, Piesman J. How can we prevent Lyme disease? N Engl J Med. 2003;2003(348):2424–30.
42. Kahl O, Janetzki C, Gray JS, Stein J, Bauch RJ. Tick infection rates with *Borrelia*: *Ixodes ricinus* versus *Haemaphysalis concinna* and *Dermacentor reticulatus* in two locations in eastern Germany. Med Vet Entomol. 1992;6(4):363–6.
43. Piesman J, Mather TN, Sinsky RJ, Spielman A. Duration of tick attachment and *Borrelia burgdorferi* transmission. J Clin Microbiol. 1987;25(3):557–8.
44. ECfDPaC (ECDC). Factsheet on Lyme borreliosis, for healthcare professionals 2018. Available from: https://ecdc.europa.eu/en/publications-data/factsheet-lyme-borreliosis-healthcare-professionals.
45. Kahl O, Janetzki-Mittmann C, Gray JS, Jonas R, Stein J, de Boer R. Risk of infection with *Borrelia burgdorferi* sensu lato for a host in relation to the duration of nymphal *Ixodes ricinus* feeding and the method of tick removal. Zentralblatt fur Bakteriologie : Int J Med Microbiol. 1998;287(1–2):41–52.
46. Stanek G, Kahl O. Chemoprophylaxis for Lyme borreliosis? Zentralblatt fur Bakteriologie : Int J Med Microbiol. 1999;289(5–7):655–65.
47. ECDC. European Centre for Disease Prevention and Control (ECDC). Synergies in community and institutional public health emergency preparedness for tick-borne diseases in the Netherlands; 2018.
48. CDC. Centers for Disease Prevention and Control (CDC). Availability of Lyme disease vaccine. MMWR Morb Mortal Weekly Rep. 1999;48(2):35–6. 43
49. Poland GA, Jacobson RM. The prevention of Lyme disease with vaccine. Vaccine. 2001;19(17–19):2303–8.
50. Poland GA. Vaccines against Lyme disease: What happened and what lessons can we learn? Clin Infect Dis. 2011;52(Suppl 3):s253–8.
51. Aronowitz RA. The rise and fall of the Lyme disease vaccines: a cautionary tale for risk interventions in American medicine and public health. Milbank Q. 2012;90(2):250–77.
52. Comstedt P, Hanner M, Schuler W, Meinke A, Lundberg U. Design and development of a novel vaccine for protection against Lyme borreliosis. PLoS One. 2014;9(11):e113294.
53. Livey I, O'Rourke M, Traweger A, Savidis-Dacho H, Crowe BA, Barrett PN, et al. A new approach to a Lyme disease vaccine. Clin Infect Dis. 2011;52(Suppl. 3):s266–70.
54. Shen AK, Mead PS, Beard CB. The Lyme disease vaccine--a public health perspective. Clin Infect Dis. 2011;52(Suppl. 3):s247–52.
55. Wressnigg N, Barrett PN, Pollabauer EM, O'Rourke M, Portsmouth D, Schwendinger MG, et al. A Novel multivalent OspA vaccine against Lyme borreliosis is safe and immunogenic in an adult population previously infected with *Borrelia burgdorferi* sensu lato. Clin Vaccine Immunol. 2014;21(11):1490–9.

56. Wressnigg N, Pollabauer EM, Aichinger G, Portsmouth D, Low-Baselli A, Fritsch S, et al. Safety and immunogenicity of a novel multivalent OspA vaccine against Lyme borreliosis in healthy adults: a double-blind, randomised, dose-escalation phase 1/2 trial. Lancet Infect Dis. 2013;13(8):680–9.
57. Stanley A, Plotkin MD. Need for a new Lyme disease vaccine. N Engl J Med. 2016;375(10):911–3.
58. Auwaerter PG, Bakken JS, Dattwyler RJ, Dumler JS, Halperin JJ, McSweegan E, et al. Antiscience and ethical concerns associated with advocacy of Lyme disease. Lancet Infect Dis. 2011;11(9):713–9.
59. Tonks A. Lyme wars. BMJ (Clin Res Ed). 2007;335(7626):910–2.

Other *Ixodes*-Borne Diseases 9

Pierre H. Boyer, Antoine Grillon, Benoît Jaulhac,
Aurélie Velay, Frédéric Schramm,
and Emilie Talagrand-Reboul

9.1 Introduction

Ticks are the most important vectors in the northern hemisphere in human and veterinary medicine [1], and Lyme borreliosis is the most frequent tick-borne disease. In addition to *Borrelia burgdorferi* sensu lato (s.l.), the causative agent of Lyme borreliosis, they can harbor many microorganisms [2]. Some of these microorganisms can be transmitted to humans and may cause disease. Fever is the most frequent symptom associated with other tick-related pathogens in Europe, in contrast to Lyme borreliosis, which causes less fever. In addition to fever, some symptoms are more specific to a particular infectious agent.

In this chapter, we review some ecological, epidemiological, and clinical aspects of the main microorganisms, apart from *B. burgdorferi* s.l., known to be transmitted

P. H. Boyer · A. Grillon · F. Schramm · E. Talagrand-Reboul (✉)
University of Strasbourg, Hôpitaux Universitaires de Strasbourg, Faculté de Médecine, Fédération de Médecine Translationnelle de Strasbourg, UR7290 Early Bacterial Virulence, Strasbourg, France
e-mail: pierreboyer@unistra.fr; a.grillon@unistra.fr; fredericschramm@unistra.fr; talagrandreboul@unistra.fr

B. Jaulhac
University of Strasbourg, Hôpitaux Universitaires de Strasbourg, Faculté de Médecine, Fédération de Médecine Translationnelle de Strasbourg, UR7290 Early Bacterial Virulence, Strasbourg, France

French National Reference Center for Borrelia, Hôpitaux Universitaires de Strasbourg, Strasbourg, France
e-mail: jaulhac@unistra.fr

A. Velay
Virology Laboratory, Hôpitaux Universitaires de Strasbourg, Strasbourg, France
e-mail: aurelie.velay@chru-strasbourg.fr

K.-P. Hunfeld, J. Gray (eds.), *Lyme Borreliosis*,
https://doi.org/10.1007/978-3-030-93680-8_9

by *Ixodes* ticks in Europe: *B. miyamotoi*, *Anaplasma phagocytophilum*, *Candidatus* Neoehrlichia mikurensis, *Rickettsia monacensis*, *Rickettsia helvetica, Francisella tularensis*, human babesiosis, and the ixodid-borne flaviviruses (Table 9.1).

9.2 *Borrelia miyamotoi*

Relapsing fever (RF) *Borrelia* are usually associated with lice and soft ticks in Africa, America, and Asia; about 20 species have been validated and additional taxa are also proposed. However, three species of RF-*Borrelia* are transmitted by hard ticks and so are called Hard Tick-Borne Relapsing Fevers (HTBRF). *B. theileri* was observed at the beginning of the 20th century by Laveran in the blood of livestock [3] and *Rhipicephalus* spp. ticks are vectors of this bacterium. *B. lonestari* has been described in *Amblyoma americanum* ticks and was initially suspected in the Southern Tick-Associated Rash Illness (STARI), but the evidence is lacking concerning the implication of this bacterium in this syndrome [4]. Finally, *B. miyamotoi* is probably the most discussed HTBRF *Borrelia* species; indeed this species was discovered in Japan in the mid 1990s in the ticks (*I. persulcatus*) and rodents (*Apodemus argenteus*) [5] and has subsequently been described in ticks belonging to the *Ixodes* genus in the Holarctic region [6]. This bacterium is, up to now, the only relapsing fever known to share the same *Ixodes* vectors as the bacteria of the *B. burgdorferi* s.l. group. Interest in this bacterium has grown since 2011 with the publication of a series of 46 Russian human cases [7] and more recently a few cases of meningoencephalitis [8–11].

9.2.1 Bacterial Features

The taxonomy of the *Borrelia* genus is currently debated [12] since the proposal by Adeolu and Gupta [13] to split the genera into two: namely *Borreliella* for the bacteria responsible for the Lyme disease, leaving the name *Borrelia* for the relapsing fever spirochetes. In this last group or genus and based on several genes (glycerophosphodiester phosphodiesterase (GlpQ), 16S rDNA, flagellin), *B. miyamotoi* clusters with the other HTBRF (*B. lonestari* and *B. theileri*).

Comparisons within the species revealed a genetic diversity for *B. miyamotoi*. Indeed, three separate clades following the geographic distribution were described [14]: the Asian (aka Siberian) type, the European, and the American type, respectively, transmitted by *I. persulcatus* and *I. pavlovskyi* (*I. ovatus*); *I. ricinus* ; *I. scapularis* and *I. pacificus*. Sequence variations have recently been described based on the sequencing of the *16S rRNA* gene in the Asian and American clades [15, 16]. Future genomic studies will be of interest to better understand *B. miyamotoi* evolutionary history and host/pathogen interaction.

Table 9.1 Key clinical and epidemiological features of human *Ixodes*-borne diseases other than Lyme borreliosis

Micro-organism	Disease	Tick vector	Main reservoir hosts	Other modes of contamination	Geographical features	Main symptoms of the disease	Fatality rate	Additional clinical/ biological features	Diagnostic strategy	Treatment
Bacteria										
B. miyamotoi	*B. miyamotoi* disease (BMD)	*I. ricinus complex*	Partially known, include: wood mice (*Apodemus* spp.), the bank vole (*M. glareolus*)	—	Temperate regions of North America, Europe & Asia	Flu-like syndrome (fever, malaise, myalgia…) which can relapse without treatment Rare cases of meningoencephalitis described	—	Elevated liver enzymes, CPK elevated. Thrombopenia and leukopenia observed in some patients	PCR on a whole blood during the febrile episode or on CSF when neurological manifestations. Serology	Ceftriaxone or Doxycycline
A. phagocytophilum	Human granulocytic anaplasmosis (HGA)	*I. ricinus complex*	Micromammals (rodents, insectivores), Large mammals (cervids, wild boar)	Blood transfusion (rare), mother-to-child (rare)	North America, Europe, Eastern Asia	Flu-like syndrome (fever, malaise, myalgia…) ± rash Complications (elderly, IC patients): septic shock, hemorrhage, multi-organ failure (heart, lungs, kidneys, liver), opportunistic infections	<1%	Anemia, thrombopenia, leucopenia, elevated liver enzymes, CRP	PCR on whole blood sampled before antibiotic administration Serology: anti-Ap IgG (IFA) with seroconversion or ≥4-fold increase in the antibody titre	Doxycycline, Rifampin
Candidatus N. mikurensis	Neoehrlichiosis	*I. ricinus, I. persulcatus*	Poorly known, include: wood mice (*Apodemus* spp.), the bank vole (*M. glareolus*)	—	Temperate regions of Europe & Asia (not described in North America)	Flu-like syndrome (fever, malaise, myalgia…) which can last for weeks Thromboembolic events in immunocompromised patients	—	Elevated white blood cell counts, increase level of inflammatory markers (CRP), elevated liver enzymes	PCR on a whole blood, no serology available	Doxycycline

(continued)

Table 9.1 (continued)

Micro-organism	Disease	Tick vector	Main reservoir hosts	Other modes of contamination	Geographical features	Main symptoms of the disease	Fatality rate	Additional clinical/biological features	Diagnostic strategy	Treatment
R. helvetica	—	*I. ricinus*	Unknown with precision. Tick itself could be a reservoir	—	Western Europe (one report from Turkey)	Febrile syndrome	Few case reports with a fatal outcome	—	PCR on whole blood Serology	Doxycycline
R. monacensis	—	*I. ricinus*	Unknown with precision	—	Western Europe	Febrile syndrome	—	—		
F. tularensis	Tularaemia	*D. andersoni* *D. variabilis* *A. americanum*	Lagomorphs, Small rodents	Inoculation by other arthropods. Direct transmission. Transmission from contaminated water or soil	Temperate regions of North America, Europe & Asia	Flu-like syndrome, other manifestations depend on the route of infection (Inoculation eschar Lymphadenopathy Oropharyngeal form Conjunctivitis…)	Without treatment mortality 8% with type A (USA) depending on the clinical form	Elevated leukocyte count, increase level of inflammatory markers	Blood culture or culture and PCR of a lesion if present. Serology	Doxycycline Fluoroquinolones Gentamicin
Parasites										
Babesia microti (Bm)	Human babesiosis	*I. ricinus* complex	Small rodents	Blood transfusion, mother-to-child (rare)	US, Europe, Asia	Flu-like syndrome (fever, malaise, myalgia…), hemolytic anemia Severe cases (splenectomized, IC patients, elderly): anemia, thrombopenia, hemorrhage, multi-organ failure (heart, lungs, kidneys, liver)	~5%	Hemolytic anemia, thrombopenia	Blood smear PCR on whole blood (species typing) Species specific serology: IgG (IFA) with high titre, positive immunoblot, seroconversion or ≥4-fold increase in the antibody titre	Atovaquone + azithromycin Quinine + clindamycin

Babesia divergens (Bd)	Human babesiosis	*I. ricinus*	Cattle	—	Europe	Mild to severe cases in splenectomised/ hyposplenic patients	>30%	Hemolytic anemia, thrombopenia		
Babesia venatorum (Bv)	Human babesiosis	*I. ricinus* complex	Roe deer	—	Europe, Asia	Mild to severe cases in splenectomized/ hyposplenic patients	5–30%	Hemolytic anemia, thrombopenia	Blood smear PCR on whole blood (species typing)	
									(Serology: no commercial kit, possible cross-reactions with *Bd* serological tests)	
Viruses										
Tick-Borne Encephalitis virus (TBEV) 3 variants: European (Eu), Siberian (Sib), Far Eastern (FE)	Tick-Borne Encephalitis (TBE)	*I. ricinus* (Eu-TBEV) *I. persulcatus* (Sib-TBEV, FE-TBEV)	Voles and mice	unpasteurized dairy products	Europe, Central and South-Eastern Asia	Prodromal phase: Flu-like syndrome (fever, headache, muscle pains…)	FE-TBEV 5–20% Eu-TBEV, Sib-TBEV ~2%	CSF lymphocytosis, increased proteinorrhachia, normal glycorrhachia	Serology: - Blood: anti-TBEV IgM+IgG (EIA) with the two isotypes positive,	Symptomatic
						acute phase (1/3): severe neurological illness (meningitis, encephalitis, meningoencephalitis)			seroconversion or ≥4-fold increase in the antibody titer	
									-CSF: IgM	(prevention: vaccine)
									(PCR on blood at the prodromal phase)	

(continued)

Table 9.1 (continued)

Micro-organism	Disease	Tick vector	Main reservoir hosts	Other modes of contamination	Geographical features	Main symptoms of the disease	Fatality rate	Additional clinical/biological features	Diagnostic strategy	Treatment
Louping-Ill virus (LIV)	Louping-ill	*I. ricinus*	British red grouse, sheep, mountain hares	Exposure to infected tissues (aerosols)	British Isles	Prodromal phase: Flu-like syndrome	rarely	—	Serology: no commercial kit, cross-reactions with TBEV serological tests	Symptomatic
						Acute phase (facultative): severe neurological illness				
Powassan virus (POWV)	Powassan	*I. scapularis* (*I. cookie*, I. *marxei*)	Rodents, mustelids, lagomorphs	—	Northern America, Far-Eastern Russia	Prodromal phase: Flu-like syndrome ± erythematous rash	10% in neuroinvasive illness	CSF lymphocytosis, increased proteinorrhachia, normal glycorrhachia	Serology: Blood: anti-POWV IgM+IgG (EIA) with seroconversion, ≥4-fold increase in the antibody titer or specific IgM confirmed after neutralizing antibody testing	Symptomatic
						Acute phase: severe neurological illness			- CSF: IgM	
									(PCR on blood at the prodromal phase, on CSF at the acute phase)	

Ap *Anaplasma phagocytophilum*, Bd *Babesia divergens*, Bm *Babesia microti*, Bv *Babesia venatorum*, CRP C-reactive protein, CSF Cerebrospinal fluid, IC Immunocompromised, IFA Immunofluorescence assay, LIV Louping-Ill virus, PCR Polymerase chain reaction, POWV Powassan virus, TBE Tick-Borne Encephalitis, TBEV Tick-Borne Encephalitis virus

9.2.2 Ecology

Little is known about *B. miyamotoi* reservoir hosts. This spirochete displays some characteristics in common with *B. burgdorferi* s.l., and it has been hypothesized that these bacteria share the same reservoir hosts. Indeed, Wagemakers et al. [17] showed by compiling several studies that there is a positive correlation between the infection rate of *B. burgdorferi* s.l. in ticks and the infection rate of *B. miyamotoi*. As ticks can feed on several hosts, *B. miyamotoi* DNA has been found in several animals from small rodents to birds and in ticks collected on wild boar (*Sus scrofa*) and roe deer (*Capreolus capreolus*) in North America, Japan, and Europe [17]. However, importantly, Kahl et al. [18] differentiate carrier hosts from reservoir hosts. Carrier hosts are hosts that harbor a particular pathogen for at least a short period but are not necessarily infective for ticks, whereas reservoir hosts are proven natural hosts of vector ticks, and ticks may become infected while feeding on them [18]. In view of these definitions, only a few animals have been experimentally proven to be reservoir hosts: the wood mouse (*Apodemus* spp.), the bank vole (*M. glareolus*) [19], and the white-footed mouse (*Peromyscus leucopus*) [20]. It has also been shown that domestic ruminants do not seem to eliminate *B. miyamotoi* from ticks [21], which may therefore have a role in its dissemination, contrary to what is observed for the bacteria of the *B. burgdorferi* s.l. group. However, the rate of transmission is too low for ticks to be the only reservoir. It should be noted that, in early reports, *B. miyamotoi* had probably been observed instead of *B. burgdorferi* s.l. in larvae [22, 23]. It has also been shown that *I. ricinus* larvae could transmit *B. miyamotoi* in a mouse model [24], suggesting that transovarial transmission of *B. miyamotoi* may occur.

9.2.3 Epidemiology

B. miyamotoi has been reported in tick vectors in the northern hemisphere, especially ticks of the *I. ricinus* complex which are known to transmit the *B. burgdorferi* s.l. complex. Indeed, the distribution of *B. miyamotoi* seems to overlap the distribution of the main species responsible for Lyme borreliosis [17]. The prevalence of ticks carrying *B. miyamotoi* is low even in areas where the disease is endemic [7, 25]. The median prevalence is 1.5% (minimum: 0–maximum: 6.4%) [7, 17].

Serological studies revealed that *B. miyamotoi* seropositivity in blood donors of the Netherlands is 2% (95% CI 0.4–5.7%) and is higher in the forestry worker population (10% (5.3–16.8%)) and in patients suspected of anaplasmosis (14.6% (9.0–21.8%)) [26]. In the United States, other serological studies showed a similar prevalence of antibodies against *B. miyamotoi* in a healthy population: 3.9% [27]. Collectively, these results suggest that humans are exposed to *B. miyamotoi* to a lesser extent compared with *B. burgdorferi* s.l. but can develop disease under certain conditions.

9.2.4 Clinical Manifestations

The typical symptomatic *B. miyamotoi* disease (BMD) was described first in Russia in 2011 [7], in America [28] and Japan [29]. More recently, some cases were identified in China [30] and in Western Europe [31, 32]. It is an acute, febrile, and viral-like syndrome occurring approximately 2 weeks after a tick bite. Without treatment, relapses (one or more) can occur in up to 11% of the patients in the Russian case series [7]. Other symptoms including headache, arthralgia, chills, myalgia, malaise, and fatigue were also observed. BMD and Human Granulocytic Anaplasmosis (HGA) have a similar clinical presentation and should be the subject of differential diagnosis. Interestingly, a patient with an asymptomatic infection proven by specific PCR was found in Austria [33].

In 2013, two cases of meningoencephalitis due to BMD were reported initially in immunocompromised patients [9, 10], another case was then diagnosed in Germany [8], and two cases more recently in Sweden [11]. The first three cases of meningoencephalitis cases appeared to show common characteristics, indeed patients were treated for non-Hodgkin lymphoma with a CHOP protocol (cyclophosphamide, doxorubicin, vincristine, and prednisolone), they were also treated with rituximab, an anti-CD20 monoclonal antibody. Interestingly, lymphocytic pleocytosis in cerebrospinal fluid (CSF) with elevated protein was observed in the three cases, as for Lyme neuroborreliosis. A slight difference was found between the three cases of *B. miyamotoi* neuroborreliosis, indeed the German case developed a more acute form than the two other cases. In Sweden, one of the two cases was also treated with rituximab (for rheumatoid arthritis), but very interestingly the other one was apparently immunocompetent [11]. As observed in the other relapsing fevers, *B. miyamotoi* exhibits neurotropism, but this seems to be expressed under particular immunosuppression conditions.

9.2.5 Laboratory Diagnosis

To date, PCR and serology have been the two diagnostic approaches, depending upon the stage and duration of infection. Antigens such as glycerophosphoryl diester phosphodiesterase (GlpQ) have proven useful, being possessed by relapsing fever members of the genus but not by the Lyme borreliosis-associated species [34]. Consequently, the serological assays based on GlpQ target all the relapsing fever *Borrelia,* but *B. miyamotoi* is the only described HTBRF species in the Northern hemisphere transmitted by the *Ixodes* genus. This sero-marker does not seem to be sensitive enough to diagnose all cases [28]. These results were confirmed by a more recent study showing the low specificity and sensitivity of GlpQ for *B. miyamotoi* diagnosis [35].

The variable major proteins (Vmps) of *B. miyamotoi* have been explored as potential antigens for serodiagnosis [36]. Interestingly, the combination of both GlpQ and a cocktail of highly immunogenic Vmps has been recently evaluated in a cohort of 182 Russian patients [37]. The sensitivity was determined to be 94.7% and the specificity 96.6% for IgM from 11 to 20 days after the disease onset. The C6

ELISA used for Lyme borreliosis diagnosis may also be interesting since it is positive in patients infected by *B. miyamotoi*, and the similarity between the C6 part of VlsE and the *B. miyamotoi* Vmps could be the basis of this cross-reactivity [38]. A new antigen has recently been described for the serodiagnosis of *B. miyamotoi*: *Borrelia* membrane antigen A (BmaA) [39, 40] which needs to be evaluated using a large cohort of patients.

During the febrile episode, molecular-based tests are prime of interest. Real-time PCR assays have been widely described based on the 16s rDNA or the flagellin gene [17]. However, the spirochetemia of *B. miyamotoi* seems to be lower than in the other relapsing fevers [28], and PCR is more likely to be positive during the fever spikes [41]. Blood smear examination does not seem to be sensitive enough for the diagnosis of *B. miyamotoi* [42]. Isolation of *B. miyamotoi* has been successful from febrile patients [43] using the Kelly-Pettenkofer Medium (MKP) with added calf serum. This technique cannot be implemented in all laboratories and is reserved for specialized laboratories or research purposes only.

9.2.6 Treatment

Treatment of BMD is based on the recommendations for treatment of Lyme borreliosis. Ceftriaxone and doxycycline have been mainly used to treat BMD, with minocycline and amoxicillin/clavulanic acid used to a lesser extent [17]. All the patients described in the medical literature recovered after the treatment and no relapse was observed after the treatment.

9.3 *Ixodes*-Borne *Anaplasmataceae*

The family of Anaplasmataceae includes six bacterial genera: *Anaplasma*, *Ehrlichia*, *Candidatus* Neoehrlichia, *Neorickettsia*, *Wolbachia*, and *Aegyptianella*. These bacteria are intracellular, associated with invertebrate hosts. Some of these bacteria may be responsible for diseases in mammals including humans. They seem to have a tropism for the reticuloendothelial cells. Here, we will focus on two *Ixodes*-borne *Anaplasmataceae* responsible for proven human disease: *Anaplasma phagocytophilum* and *Candidatus* Neoehrlichia mikurensis.

9.3.1 *Anaplasma phagocytophilum*

Human granulocytic anaplasmosis (HGA) is a tick-borne acute febrile bacterial infection caused by a Rickettsiales species, *Anaplasma phagocytophilum* (*Ap*), which embraces three former taxa: *Ehrlichia phagocytophila*, *E. equi*, and human granulocytic ehrlichiosis (HGE) agent. Veterinary forms of the disease were first described in the 1930s in European sheep and cattle [44] and then in American horses and dogs in 1969 and 1982, respectively [45, 46]. Since the preliminary reports, the mode of transmission by *Ixodes ricinus* tick bite was discovered and intracytoplasmic rickettsia-like bacterial bodies were observed after Romanowsky staining within granulocytes and monocytes in blood films from infected sheep [47]. The first human clinical descriptions were performed later in the United States in 1994 and in Europe in 1997 [48, 49].

9.3.1.1 Bacterial Characteristics

As a member of the Rickettsiales, *Ap* is an obligate intracellular bacterium of eukaryotic cells. The only vectors known for *Ap* are the ticks of the *I. ricinus* complex. In rare cases, *Ap* can be directly transmitted by blood in the context of transfusion organ transplant and from mother to child during pregnancy [50]. The bacteria exist in two morphological forms: large reticulate and small dense-core cells, both are present in intravacuolar colonies (compact inclusions) or "morulae." These two forms divide by binary fission. The size of individual cells and morula are around 0.3μm and 2μm in diameter, respectively, but they can vary highly in shape and size. The structure of its wall is related to the Gram-negative bacteria but lipopolysaccharide and peptidoglycan are absent [51]. The bacterium does not grow using cell-free media but can be cultivated *in vitro* in human granulocyte (HL-60) or tick cell lines [51, 52].

9.3.1.2 Zoonotic Transmission and Hosts

Anthropophilic ticks belonging to the *I. ricinus* complex are the only known vectors of HGA and the vectorial competence of the species *I. ricinus*, *I. scapularis*, *I. pacificus*, and *I. persulcatus* have been experimentally proven as well as transstadial transmission. Transovarial transmission does not occur [46].

After ingestion of *Ap* with the blood meal on an infected host, these latter bacteria colonize the digestive epithelium of the tick and migrate to the salivary glands. Like *B. burgdorferi* s.l., *Ap* are released in the tick saliva during the next blood meal on a naive host. Ixodid saliva modulates the myeloid pro-inflammatory response to the intracellular bacteria during the pathogen transmission, and the pathogen requires a time of tick attachment of at least 4 to 24 h for transmission to occur [50]. No vectors apart from ticks of the *I. ricinus* complex have been identified but DNA has been detected in other tick species: *I. hexagonus*, *I. ventalloi*, *I. trianguliceps*, *I. dentatus*, *I. ovatus*, *I. nipponensis*, *Amblyomma americanum*, *Dermacentor* spp., and *Haemaphysalis* spp. [53].

Several epidemiological cycles have been proposed for the circulation of *Ap* depending on regions and pathogen strains. Micromammals, including rodents and insectivores, and large mammals, including cervids and wild boar, may act as reservoirs of *Ap* [53]. Analysis of *Ap* genetic diversity has revealed the existence of several distinct lineages within the species, some of which are involved in specific infection cycles with preferential association with some potential host reservoirs. For example, in a study of 188 European *Ap* strains from different host species of various geographic origins, sequences of *ankA* gene from human and domestic animal samples exclusively belonged to one clade, and sequences from roe deer samples occurred in three other clades. Sheep, cattle, and red deer (*Cervus elaphus*) strains clustered in both the first clade and in "roe deer" clades. The absence of roe deer-associated sequences in the first clade suggests that roe deer do not act as a reservoir for human pathogenic strains in Europe [54]. Moreover, at least two *Ap* variants can simultaneously circulate in some hosts, as shown in cattle herds in France [55]. Host specificity in the lifecycle of *Ap* is also demonstrated by the strain Ap-V1, nonpathogenic for humans, which infects ruminants and is transmitted by *I. scapularis*. The strains involved in HGA are also responsible for infections in canids, horses, and ruminants [56]. Large-scale genetic studies have confirmed this type of population structure in distinct genetic clusters by multi-locus sequencing [57, 58]. Using this methodology, Langenwalder et al. (2020) argue that hedgehogs and wild boars may act as reservoirs for human infections in Europe [58].

9.3.1.3 Epidemiology

The distribution zone of the disease corresponds to the regions inhabited by members of the anthropophilic *I. ricinus* complex ticks in the northern hemisphere. Therefore, cases of HGA are reported in North America, Europe, and East Asia.

In North America, the disease has been described in the United States, Canada, and more recently in Mexico [59]. The vectors are, as for the *B. burgdorferi* s.l. complex, *I. scapularis* across the eastern United States and *I. pacificus* along the west coast. The number of US reported cases has increased steadily since the first year of notification in 2000 [60], probably at least in part due to better physician knowledge of the disease, and also possibly due to local increases in the level of exposure as this has been suggested by Russel et al. (2021) in a particular region of growing incidence during 2010–2018 [61]. From 2008 to 2012, passive surveillance data indicated an average annual incidence of 6.3 cases per million population. The highest incidences were recorded in the northeastern and upper Midwestern states with more than 130 cases per million population per year in some regions [60]. In Europe, the disease occurs at a much lower incidence than in North America but is widely distributed. Cases have been reported from many countries, including Slovenia, Norway, Sweden, the Netherlands, Poland, Austria, Switzerland, Italy, Spain, France, Greece, and Russia. In Asia, the disease is present in China, Mongolia, South Korea, and Japan. The vectors of HGA are, as for the *B. burgdorferi* s.l. complex, *I. ricinus* in Europe and *I. persulcatus* in Eastern Europe and in Asia. Serological surveys have revealed that a large proportion of people have encountered the bacteria without any history of reported infection, probably due to subclinical or milder forms of HGA. A recent meta-analysis concluded that overall seroprevalences were 13.8% and 5.0% in high-risk populations and general population, respectively [62].

Depending on the studies, the molecular detection rate of *Ap* among questing ticks varies between less than 1% and up to 20% in *I. ricinus* and 22% in *I. persulcatus*. These highly variable prevalence data are under the influence of the study area, the molecular method used, and whether nymphal or adult stages are investigated [53].

9.3.1.4 Pathogenesis and Host Response

After transmission by the tick bite, the infection is disseminated by the peripheral blood to hematopoietic organs, mainly the bone marrow in humans. *Ap* can infect myeloid cells at all stages of maturation. The intracellular pathogenic behavior of

Ap is enabled by its ability to modulate the actin cytoskeleton of eukaryotic cells from ticks and vertebrates, involving possibly an actin filament-associated *Ap* protein that was recently identified [63]. Bacteria are internalized in the target cell into phagosomal vesicles within the cytoplasm, then, they take a non-infectious reticulate form and replicate to form a microcolony or "morula" (Fig. 9.1). To promote their intracellular survival within host cells, bacteria inhibit the fusion of the phagosome with lysosomes and thereby avoid acidic degradation. The propagation of the infection occurs with the release of bacteria from infected cells and the formation of new infectious dense-core forms.

Innate immune induction in response to *Ap* infection leads to inflammatory lesions in tissues which result in the severe clinical manifestations of HGA [64].

9.3.1.5 Clinical Manifestations

After the infecting tick bite, the incubation period lasts generally from 1 to 3 weeks [65]. The clinical presentation is frequently mild or moderate, with influenza-like symptoms such as acute fever, malaise, myalgia, headaches, and/or arthralgia. Nonspecific biological signs are also frequent: leukopenia, thrombocytopenia, and elevation in liver enzymes (AST, ALT). In some cases, the febrile illness can be associated with gastrointestinal symptoms (nausea, vomiting, and diarrhea), stiff neck, cough, confusion, non-pruritic rash, anemia, and/or elevated serum creatinine. Rashes are uncommon (<10%). The milder forms resolve in 10 days even without antibiotic treatment [50]. However, the illness may be severe especially in older people, in immunocompromised patients (HIV, chemotherapy, treatment…) and/or when the antibiotic administration is delayed. The reported complications include renal or respiratory failure, septic shock, disseminated intravascular coagulation and hemorrhage, rhabdomyolysis, myocarditis, serious opportunistic infections

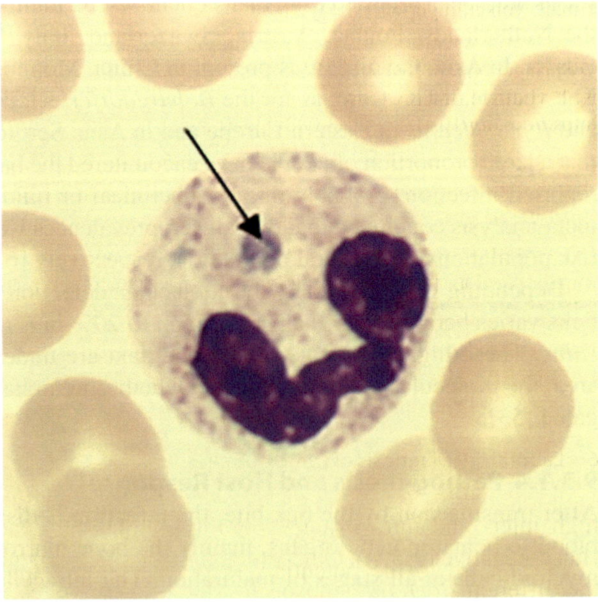

Fig. 9.1 Intragranulocytic morula (arrow) on an MGG stained peripheral blood smear in a patient suffering from human granulocytic anaplasmosis (photo credit: Dr C. Koebel, Bacteriology Laboratory, Hôpitaux Universitaires de Strasbourg, Strasbourg, France)

(HSV, *Candida* or *Aspergillus*—causing invasive infections), and macrophage activation-like syndrome. Meningitis or encephalitis is rare (<0.3%). In the United States, the estimated hospitalization rate is high (approximately 36% of cases). Overall, the case fatality rate of HGA is less than 1% [53]. HGA appears more common in adults than in children and there are rare case reports of a more complicated clinical course in children [66].

9.3.1.6 Laboratory Diagnosis

A suspected diagnosis of HGA is made on (1) clinical suspicion including fever, (2) recent tick bite or tick exposure in endemic areas especially during spring and summer months, and (3) nonspecific biological signs (mild anemia, thrombocytopenia, leukopenia, elevated liver enzymes, elevated C-reactive protein, and/or elevated serum creatinine). Biological confirmation of the diagnosis relies either on the detection of *Ap* in blood, by specific PCR (or by culture), or serological evidence (seroconversion or fourfold or greater increase in the serum antibody titer). An isolated or stable positive antibody titer or the detection of intracytoplasmic morulae in peripheral blood smears are not specific or sensitive enough to establish the definitive etiologic diagnosis of HGA [50, 65, 67].

Blood smear microscopy. In the initial fever period, intracytoplasmic morulae of *Ap* can be seen within neutrophil granulocytes after microscopic examination of peripheral blood films using May-Grunwald Giemsa or Wright stain (Fig. 9.1). Due to the low level of infected cells in the blood, this method is time-consuming and has poor sensitivity (only up to 20%) even for trained staff [50, 67].

Blood culture. *Ap* does not grow in routine blood culture and requires HL-60 cell lines for its *in vitro* cultivation. This technique is only used in specialized laboratories.

Serological tests. The reference method is based on an indirect immunofluorescence assay (IFA) for the detection of specific immunoglobulin G antibodies. Usually, a first sample is collected during the febrile illness and a second one 3–4 weeks later to detect seroconversion or fourfold or greater increase in the serum antibody titer [65]. Thereby serological tests offer mostly a retrospective diagnosis of HGA. Specific *Ap* antibodies can be detected for months or years after the acute illness. Immunoglobulin M serology is not recommended given the high rate of false-positive results.

PCR assays. Currently, polymerase chain reaction (PCR) testing of whole blood is considered the gold standard for the diagnosis of HGA. Different homemade and commercial methods have been developed using different targets [65, 68]. Sensitivity is highest in the acute phase until 10 days after the onset of the illness without treatment and quickly decreases after antibiotic administration (within 24–48 h). Given the variable and possibly intermittent occurrence of bacteremia, a negative result does not firmly rule out the diagnosis of *Ap* [67].

9.3.1.7 Treatment

Antibiotic therapy should be considered for patients presenting an acute febrile illness compatible with HGA, especially with bicytopenia and/or elevated liver enzymes. Due to the potentially serious complications, treatment should not be delayed until laboratory testing has been completed [50]. Doxycycline and rifamycins have an excellent *in vitro* activity against *Ap*. In contrast, these bacteria are not susceptible to β-lactams, aminoglycosides, macrolides, or chloramphenicol [52]. Doxycycline for 7–10 days is the first treatment choice in HGA in adults and children (including <8 y. o.). Rifampin is an effective alternative treatment in case of a severe allergy or during pregnancy or in children suffering from mild forms. The clinical improvement is generally prompt after the beginning of antibiotics in 24 to 48h. With early administration, this treatment prevents the severe complications of HGA. There are no reported cases that are refractory to treatment or reports on chronic infection [50].

9.3.2 *Candidatus* Neoehrlichia mikurensis

9.3.2.1 Introduction-Bacterial Features

Candidatus Neoehrlichia mikurensis was first identified and described in 2004 from rats and ticks of the Mikura island in the south of the Japanese Archipelago [69]. This bacterium was previously detected in ticks in Europe [70–72] and was initially named *Candidatus* Ehrlichia walkerii by Brouqui et al. in 2003 [70]. However, genetic analysis based on the 16s rDNA and the *groEL* gene sequencing revealed that it belongs to a new cluster in the *Anaplasmataceae* family. *Can.* N. mikurensis are Gram-negative pleomorphic cocci of 0.5–1.2 μm of diameter. As the other members of this family, *Can.* N. mikurensis is a strict intracellular bacterium that seems to parasitize endothelial cells as membrane-bound inclusions [69]. This tropism for the endothelial cells has recently been confirmed by the cultivation of the bacteria in endothelial cell lines [73]. Sequencing of the *groEL* and *16S rRNA* genes of isolates from rodents, dogs, and humans in Japan, Siberia, Germany, Switzerland, and the Netherlands identified three groups of variants for the groEL gene occurring in Siberia, Germany, and Japan, respectively [74]. Studies led by Li, *et al.* revealed the population of *Can.* N. mikurensis is structured in four groups according to it's geographic distribution [75].

9.3.2.2 Ecology and Epidemiology

I. ricinus, *I. persulcatus*, *I. ovatus*, *I. frontalis*, *I. hexagonus*, *D. reticulatus*, and *Haemaphysalis concinna* have been reported to be carrier-ticks of *Can.* N. mikurensis. Interestingly, rates of infection of *Can.* N. mikurensis are the highest among the *Ixodes* species, suggesting that these are the primary vectors. No other *Ixodes* spp. have been identified as carriers [76]. *Can.* N. mikurensis has been detected in ticks in the northern hemisphere in Western and Eastern Europe, in Asia, and Japan, but interestingly it has not been detected in the United Kingdom or in North America. The prevalence of *Can.* N. mikurensis among ticks was reported as increasing in the Netherlands between 2006 and 2010 [77]. The organism, however, appears to be present in ticks for longer periods of time at a low prevalence, as it was found in ticks already collected in 1960 [78]. The median prevalence among ticks is 3.95% (minimum: 0.08% maximum: 22%). Nymphs and adults ticks have been repeatedly reported as carriers, and transovarial transmission seems to be exceptional [79], so a reservoir host is apparently essential for the bacteria to be maintained in nature. Several small rodents are suspected as reservoir hosts for *Can.* N. mikurensis: voles, wood mice, rats, and chipmunks [76]. But only *Myodes glareolus* (bank vole) and *Apodemus* spp. (wood mouse) have been shown to be reservoir hosts by transmission experiments [19].

9.3.2.3 Clinical Manifestations

So far, around a hundred symptomatic and subclinical human cases of infection have been reported (Table 9.2) [80–82]. Initially, infection with *Can.* N. mikurensis was reported in patients with immunocompromised backgrounds [83]. Most reports corroborated this last fact, indeed patients infected with *Can.* N. mikurensis suffered from hematological malignancy (CLL, mantle cell lymphoma, post-transplant lymphoproliferative disorder) or autoimmune disorders, and had been treated with immunosuppressive or cytotoxic drugs (particularly anti-CD20 Rituximab), and/or had been splenectomized [74, 83–87]. However, the bacterium has also been reported in apparently immunocompetent, but clinically symptomatic patients [33, 85, 88–90] (Table 9.2).

The clinical picture of neoehrlichiosis includes high fever that can relapse or occur in spikes, and last for several days. Fever occurs predominantly at night. Several other manifestations have been observed, usually occurring together with fever: chills and malaise, joint and/or muscle pain [91]. Nonproductive cough and dyspnea have also been reported [74, 88]. A cutaneous erysipelas-like rash was described in several reports [83, 92]. It is noteworthy that thromboembolic events including deep vein thrombosis were reported in a significant number of papers, especially in a cohort of 11 immunocompromised patients published by Grankvist et al. in which 6 had vascular and thromboembolic events, including in 4 with, a deep vein thrombosis [85]. These vascular events seem to be very frequent (occurring in more than 50 % of the cases). Also, in a recently published cohort of 40 patients with documented neoehrlichiosis, 24 of these individuals presented with a thromboembolic event including deep vein thrombosis, pulmonary embolism, repeated thrombophlebitis, transitory ischemic attacks, and arteritis [93].

Table 9.2 Human infections with *Candidatus N. mikurensis*

	Symptomatic infection	
Asymptomatic infection	Immunocompetent patients	Immunocompromised patients
Welc-Faleciak et al. [81]: $n = 5$	von Loewenich et al. [74]: $n = 1$	Welinder-Olsson et al. [83]: $n = 1$
Jahfari et al. [80]: $n = 7$	Fehr et al. [88]: $n = 1$	von Loewenich et al. [74]: $n = 1$
Lenart et al. [90]: $n = 1$	Li et al. [89]: $n = 7$	Pekova et al. [84]: $n = 2$
Markowicz et al. [33]: $n = 11$	Grankvist et al. [85]: $n = 2$	Grankvist et al. [92]: $n = 11$
	Höper et al. [93]: $n = 10$	Dadgar et al. [86]: $n = 1$
	Boyer et al. [82]: $n = 2$	Höper et al. [93]: $n = 30$
		Boyer et al. [82]: $n = 2$

9.3.2.4 Laboratory Diagnosis

Few variations in biological parameters were observed in infected patients. The C-reactive protein and procalcitonin levels were elevated. There was also neutrophil leukocytosis, thrombocytopenia, and hyponatremia [92, 94].

As a high number of copies has been described in patients with neoehrlichiosis, the polymerase chain reaction is the primary tool for the etiological diagnosis of *Can.* N. mikurensis infection, using whole blood (EDTA and citrated blood) and bone marrow as a diagnostic sample material [76]. Specific PCRs targeting the *16s rRNA* or the *groEL* gene are described in the literature [76, 80]. A multiplex PCR has been developed with specific probes for the *Anaplasmataceae* family, *Neoehrlichia* genus, and *Can.* N. mikurensis, enabling the detection of all three targets in a single reaction [83]. Also a cell culture method has recently been published, but its use seems to be limited to research laboratories [73].

So far, there is no serological diagnosis for the diagnosis of *Can.* N. mikurensis infection. However, serum antibody cross-reactivity against *Ehrlichia* spp., *Anaplasma* spp., and *Rickettsia* spp. can be observed [83, 89, 95]. To our knowledge, *Can.* N. mikurensis has not been detected directly in blood smears.

9.3.2.5 Treatment

Up to now no clinical trial or study has been conducted comparing the relative effectiveness of several antibiotics on *Can.* N. mikurensis infection. Since it is an intracellular bacterium, closely related to bacteria of the *Ehrlichia* and *Anaplasma* genera, the choice of the antimicrobial substance should be restricted to antibiotics with good intracellular penetration, i.e. doxycycline which is recommended for the treatment of both, anaplasmosis and ehrlichiosis [60].

In several case reports, doxycycline for 2–3 weeks at the usual dose of 200 mg/24 h was employed successfully [91]. Rifampicin (300–450 mg twice a day) can be used as an alternative to doxycycline or applied as part of a combination therapy [88]. After 5 days of treatment, patients usually recover and PCR investigations after treatment yield a negative result for *Can.* N. mikurensis [91]. Symptomatic treatment of patients is strongly required due to the possible occurrence of thrombembolism.

9.4 *Ixodes*-Borne Rickettsiosis

Historically, "rickettsia" has been used to describe multiple small uncultivable (or not yet cultivated) rods that had not been otherwise identified. Successive taxonomic changes have been proposed for this disparate group. The *Rickettsiaceae* family now includes two genera, namely, *Rickettsia* and *Orientia* [96]. Historically, the *Rickettsia* genus has been subdivided into the typhus group, which includes two species (*R. prowazekii* and *R. typhi*) and the spotted fever group (SFG), which includes several species, some of which may be responsible for human diseases. Their taxonomy is still debated. Moreover, several subgroups have emerged from the SFG, namely, *R. rickettsii*, *R. massiliae*, *R. helvetica*, and *R. akari* groups [97].

Several bacteria belonging to the *Rickettsia* genus are associated with hematophagous arthropods and among the 31 *Rickettsia* species and the numerous currently uncharacterized *Rickettsia* spp. [97], around 10 species are associated with ticks belonging to the *Ixodes* genus.

In Europe, two *Rickettsia* species are carried by *I. ricinus,* namely *R. helvetica* and *R. monacensis*, both of which belong to the Spotted Fever Group.

9.4.1 *Rickettsia helvetica*

9.4.1.1 Clinical Picture

Rickettsia helvetica was isolated from *Ixodes ricinus* in Switzerland in 1979 by Willy Burgdorfer and was later recognized as a distinct species [98]. Since its discovery and until 1999, it was considered to be non-pathogenic, but then human infections were increasingly described at the turn of the twenty-first century. It is now generally accepted that *R. helvetica* infection can result in post-tick bite febrile syndromes that can persist from days to weeks after the onset also in apparently immunocompetent patients [99]. Cutaneous involvement is not typically found but some patients have been described with an inoculation eschar [100, 101]. A maculopapular rash on the back and chest was also described in a case series and a case report [102, 103]. Other clinical pictures remain more dubious since they have all been observed by just a single team in Sweden. According to this report, *R. helvetica* could be responsible for meningitis also, since it has been found in the CSF alone or accompanied by the herpes simplex virus 2 [104, 105]. Notably, Koetsveld et al. published molecular evidence of *R. helvetica* and *R. monacensis* in the CSF of patients suspected of Lyme neuroborreliosis, but the implication of this coinfection for the symptoms or the effect of these bacteria on the clinical course of Lyme neuroborreliosis is not clear [106]. It has also been hypothesized that *R. helvetica* could be responsible for myocarditis associated with sudden death [107] but these findings have not been corroborated by other findings.

Interestingly, seroconversion in the absence of symptoms has been reported in 22.2% of a cohort of 35 persons in the Gotland (Sweden) where *I. ricinus* is highly endemic [101]. Contact with the infection has also been indicated in France where the seroprevalence was reported to be 9.2% in forestry workers [99]. Compared to this high seroprevalence, clinical cases remain rare, obviously supporting the fact that *R. helvetica* is of low pathogenicity for humans. A recent study showed that *R. helvetica* has both, nonfunctional virulence proteins and a low level of expression of proteins that are usually essential for virulence in other *Rickettsia* spp. [108].

9.4.1.2 Ecology and Epidemiology

R. helvetica has been found in ticks across Europe (from Great Britain and France to the Baltic countries and Ukraine, through Denmark, Germany, and Poland). In addition, it has also been found in countries around the Mediterranean Sea [109]. In western Europe, *I. ricinus* is probably the most important vector for *R. helvetica* because the carrying rate for this species is higher than in others [110]. The infection rate of ticks reported in the literature varies from 4.7% in Slovakia to 17.4% in

Sweden [109], and some authors even mention a rate of 36.8% in endemic foci [99]. These data, however, are difficult to compare because these studies deal with various tick stages. In addition, data on female adult ticks are not completely representative for the acarological risk for humans bitten by *I. ricinus*, since *R. helvetica* has been observed in all tick stages suggesting transovarial transmission [111]. Other studies noted an increase in prevalence depending on the stage, thereby suggesting the existence of an animal reservoir for *R. helvetica* [109].

The identity of such animal reservoirs of *R. helvetica*, however, is unclear. Several animals have been investigated, for example, wild boar and roe deer [112, 113] with carrier rates of 6.5–19.0%. However, it has not been demonstrated that ticks can acquire *R. helvetica* from these animals, though it was demonstrated that the prevalence of *R. helvetica* was higher in ticks from roe deer and dogs [114]. As for other *Ixodes*-borne microorganisms, small rodents have been presumed to be a reservoir host for *R. helvetica* because small rodents are hosts for tick larvae and nymphs [115]. Indeed, *R. helvetica* has been detected to a variable extent in *Apodemus* spp. mice and voles of different geographic origins [116, 117]. According to the study of Burri et al., *A. sylvaticus* and *Myodes glareolus* are unable to transmit *R. helvetica* to ticks [19].

Several bird species can be rickettsiemic [109] and similar to small rodents, birds are hosts for immature stages of ticks, but the reservoir competence of birds for *R. helvetica* has not been demonstrated yet.

9.4.2 *Rickettsia monacensis*

This species was described and isolated for the first time in Germany from *I. ricinus* ticks [118]. *R. monacensis* has been observed in different European countries: Poland, Germany, Hungary, Slovakia, France, and Ukraine as well as in Algerian ticks [109]. The prevalence of *R. monacensis* in questing ticks is variable, but it seems that it is lower than that of *R. helvetica*. It varies from 0.3% to 52.9%, but most prevalences are low and high prevalences could be linked to an area with a particular epidemiology. The animal reservoir of *R. monacensis* is currently unknown.

Initially considered to be a nonpathogenic species, cases of human disease have been described in Spain and Italy [109]. Symptoms include high fever, headache, and arthralgia. Inoculation ulcers may be present or not. If symptoms are present, the clinical picture may be reminiscent of Mediterranean Spotted fever.

9.4.3 Laboratory Diagnosis

The best sample for a direct diagnosis of a spotted fever group *Rickettsia* infection is a skin biopsy or a swab from the site of the inoculation ulcer or rash. The diagnosis can also be made, but with less sensitivity, from a blood sample. Immunofluorescence-based serological methods, which are important in the diagnosis of rickettsiosis, are performed in reference centers. To facilitate interpretation of the results, two sera should be taken, one at the time of the acute episode and the other at a later time [119].

9.5 *Francisella tularensis*

9.5.1 Bacterial Features

F. tularensis is a small Gram-negative rod, responsible for tularemia, and occurs in the northern hemisphere, in the holarctic region. This species is subdivided into four subspecies: *F. tularensis* subsp. *tularensis* (also known as type A strains), subsp. *holarctica* (type B strains), *subsp. mediasiatica,* and *subsp. novicida*. Tularemia clinical cases are mainly related to the *tularensis* and *holarctica* subspecies [120]. *F. tularensis tularensis* is primarily reported in North America, but isolates from the environment or arthropods have been identified also in Europe [121].

F. tularensis has an extensive wild animal reservoir: mammals, amphibians, birds, reptiles, and fishes can carry this bacterium. However, small rodents (mice, rats, voles, beavers, lemmings, etc.) and lagomorphs (rabbits, hares) are probably the main animal reservoirs [122]. *F. tularensis* can survive for several weeks in the soil or the aquatic environment, which can lead to contamination [123]. Finally, arthropods are a potential reservoir of *F. tularensis*, in particular mosquitoes, which become infected during their aquatic larval stage from an aquatic reservoir. No human-to-human transmission has been described to date [120]. Transmission by ticks will be discussed hereafter.

9.5.2 Tick Transmission of *F. tularensis*

Since its discovery at the beginning of the 20th century, isolation of *F. tularensis* was possible from *Dermacentor andersoni*, and a case of a patient who developed tularemia after a tick bite was reported by Parker, Spencer, and Francis in 1924 [124]. Evidence for transmission from animal to animal by ticks was also provided in the first studies on this bacterium [124]. In contrast to what is observed for mosquitoes and deer flies, which are also vectors of *F. tularensis*, ticks can participate in the maintenance of *F. tularensis* in the environment for a long period [125]. The bite of *Dermacentor andersoni, D. variabilis*, or *Amblyomma americanum* is the most common route of contamination in North America [125]. In France, approximately 20% of tularemia cases have been reported to be caused by a tick bite [126], but the study did not specify the species of tick concerned. Similarly, three cases of ulceroglandular tularemia from the Bade-Wurtemberg region have been reported with the origin of a presumed tick bite [127]. Serological data on forestry workers suggest a very low rate of transmission by ticks in areas of high *I. ricinus* endemicity [128].

Transstadial transmission of *F. tularensis* seems to occur under laboratory conditions in the established North American vectors, *Dermacentor andersoni, D. variabilis*, and *Amblyomma americanum* [125].

Concerning *I. ricinus*, the percentage of ticks carrying *F. tularensis* is very low and seems to be lower than for *Dermacentor* species. Transstadial transmission occurs for *F. tularensis* in *I. ricinus* [129–131], unfortunately, the scientific quality of these papers cannot be fully appreciated since they are published only in Slovak. Transovarial transmission does not occur in *Dermacentor reticulatus,* nor in *Ixodes ricinus* [132].

Finally, using an experimental model consisting of tick cell lines, some authors suggest that the cell line of *I. scapularis*, is less permissive of *F. tularensis* infection than that of *D. andersoni* [133]. Future experiments highlighting the vector competence of *I. ricinus* for *F. tularensis,* would shed light on the transmission of this bacterium in Europe.

9.5.3 Clinical Pictures

The mean incubation of tularemia is 3–5 days, with a maximum of 2 weeks [120]. The first clinical manifestations are not very specific, evoking a flu-like syndrome (moderate fever, headache, arthralgia, myalgia, dry cough, sometimes diarrhea).

After the prodromal phase, the clinical manifestations of tularemia depend on the route of inoculation of bacteria and are classically grouped into six clinical forms. The ulceroglandular form, the most classic form, corresponds to a cutaneous lesion at the site of inoculation (papule, vesicle) which evolves rapidly towards a cutaneous ulcer [134]. Adenopathy arises rapidly in the lymphatic drainage area of the ulcer. This is the typical clinical picture that can be observed after a tick bite. Localized lymphadenopathy without skin lesions may be observed spontaneously or after healing of the cutaneous ulcer, and corresponds to the glandular form.

Other clinical manifestations can be observed: the oculoglandular form (syndrome of Parinaud) corresponds to conjunctival self-inoculation of *F. tularensis* after the handling of an infected animal; the oropharyngeal form, which occurs after oral inoculation (manual transmission, or ingestion of water or contaminated food); the pulmonary form, which may be primary after inhalation of a contaminated aerosol or secondary after hematogenous diffusion of bacteria; the typhoid form, which is characterized by severe systemic infection, with an acute influenza-like syndrome and often neurological signs (confusion, prostration), but without a visible inoculation site and without clinical signs of focal infection (especially without adenopathy) [120].

9.5.4 Laboratory Diagnosis

9.5.4.1 Direct Diagnosis

Direct diagnosis can be performed by culture or by nucleic acid amplification, which is more sensitive for the detection of *F. tularensis*. Direct diagnosis can be performed on different matrices according to the clinical presentation: blood, lymph node samples, skin biopsy, conjunctival and oropharyngeal specimens [120]. Blood specimens are less sensitive for the detection of *F. tularensis* than other matrices since the bacterium is not always present in the blood.

F. tularensis is a fastidious bacterium that requires enriched media such as chocolate agar plates or in a blood culture system (Fig. 9.2). *F. tularensis* culture must be performed under appropriate biosafety conditions. Identification is no longer a problem since the implementation of matrix-assisted laser desorption/ionization time-of-flight mass spectrometry in clinical microbiology laboratories [120].

9.5.4.2 Indirect Diagnosis

Diagnosis of tularemia is mainly based on serological assay using microagglutination or indirect immunofluorescence techniques. Antibodies can be detected one or two weeks after the disease onset, reach a peak around 3–4 weeks, and may persist for months to years [120].

9.5.4.3 Case Definitions

According to the World Health Organization [135], cases can either be suspect, presumptive or confirmed. For suspected cases, "an exposure history consistent with risks known to be associated with tularemia together with clinical symptoms compatible with tularaemia" are required. Presumptive cases are defined as: "suggestive clinical symptoms and a clinical sample that tests positive for tularaemia by antigen or DNA detection. A single positive serum is also considered presumptive." Finally, confirmed cases are defined as: "Recovery of an isolate and identification of the culture as *F. tularensis* by antigen or DNA detection. Alternatively, paired serum specimens with a fourfold difference in titer (tube or microagglutination assay) or significantly (ELISA), with at least one serum positive, are also considered confirmatory" which suggests that a positive culture must be obtained for the confirmed case definition.

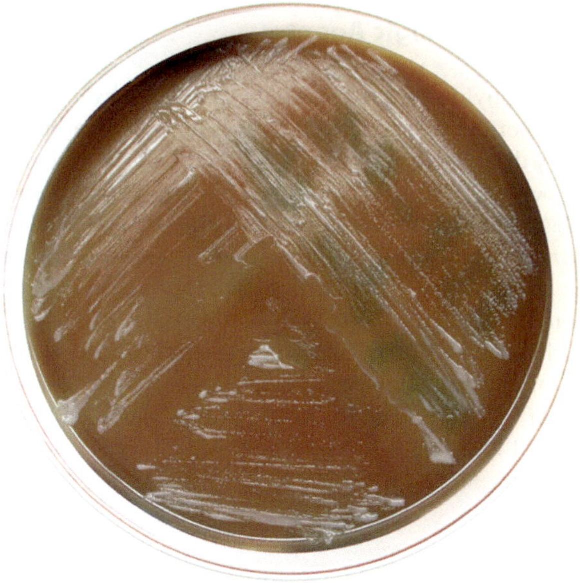

Fig. 9.2 Pure *F. tularensis* culture on a chocolate agar plate (photo credit : Dr F. Schramm, Bacteriology Laboratory, Hôpitaux Universitaires de Strasbourg, Strasbourg, France)

9.5.5 Treatment

F. tularensis is naturally resistant to beta-lactams because of its intracellular multiplication in macrophages and the production of a class A beta-lactamase [136, 137]. Aminoglycosides (streptomycin and gentamicin), tetracyclines (especially doxycycline), and fluoroquinolones (ciprofloxacin, levofloxacin, and moxifloxacin) are the most active antibiotics *in vitro*. Macrolides are active *in vitro* only on strains of type A and B biovar 1; B biovar 2 are naturally resistant [120].

Fluoroquinolones and tetracyclines are used for mild cases of tularemia. Interestingly, more relapses were observed with treatment by doxycycline (10–15%) than with ciprofloxacin (5–10%) [138]. Streptomycin is considered to be the reference molecule in the treatment of severe forms of tularemia, with success rates close to 100%. As this antibiotic is no longer available in most countries, the administration of gentamicin (3 mg/kg daily, in one or two intravenous infusions) is currently recommended in severe forms, alone or in combination with a fluoroquinolone [120].

9.6 Human Babesiosis

The name "Babesia" comes from Victor Babes who, in 1888, was the first microbiologist to identify the intraerythrocytic protozoan in the blood of Romanian cattle and sheep suffering from febrile and severe hemolytic illness of unknown cause. In 1893, the parasite was described as the agent of the tick-borne Texas fever in US cattle. Thereby, babesiosis (or "piroplasmosis") was the first identified arthropod-borne disease. The first case of human babesiosis was reported by Skrabalo and Deanovic in 1957. This was a fatal case in an asplenic Croatian herdsman [139].

9.6.1 Etiologic Agents

In the phylum *Apicomplexa*, the genus *Babesia* embraces more than 100 species of tick-borne intraerythrocytic protozoans. Numerous species are involved in veterinary diseases (e.g., *B. bigemina* and *B. bovis*, responsible for the worldwide bovine babesiosis). To date, three species are mainly responsible for human babesiosis: *Babesia microti* (United States, Europe, Asia), *B. divergens* (Europe), and *B. venatorum* (Europe, Asia). These three species are transmitted by ixodid ticks. *B. duncani*, transmitted by the tick *Dermacentor albipictus* and restricted to the North American Pacific coast, is a fourth species of *Babesia* sp. involved in human cases [140]. Several other undescribed species have occurred in very rare cases [141]. *B. microti* is a member of a species complex that is phylogenetically quite distant from the *Babesia* sensu stricto group, which includes *B. divergens* and *B. venatorum* [142].

9.6.2 Life Cycle, Zoonotic Transmission, and Hosts

In Europe, *B. divergens*, *B. microti, and B. venatorum* are transmitted by *I. ricinus*. In the United States, *B. microti* is transmitted by *I. scapularis*. *I. persulcatus* is the vector of *B. microti* and *B. venatorum* in Asia [143]. The cycle of *Babesia* spp. begins with sporozoite formation called "sporogony" which takes place in the salivary glands of the tick vector. When the infected tick feeds on a naive vertebrate host, the sporozoite (infective forms) are inoculated along with tick saliva. Sporozoites migrate to the blood vessels and actively penetrate the red blood cells within which the vegetative form or "trophozoites" develop. Trophozoites undergo intraerythrocytic division forming "merozoites" that are intermittently released into the circulation and can then infect new cells [144]. Some forms resulting from merozoite invasion do not divide but develop into gametocytes that are the transmission stages from the vertebrate host to the tick vector. In most *Babesia* spp., the parasites persist from one feeding tick stage to the next and, in the group *B. microti*, they are then transmitted transstadially. Transovarial transmission only occurs in the *Babesia* sensu stricto group [145]. The main reservoir hosts are small rodents for *B. microti*, cattle for *B. divergens,* and roe deer in the case of *B. venatorum* [141, 146, 147]. The transmission of infection to a vertebrate host requires at least 48h of tick attachment in the case of a single nymph infected by *B. microti* [148]. Cases of human-to-human *B. microti* babesiosis transmitted by blood transfusion have been reported since 1979 [149], and there are rare documented cases of mother-to-child transmission [150].

9.6.3 Epidemiology

Human babesiosis caused by *B. microti* is endemic in the United States with 900–1800 annual cases notified to the CDC from 2011 to 2014, corresponding to an incidence rate of around 0.8 per 100,000 population with most of the cases reported in the northeastern (Rhode Island, Massachusetts and Connecticut with 16.3, 8.0 and 5.7 cases/100,000 population in 2014, respectively) and in the Midwest of the country [151]. The incidence of transfusion-transmitted babesiosis is estimated to be about 1–2% of the total of human cases [152].

The epidemiology of human babesiosis in Europe is not well known. While bovine *B. divergens* babesiosis is widely distributed in Europe, as is the tick vector *I. ricinus*, fewer than 50 human cases of babesiosis have been published to date, primarily severe cases in immunocompromised patients [141, 153]. *B. venatorum* infections are rarely reported in Europe; only sporadic cases have been described in Austria, Italy, Germany, and Sweden with milder forms than *B. divergens* infections [141, 153]. *B. microti* is also widespread in ticks in Europe (e.g., [154, 155]), but human disease is reported very rarely [156, 157]. Seroprevalence in Europe varies depending on the studied region from 2 to 23% and is higher in the tick-exposed population [158].

In Asia, *B. venatorum* is reported as endemic in the northeastern region of China, and human cases of *B. microti*-babesiosis have been reported in China, Taiwan, and Japan [141].

9.6.4 Clinical Manifestations

In human babesiosis, the clinical manifestations mainly arise from the lysis of infected erythrocytes. The incubation period lasts generally from 1 to 4 weeks whatever the transmission route (tick bite or transfusion). Asymptomatic human infections are frequent in the United States. Given the results of the seroprevalence surveys, and the low number of published cases, *Babesia* infections in Europe may also be asymptomatic [158]. Moderate symptomatic cases in the United States show flu-like symptoms including fever, sweats, chills, headaches, myalgia, articulation pains, fatigue, and more or less marked hemolytic anemia signs such as jaundice, hemoglobinuria, hepatomegaly, and/or splenomegaly [141, 159]. Severe disease can occur in splenectomized, elderly, or immunocompromised patients. In these cases, the complications of babesiosis are severe anemia and/or thrombocytopenia, disseminated intravascular coagulation, macrophage activation syndrome, unstable blood pressure, and multi-organ failures (heart, lungs, kidneys, liver). In Europe, *B. divergens* and *B. venatorum* cause severe and mild to severe infections, respectively, and almost all cases have occurred in splenectomized or hyposplenic patients [141, 153]. Despite adapted treatment, the clinical presentation can be prolonged in fragile patients. The fatality rate of symptomatic infection reaches around 5% in *B. microti* cases and >30% in *B. divergens* cases [141].

9.6.5 Laboratory Diagnosis

According to the CDC, the diagnosis of babesiosis relies on (1) clinical suspicion driven by objective signs (fever, anemia, thrombocytopenia) and subjective symptoms (chills, sweats, headaches, myalgia, arthralgia) and (2) microbiological evidence embracing direct detection of the parasite in biological samples and indirect serological tests. *Babesia* serology is not specific enough, nor sensitive at the time of the acute illness, to provide diagnostic confirmation and is only supportive biological evidence (e.g., [141]). Thereby, human babesiosis is confirmed when clinical suspicion is supported by direct detection (blood smears, DNA detection, or *in vivo* cultivation) of *Babesia* spp. while a case is probably when there is at least one objective sign and a positive serological result. In 2018, the US Food and Drug administration approved donor screening concerning blood, organ, and tissues samples based on *B. microti* testing by Array Fluorescent ImmunoAssay (AFIA) serological testing and by PCR assays on whole blood (both Imunogen® assays) [160, 161].

Blood hematological and biochemical analysis. Among the unspecific biological signs, regenerative anemia due to hemolysis, and thrombocytopenia are generally seen in human babesiosis and others may occur proteinuria, hemoglobinuria, and elevated blood urea nitrogen, creatinine, bilirubin, and liver enzymes [141, 153].

Blood smear microscopy. In the acute phase, intraerythrocytic parasites may be observed in Giemsa or Wright stained blood smears. The examination of blood smears for this purpose should be conducted by experienced technicians. Typically, *Babesia* are shown as intraerythrocytic round trophozoites or piriform merozoites (Fig. 9.3). Groups of 4 elements (tetrads), although rare, are characteristic of the *B. microti*-group parasites. This diagnostic feature is particularly difficult to observe because the parasitemia may be very low and the morphology of trophozoites can be misleading (e.g., mistaken for *Plasmodium falciparum* or artifacts) [162].

PCR assays. During the acute parasitemic phase, the DNA of *Babesia* may be detected in whole blood. The molecular biology assays are specific to each *Babesia* species. The *18S ribosomal RNA* gene is a possible target for gene amplification [160]. The sensitivity of these methods (from 0.1 to 10 parasites/μL of blood) is better than blood smear examination [141].

Serological Tests. Immunofluorescence assays (IFA) are the most widely used serological tests for the determination of human exposure to *Babesia* spp. The serology is often not contributive for acute cases of babesiosis but can offer a retrospective diagnosis [153]. A high titer (≥1:256) or a positive IgG immunoblot are supportive biological evidence of babesiosis, while seroconversion or fourfold or greater increase in the serum antibody titer confirms the diagnosis [141, 160].

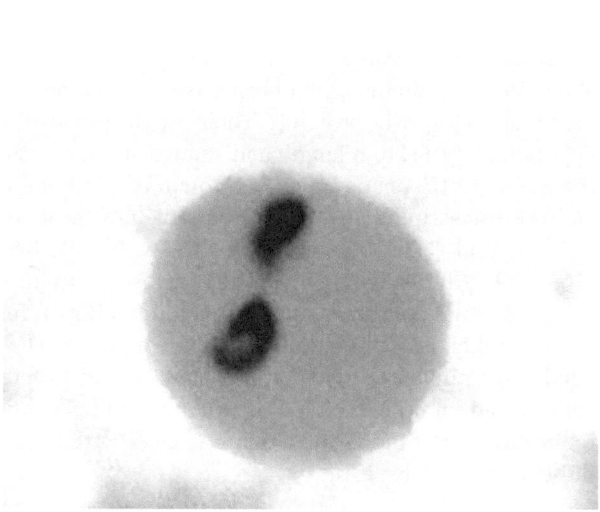

Fig. 9.3 Piriform parasitic inclusion of *Babesia* venatorum in an infected erythrocyte (photo credit : Pr K.-P. Hunfeld, Institute of Medical Microbiology & Infection Control, Hospital of the Johann Wolfgang Goethe-University Frankfurt am Main, Germany)

9.6.6 Treatment

The specific treatment is generally a combination of either atovaquone plus azithromycin, or quinine plus clindamycin over 7–10 days. Supportive treatment may be needed in severe illness: for example, vasopressors, blood transfusions, exchange transfusions (if parasitemia >10%, hemoglobin <10 g/dL or organ failure), mechanical ventilation or dialysis [141, 153].

9.7 Ixodid-Borne Flaviviruses

Louping ill is a sheep disease known since the 18th century in Scotland (United Kingdom) and was suspected to be transmitted by the tick *Ixodes ricinus* when the causative agent, louping ill virus (LIV), was first isolated in 1929 from infected animals [163]. Its name describes the neurological deleterious effects of the virus because "loup" means "to spring into the air" in the ancient Scots language. The first human cases were reported in 1934 [164]. Only a few years after the description of a novel human encephalitis disease in 1931 in Austria, the causative virus (Tick-Borne Encephalitis virus, TBEV) described as "Russian spring and summer encephalitis virus" was discovered in 1937 in Far-Eastern Russia [165]. The central European variant was shown to be transmitted by *I. ricinus* in 1949 [166]. The third human-associated *Ixodes*-borne flavivirus is Powassan virus (POWV), which was named with reference to the Canadian town where it caused a fatal case of encephalitis in a child in 1958 [167].

9.7.1 Virology

Like numerous other mosquito or tick-borne viruses, TBEV, LIV, and POWV are classified in the genus *Flavivirus*, family *Flaviviridae*. They are enveloped viruses about 50 nm in diameter, harboring two surface proteins, the envelope (E) and the membrane (M/prM) proteins. Their single positive-stranded RNA genomes are approximately 11kb in length and share a similar organization with one open reading frame (ORF) encoding a polyprotein of 3414 amino acids that is processed co- and posttranscriptionally into three structural proteins (C, M, and E) and seven nonstructural (NS) proteins (NS1, NS2A, NS2B, NS3, NS4A, NS4B, and NS5) [168, 169]. After attachment and endocytosis, the virus enters the target cell (tick or vertebrate) and changes its conformation to allow a fusion process and the release of the viral capsid within the host cell cytoplasm. The viral RNA is directly translated into a polyprotein, which is processed into structural and NS proteins by both cellular and viral proteases. The structural and NS proteins participate in the RNA replication. After the virion assembly, viral particles are released from the host cell through exocytosis [170].

9.7.2 Ticks, Hosts, and Reservoirs

TBEV, LIV, and POWV are transmitted by hard ticks belonging to the genus *Ixodes* (see part "Epidemiology and transmission" for more information about the tick species involved in the human disease). The transmission of TBEV occurs mainly in the absence of systemic viremia through infected leukocytes migrating to skin with a preferential localization at the blood meal place, enabling transmission from vertebrates to ticks and between co-feeding ticks (Labuda's paradigm). In this way, ticks seem to be both vectors and reservoirs of the virus, while the vertebrates are intermediate hosts acting as transporters [171]. Non-viremic transmission by co-feeding has also been described for LIV [172]. Transstadial transmission from larva to nymph or adult (TBEV, LIV) and transovarial transmission from adult female to egg (TBEV) were also reported for these flaviviruses [168, 173]. Tick saliva factors enhance pathogen transmission by their role as immunomodulators of the host innate immune defenses. This saliva-assisted transmission has been experimentally proven for TBEV and POWV, for which the transmission rate was higher and the infection course was more deleterious when the inoculation of virus was supplemented by salivary gland extract [174]. Humans are an accidental and dead-end host of the three *Ixodes*-borne flaviviruses. The time of tick attachment required to transmit flaviviruses to humans, from a few minutes to a few hours, is very quick compared with other tick-borne pathogens such as *Borrelia burgdorferi* sensu lato or *Anaplasma phagocytophilum* [174, 175].

Many vertebrate species can be infected by the TBEV, but their relative importance as viral reservoir compared to ticks, especially for rodents, is not fully elucidated [176]. The LIV is mostly transmitted to ticks by British red grouse, sheep, and mountain hares [177]. The ecological cycles of POWV involve small-to-medium mammals: rodents, mustelids, and lagomorphs [175].

9.7.3 Pathogenesis and Host Response

In addition to being transmitted by *Ixodes* ticks, TBEV, POWV, and LIV also display the same neurotropism. The pathogenesis mechanisms have been mostly studied in the case of TBEV. After inoculation into the host during the tick bite, the first replication cycles of the virus might occur locally in the skin, in dendritic cells for TBEV, and in macrophages and fibroblasts for POWV. Tick saliva exhibits immunomodulatory properties that decrease the local inflammatory process. Due to their pattern recognition receptors, dendritic cells can recognize the virus and subsequently initiate a type I IFN response. The viral replication continues in the lymph nodes. Then, a short phase of viremia leads to virus dissemination especially in the central system nervous (CNS) after crossing the blood–brain barrier. Acting as antigen-presenting cells, dendritic cells also induce the adaptive immune response that begins at the end of the viremic phase. In the brain tissue, viruses mainly replicate in neurons [169, 175, 178].

9.7.4 TBE Virus

9.7.4.1 Epidemiology and Transmission

Tick-borne encephalitis is widely distributed in Central, Eastern, and Northern Europe and in Central and South-Eastern Asia. Phylogenetic analysis of TBEV revealed the existence of three geographically restricted subtypes: European (TBEV-Eu), Siberian (TBEV-Sib), and Far Eastern (TBEV-FE) [179]. The TBEV-Eu subtype is transmitted by *I. ricinus*, while the TBEV-Sib and the TBEV-FE subtypes are transmitted by *I. persulcatus* [180]. TBE is the second most prevalent tick-borne disease after Lyme borreliosis in Europe with around 2000–3000 annual cases reported in the EU. The highest incidences of TBE cases in 2016 were reported in the Baltic states (Lithuania, Latvia, and Estonia with 21.9, 10.4, and 6.2 cases/100,000 hab., respectively), in Central Europe (Czech Republic, Slovenia, Slovakia, and Austria with 5.4, 4.0, 3.2 and 1.1 cases/100,000 hab., respectively) and in Scandinavia (Sweden and Finland with 2.4 and 1.1 cases/100,000 hab., respectively) [181]. In Europe, TBEV infections occur mainly (93%) during the warmest months of the year between May and October corresponding to the peak of tick activity [181]. In rare cases, TBEV can be transmitted by the consumption of unpasteurized milk products [181].

9.7.4.2 Clinical Manifestations

The incubation period ranges from 7 to 14 days. The disease has a biphasic evolution with firstly a prodromal phase consisting of a flu-like syndrome (fever, headache, muscle pains) over 2 to 4 days which is followed in about a third of cases up to one week later by a severe neurological illness phase, with febrile meningitis, encephalitis, or meningoencephalitis. In the prodromal phase various symptoms, which may include fever, malaise, anorexia, muscle pains, headache, nausea, and vomiting, occur. TBEV-FE strains cause the most severe form of CNS disorder with recorded case fatality rates of 5–20%, while TBE mortality rate is estimated at approximately 2% for Eu-TBEV and Sib-TBEV subtypes. Neurological sequelae are frequent in the neuroinvasive forms [169, 178, 182].

9.7.4.3 Laboratory Diagnosis

According to the ECDC/EU definition, the confirmation of a TBE case is based on (1) clinical suspicion (meningitis, meningoencephalitis, or meningoencephalomyelitis), and (2a) serological evidence in the serum or in the CSF, or (2b) a TBEV isolation or (2c) positive detection of TBEV nucleic acid in a clinical specimen [183].

CSF cellular and biochemical analysis. The CSF analysis in TBE cases shows generally a pleocytosis ranging from 6 to 1200 mononuclear cells/μL with a moderate increase in proteinorrachia and normal levels of glucose and lactate [184].

Serological testing. Serological confirmation is based either on the presence of TBE-specific IgM and IgG antibodies in the serum, or seroconversion, or fourfold or greater increase in the serum antibody titer, or the presence of IgM in the CSF. TBE-specific antibodies can be detected in the serum since in the acute illness phase of the disease IgM antibodies are present for the first few several months and, after a few weeks protecting IgG occurs and are maintained in the long term. The commercialized enzyme-linked immunosorbent assays (ELISA) have generally a great diagnostic sensitivity but there are cross-reactions among flaviviruses (Yellow fever, Dengue, West Nile virus), that should be eliminated by a confirmation neutralization assay mainly in regions where several flaviviruses are found. The intrathecal synthesis of TBE-specific antibodies is needed to confirm the TBE cases of vaccinated patients [184].

Direct detection. The detection of TBEV nucleic acids in blood by RT-PCR assays is a sensitive diagnostic method but only at the prodromal stage corresponding to the viremic phase [184].

9.7.4.4 Treatment and Prevention

There is no specific treatment for TBEV, but four inactivated vaccines are currently available to prevent the infection. Two vaccines against European strains are mainly used in Europe (Encepur® and FSME-Immun®). The two others against Far Eastern strains are mainly used in Russia (TBE-Moscow and EnceVir®). Vaccination against TBE is recommended for the general population in highly endemic areas (incidence ≥5 cases/100,000 pop.) and in targeted at-risk populations (e.g., forest workers) in other areas. In TBE confirmed cases, supportive care, based on the severity of the disease, should be administered including reduction of the brain edema, pain medication, seizure treatment, and assisted ventilation [175, 184].

9.7.5 Louping Ill Virus

9.7.5.1 Epidemiology and Transmission

LIV is transmitted by the European tick *I. ricinus* and has been mainly detected in the British Isles, and also in Norway and Denmark. In sheep, it causes a febrile disease leading to fatal encephalomyelitis. Variants of the virus have been detected in Spain, Turkey, and Greece. LIV infections in humans are very rare. Fewer than 50 human cases have been reported since 1934, the majority of whom have occurred in laboratory workers, veterinarians, abattoir workers, and butchers who were exposed to infected tissues or aerosols [185].

The clinical presentation of LIV infection is very similar to that caused by TBEV, with a prodromal phase and then a severe neurological illness phase. LIV infections are rarely fatal in humans [168]. Serological surveys suggest that subclinical or milder forms may exist because a significant percentage of exposed persons have positive serology (e.g., 8% of abattoir workers) [186].

9.7.5.2 Laboratory Diagnosis

LIV-seropositive sera exhibit cross reactions with TBEV assays because the two viruses are very closely related. Therefore, TBEV serology can be utilized as a diagnostic method for human LIV infection in the specific areas where the virus is circulating (UK and Ireland) [187].

9.7.5.3 Treatment

There is no specific treatment against LIV. Vaccination is available for animals but not for humans [168].

9.7.6 Powassan Virus

9.7.6.1 Epidemiology and Transmission

POWV is present in Northern America (Canada and the United States primarily in the northeastern) and in Far-eastern Russia in the Primorsky Krai region. Fewer than 50 cases have been reported in the United States in the 20th century, but there has been an increasing number of human cases in the last decade with an average of 9 annual cases (min. 1- max. 22) from 2006 to 2016. Cases have been mostly recorded in Minnesota, Wisconsin, New York State, and Massachusetts [188]. There is a seasonal distribution of POWV infections in the United States with most human cases reported from May to November, corresponding to the highest activity of ticks [188].

It is supposed that tick species involved in the maintenance of POWV in enzoonotic cycles are different from the tick species responsible for the transmission to humans. In America, the three species of tick thought to be the vectors of the virus are *I. cookie*, *I. marxei*, and *I. scapularis*, but this last is more anthropophilic than the two other species and by far the most involved in human cases. In Russia, the putative vector ticks of POWV are *I. persulcatus*, *Dermacentor silvarum*, *Haemaphysalis japonica*, and *Haemaphysalis longicornis* [175].

9.7.6.2 Clinical Manifestations

The infection is frequently inconspicuous [175]. When the disease is symptomatic, the incubation period ranges from 7 to 30 days [175, 178]. As for TBE, the infection caused by POWV comprises two phases. The prodromal phase includes a variety of flu-like symptoms such as fever, headache, malaise, fatigue, confusion, myalgia, gastrointestinal symptoms, and also a facultative erythematous rash. The acute phase of the disease is encephalitis, meningitis, or meningoencephalitis. Symptoms of this neuroinvasive illness are fever, headache, altered sensorium, aphasia, paralysis, movement disorders, seizures (children), and visual disorders. The fatality rate is about 10% in neuroinvasive diseases. Long-lasting neurological sequelae are described in half of the survivors, including headaches, muscle disorders, and memory dysfunctions [188, 175].

9.7.6.3 Laboratory Diagnosis

When clinical presentation and epidemiological data lead to a suspicion of POWV infection, the CDC laboratory criteria for the diagnosis are: (1) either an indirect detection of POWV by serological tests revealing a 4-fold or greater increase in the serum specific antibody titer, or the presence of specific IgM antibodies in serum with a confirmation of the virus specificity by neutralizing antibody testing, or the presence of specific IgM antibodies in the CSF and the absence of IgM antibodies for other arboviruses circulating in the area of exposure, or (2) direct detection of the virus by its isolation, or by antigenic or molecular methods from tissues, blood, CSF or other body fluid [175].

CSF cellular and biochemical analysis. In neuroinvasive disease, the CSF analysis shows frequently moderate lymphocytic pleocytosis (<500 cells/μL) and an increase in proteinorachia with a normal glycorachia [175].

Serological testing. IFA, ELISA, or multiplex microsphere-based immunoassays (MIA) are currently used to perform POWV-specific serological tests in serum or CSF.

RT-PCR assays. The direct detection of viral RNA can be valuable for the diagnosis in serum during the short initial phase of viremia or in the CSF at the acute illness phase [175], but the negative predictive value of these tests is low.

9.7.6.4 Treatment

There are currently no specific treatments or vaccines against POWV. The therapeutic approach is supportive including respiratory assistance, reduction of cerebral edema, pain medication, antiemetic treatment, rehydration, and anti-epileptic drugs [178, 188].

9.8 Human Co-infections by Several *Ixodes*-Borne Pathogens

Tick vectors can carry several microorganisms simultaneously that potentially cause diseases in humans, as reported by numerous surveys relying on molecular evidence [2]. In tick-exposed subjects, the risk of co-exposure and/or successive exposure is obviously higher than in the general population, as observed in the case model of forestry workers and shown by serological tools [128]. The simultaneous transmission of *B. burgdorferi* and *B. microti* by individual nymphs of *I. scapularis* has been experimentally shown in hamsters [189]. Conversely, with the current knowledge, there is a low level of evidence that the vector competence of ticks includes the simultaneous transmission of several microorganisms to humans. If co-transmissions occur, the infection by one of the two putatively pathogenic microorganisms or both can be interrupted in the very early stage and does not lead to human disease [190]. Jahfari et al. [80] provided evidence that among patients suffering only from Lyme borreliosis erythema migrans, 2.7% were coinfected with *Can.* N. mikurensis or *A. phagocytophilum* or *Babesia divergens* or *B. miyamotoi* without specific additional symptomatology. Few cases of concomitant infection or "co-disease" have been reported so far. Pathogenic interactions between tick-borne diseases have been described, as for example in a murine model of concurrent babesiosis and Lyme disease where it seems that *B. microti* enhanced the severity of borreliosis symptoms [191]. Coinfection ought to be considered in patients from highly endemic regions of tick-borne pathogens and who present with more serious symptoms than those commonly seen with Lyme borreliosis, especially fever for more than 48 h in spite of proper antibiotic therapy or unexplained cytopenia [192]. Finally, even if coinfections of ticks may result in coexposure of at-risk people, the incidence of coinfection and codisease in humans remains to be evaluated.

References

1. Dantas-Torres F, Chomel BB, Otranto D. Ticks and tick-borne diseases: a One Health perspective. Trends Parasitol. 2012;28:437–46. https://doi.org/10.1016/j.pt.2012.07.003.
2. Moutailler S, Valiente Moro C, Vaumourin E, Michelet L, Tran FH, Devillers E, et al. Co-infection of ticks: the rule rather than the exception. PLoS Negl Trop Dis. 2016;10(3):e0004539. https://doi.org/10.1371/journal.pntd.0004539.
3. Laveran A. Sur la spirillose des bovidés. Compte Rendu de l'Académie des Sciences (Paris). 1903:939–41.
4. Talagrand-Reboul E, Boyer PH, Bergström S, Vial L, Boulanger N. Relapsing fevers: neglected tick-borne diseases. Front Cell Infect Microbiol. 2018;8:98. https://doi.org/10.3389/fcimb.2018.00098.
5. Fukunaga M, Takahashi Y, Tsuruta Y, Matsushita O, Ralph D, McClelland M, et al. Genetic and phenotypic analysis of *Borrelia miyamotoi* sp. nov., isolated from the ixodid tick *Ixodes persulcatus*, the vector for Lyme disease in Japan. Int J Syst Bacteriol. 1995;45:804–10. https://doi.org/10.1099/00207713-45-4-804.
6. Krause PJ, Fish D, Narasimhan S, Barbour AG. *Borrelia miyamotoi* infection in nature and in humans. Clin Microbiol Infect. 2015;21:631–9. https://doi.org/10.1016/j.cmi.2015.02.006.
7. Platonov AE, Karan LS, Kolyasnikova NM, Makhneva NA, Toporkova MG, Maleev VV, et al. Humans infected with relapsing fever spirochete *Borrelia miyamotoi*, Russia. Emerg Infect Dis. 2011;17:1816–23. https://doi.org/10.3201/eid1710.101474.
8. Boden K, Lobenstein S, Hermann B, Margos G, Fingerle V. *Borrelia miyamotoi*-associated neuroborreliosis in immunocompromised person. Emerg Infect Dis. 2016;22:1617–20. https://doi.org/10.3201/eid2209.152034.
9. Gugliotta JL, Goethert HK, Berardi VP, Telford SR. Meningoencephalitis from *Borrelia miyamotoi* in an immunocompromised patient. N Engl J Med. 2013;368:240–5. https://doi.org/10.1056/NEJMoa1209039.
10. Hovius JWR, de Wever B, Sohne M, Brouwer MC, Coumou J, Wagemakers A, et al. A case of meningoencephalitis by the relapsing fever spirochaete *Borrelia miyamotoi* in Europe. Lancet. 2013;382:658. https://doi.org/10.1016/S0140-6736(13)61644-X.
11. Henningsson AJ, Asgeirsson H, Hammas B, Karlsson E, Parke Å, Hoornstra D, et al. Two cases of *Borrelia miyamotoi* meningitis, Sweden, 2018. Emerg Infect Dis. 2019;25:1965–8. https://doi.org/10.3201/eid2510.190416.
12. Margos G, Gofton A, Wibberg D, Dangel A, Marosevic D, Loh S-M, et al. The genus *Borrelia* reloaded. PLoS ONE. 2018:13. https://doi.org/10.1371/journal.pone.0208432.
13. Adeolu M, Gupta RS. A phylogenomic and molecular marker based proposal for the division of the genus *Borrelia* into two genera: the emended genus *Borrelia* containing only the members of the relapsing fever *Borrelia*, and the genus *Borreliella* gen. nov. containing the members of the Lyme disease *Borrelia* (*Borrelia burgdorferi* sensu lato complex). Antonie Van Leeuwenhoek. 2014;105:1049–72. https://doi.org/10.1007/s10482-014-0164-x.
14. Mukhacheva TA, Salikhova II, Kovalev SY. Multilocus spacer analysis revealed highly homogeneous genetic background of Asian type of *Borrelia miyamotoi*. Infect Genet Evol. 2015;31:257–62. https://doi.org/10.1016/j.meegid.2015.02.009.
15. Cook VJ, Fedorova N, Macdonald WP, Lane RS, Barbour AG. Unique strain of *Borrelia miyamotoi* in *Ixodes pacificus* ticks, California, USA. Emerg Infect Dis. 2016;22 https://doi.org/10.3201/eid2212.152046.
16. Iwabu-Itoh Y, Bazartseren B, Naranbaatar O, Yondonjamts E, Furuno K, Lee K, et al. Tick surveillance for *Borrelia miyamotoi* and phylogenetic analysis of isolates in Mongolia and Japan. Ticks Tick-Borne Dis. 2017;8:850–7. https://doi.org/10.1016/j.ttbdis.2017.06.011.
17. Wagemakers A, Staarink PJ, Sprong H, Hovius JWR. *Borrelia miyamotoi*: a widespread tick-borne relapsing fever spirochete. Trends Parasitol. 2015;31:260–9. https://doi.org/10.1016/j.pt.2015.03.008.
18. Kahl O, Gern L, Eisen L, Lane RS. Ecological research on *Borrelia burgdorferi* sensu lato: terminology and some methodological pitfalls. Lyme Borreliosis Biol. Epidemiol. Control, CABI; 1st ed.; 2002, p. 29–46.

19. Burri C, Schumann O, Schumann C, Gern L. Are *Apodemus* spp. mice and *Myodes glareolus* reservoirs for *Borrelia miyamotoi, Candidatus* Neoehrlichia mikurensis, *Rickettsia helvetica, R. monacensis* and *Anaplasma phagocytophilum*? Ticks Tick-Borne Dis. 2014;5:245–51. https://doi.org/10.1016/j.ttbdis.2013.11.007.
20. Scoles GA, Papero M, Beati L, Fish D. A relapsing fever group spirochete transmitted by *Ixodes scapularis* ticks. Vector Borne Zoonotic Dis Larchmt N. 2001;1:21–34.
21. Richter D, Matuschka F-R. Elimination of lyme disease spirochetes from ticks feeding on domestic ruminants. Appl Environ Microbiol. 2010;76:7650–2. https://doi.org/10.1128/AEM.01649-10.
22. Zhioua E, Aeschlimann A, Gern L. Infection of Field-collected *Ixodes ricinus* (Acari: Ixodidae) larvae with *Borrelia burgdorferi* in Switzerland. J Med Entomol. 1994;31:763–6. https://doi.org/10.1093/jmedent/31.5.763.
23. Burgdorfer W, Barbour AG, Hayes SF, Péter O, Aeschlimann A. Erythema chronicum migrans--a tickborne spirochetosis. Acta Trop. 1983;40:79–83.
24. van Duijvendijk G, Coipan C, Wagemakers A, Fonville M, Ersöz J, Oei A, et al. Larvae of *Ixodes ricinus* transmit *Borrelia afzelii* and *B. miyamotoi* to vertebrate hosts. Parasit Vectors 2016;9:97. https://doi.org/10.1186/s13071-016-1389-5.
25. Boyer PH, Koetsveld J, Zilliox L, Sprong H, Talagrand-Reboul É, Hansmann Y, et al. Assessment of *Borrelia miyamotoi* in febrile patients and ticks in Alsace, an endemic area for Lyme borreliosis in France. Parasit Vectors. 2020;13:199. https://doi.org/10.1186/s13071-020-04071-9.
26. Jahfari S, Herremans T, Platonov AE, Kuiper H, Karan LS, Vasilieva O, et al. High seroprevalence of *Borrelia miyamotoi* antibodies in forestry workers and individuals suspected of human granulocytic anaplasmosis in the Netherlands. New Microbes New Infect. 2014;2:144–9. https://doi.org/10.1002/nmi2.59.
27. Krause PJ, Narasimhan S, Wormser GP, Barbour AG, Platonov AE, Brancato J, et al. *Borrelia miyamotoi* sensu lato seroreactivity and seroprevalence in the Northeastern United States. Emerg Infect Dis. 2014;20:1183–90. https://doi.org/10.3201/eid2007.131587.
28. Molloy PJ, Telford SR, Chowdri HR, Lepore TJ, Gugliotta JL, Weeks KE, et al. *Borrelia miyamotoi* disease in the Northeastern United States: a case series. Ann Intern Med. 2015;163:91–8. https://doi.org/10.7326/M15-0333.
29. Sato K, Takano A, Konnai S, Nakao M, Ito T, Koyama K, et al. Human infections with *Borrelia miyamotoi*, Japan. Emerg Infect Dis. 2014;20:1391–3. https://doi.org/10.3201/eid2008.131761.
30. Jiang B-G, Jia N, Jiang J-F, Zheng Y-C, Chu Y-L, Jiang R-R, et al. *Borrelia miyamotoi* infections in humans and Ticks, Northeastern China. Emerg Infect Dis. 2018;24:236–41. https://doi.org/10.3201/eid2402.160378.
31. Hoornstra D, Koetsveld J, Sprong H, Platonov AE, Hovius JW. *Borrelia miyamotoi* disease in an immunocompetent patient, Western Europe. Emerg Infect Dis. 2018;24:1770–2. https://doi.org/10.3201/eid2409.180806.
32. Tobudic S, Burgmann H, Stanek G, Winkler S, Schötta A-M, Obermüller M, et al. Human *Borrelia miyamotoi* Infection, Austria. Emerg Infect Dis. 2020;26:2201–5. https://doi.org/10.3201/eid2609.191501.
33. Markowicz M, Schötta A-M, Höss D, Kundi M, Schray C, Stockinger H, et al. Infections with tickborne pathogens after tick bite, Austria, 2015–2018. Emerg Infect Dis. 2021;27 https://doi.org/10.3201/eid2704.203366.
34. Schwan TG, Schrumpf ME, Hinnebusch BJ, Anderson DE, Konkel ME. GlpQ: an antigen for serological discrimination between relapsing fever and Lyme borreliosis. J Clin Microbiol. 1996;34:2483–92.
35. Reiter M, Stelzer T, Schötta AM, Markowicz M, Leschnik M, Harsch A, et al. Glycerophosphodiester phosphodiesterase identified as non-reliable serological marker for *Borrelia miyamotoi* disease. Microorganisms. 2020;8:E1846. https://doi.org/10.3390/microorganisms8121846.
36. Wagemakers A, Koetsveld J, Narasimhan S, Wickel M, Deponte K, Bleijlevens B, et al. Variable major proteins as targets for specific antibodies against *Borrelia miyamotoi*. J Immunol. 2016;196:4185–95. https://doi.org/10.4049/jimmunol.1600014.

37. Koetsveld J, Kolyasnikova NM, Wagemakers A, Stukolova OA, Hoornstra D, Sarksyan DS, et al. Serodiagnosis of *Borrelia miyamotoi* disease by measuring antibodies against GlpQ and variable major proteins. Clin Microbiol Infect. 2018;24:1338.e1–7. https://doi.org/10.1016/j.cmi.2018.03.009.
38. Sudhindra P, Wang G, Schriefer ME, McKenna D, Zhuge J, Krause PJ, et al. Insights into *Borrelia miyamotoi* infection from an untreated case demonstrating relapsing fever, monocytosis and a positive C6 Lyme serology. Diagn Microbiol Infect Dis. 2016; https://doi.org/10.1016/j.diagmicrobio.2016.06.015.
39. Harris EK, Harton MR, de Mello Marques MA, Belisle JT, Molins CR, Breuner N, et al. Immunoproteomic analysis of *Borrelia miyamotoi* for the identification of serodiagnostic antigens. Sci Rep. 2019;9:16808. https://doi.org/10.1038/s41598-019-53248-5.
40. Harris EK, Brandt KS, Van Gundy TJ, Goodrich I, Wormser GP, Armstrong BA, et al. Characterization of a *Borrelia miyamotoi* membrane antigen (BmaA) for serodiagnosis of *Borrelia miyamotoi* disease. Ticks Tick-Borne Dis. 2020;11:101476. https://doi.org/10.1016/j.ttbdis.2020.101476.
41. Karan L, Makenov M, Kolyasnikova N, Stukolova O, Toporkova M, Olenkova O. Dynamics of spirochetemia and early PCR detection of *Borrelia miyamotoi*. Emerg Infect Dis. 2018;24:860–7. https://doi.org/10.3201/eid2405.170829.
42. Telford SR, Goethert HK, Molloy PJ, Berardi V. Blood smears have poor sensitivity for confirming *Borrelia miyamotoi* disease. J Clin Microbiol. 2019; https://doi.org/10.1128/JCM.01468-18.
43. Koetsveld J, Kolyasnikova NM, Wagemakers A, Toporkova MG, Sarksyan DS, Oei A, et al. Development and optimization of an *in vitro* cultivation protocol allows for isolation of *Borrelia miyamotoi* from patients with hard tick-borne relapsing fever. Clin Microbiol Infect. 2017;23:480–4. https://doi.org/10.1016/j.cmi.2017.01.009.
44. Woldehiwet Z. *Anaplasma phagocytophilum* in ruminants in Europe. Ann N Y Acad Sci. 2006:1078, 446–60. https://doi.org/10.1196/annals.1374.084.
45. Madewell BR, Gribble DH. Infection in two dogs with an agent resembling *Ehrlichia equi*. J Am Vet Med Assoc. 1982;180:512–4.
46. Dumler JS, Barbet AF, Bekker CP, Dasch GA, Palmer GH, Ray SC, et al. Reorganization of genera in the families Rickettsiaceae and Anaplasmataceae in the order Rickettsiales: unification of some species of *Ehrlichia* with *Anaplasma*, *Cowdria* with *Ehrlichia* and *Ehrlichia* with *Neorickettsia*, descriptions of six new species combinations and designation of *Ehrlichia equi* and "HGE agent" as subjective synonyms of *Ehrlichia phagocytophila*. Int J Syst Evol Microbiol. 2001;51:2145–65. https://doi.org/10.1099/00207713-51-6-2145.
47. Foggie A. Studies on the infectious agent of tick-borne fever in sheep. J Pathol Bacteriol. 1951;63:1–15.
48. Chen SM, Dumler JS, Bakken JS, Walker DH. Identification of a granulocytotropic *Ehrlichia* species as the etiologic agent of human disease. J Clin Microbiol. 1994;32:589–95.
49. Petrovec M, Lotric Furlan S, Zupanc TA, Strle F, Brouqui P, Roux V, et al. Human disease in Europe caused by a granulocytic *Ehrlichia* species. J Clin Microbiol. 1997;35:1556–9.
50. Bakken JS, Dumler JS. Human granulocytic anaplasmosis. Infect Dis Clin North Am. 2015;29:341–55. https://doi.org/10.1016/j.idc.2015.02.007.
51. Popov VL, Han VC, Chen SM, Dumler JS, Feng HM, Andreadis TG, et al. Ultrastructural differentiation of the genogroups in the genus *Ehrlichia*. J Med Microbiol. 1998;47:235–51. https://doi.org/10.1099/00222615-47-3-235.
52. Dumler JS, Rikihisa Y, Dasch GA. *Anaplasma*. Bergeys Man. Syst. Archaea Bact. American Cancer Society; 2005. p. 1–15. https://doi.org/10.1002/9781118960608.gbm00903.
53. Stuen S, Granquist EG, Silaghi C. *Anaplasma phagocytophilum*--a widespread multi-host pathogen with highly adaptive strategies. Front Cell Infect Microbiol. 2013;3:31. https://doi.org/10.3389/fcimb.2013.00031.
54. Scharf W, Schauer S, Freyburger F, Petrovec M, Schaarschmidt-Kiener D, Liebisch G, et al. Distinct host species correlate with *Anaplasma phagocytophilum ankA* gene clusters. J Clin Microbiol. 2011;49:790–6. https://doi.org/10.1128/JCM.02051-10.

55. Lagrée A-C, Rouxel C, Kevin M, Dugat T, Girault G, Durand B, et al. Co-circulation of different *A. phagocytophilum* variants within cattle herds and possible reservoir role for cattle. Parasit Vectors. 2018;11:163. https://doi.org/10.1186/s13071-018-2661-7.
56. Battilani M, De Arcangeli S, Balboni A, Dondi F. Genetic diversity and molecular epidemiology of *Anaplasma*. Infect Genet Evol J Mol Epidemiol Evol Genet Infect Dis. 2017;49:195–211. https://doi.org/10.1016/j.meegid.2017.01.021.
57. Huhn C, Winter C, Wolfsperger T, Wüppenhorst N, Strašek Smrdel K, Skuballa J, et al. Analysis of the population structure of *Anaplasma phagocytophilum* using multilocus sequence typing. PLoS One. 2014;9:e93725. https://doi.org/10.1371/journal.pone.0093725.
58. Langenwalder DB, Schmidt S, Silaghi C, Skuballa J, Pantchev N, Matei IA, et al. The absence of the *drhm* gene is not a marker for human-pathogenicity in European *Anaplasma phagocytophilum* strains. Parasit Vectors. 2020;13:238. https://doi.org/10.1186/s13071-020-04116-z.
59. Sosa-Gutierrez CG, Cervantes-Castillo MA, Laguna-Gonzalez R, Lopez-Echeverria LY, Ojeda-Ramírez D, Oyervides M. Serological and molecular evidence of patients infected with *Anaplasma phagocytophilum* in Mexico. Dis Basel Switz. 2021;9:37. https://doi.org/10.3390/diseases9020037.
60. Biggs HM. Diagnosis and management of Tickborne Rickettsial diseases: Rocky Mountain Spotted fever and other spotted fever Group Rickettsioses, Ehrlichioses, and Anaplasmosis — United States. MMWR Recomm Rep. 2016;65 https://doi.org/10.15585/mmwr.rr6502a1.
61. Russell A, Prusinski M, Sommer J, O'Connor C, White J, Falco R, et al. Epidemiology and spatial emergence of anaplasmosis, New York, USA, 2010–2018. Emerg Infect Dis. 2021;27:2154–62. https://doi.org/10.3201/eid2708.210133.
62. Wang F, Yan M, Liu A, Chen T, Luo L, Li L, et al. The seroprevalence of *Anaplasma phagocytophilum* in global human populations: a systematic review and meta-analysis. Transbound Emerg Dis. 2020; https://doi.org/10.1111/tbed.13548.
63. Tang H, Zhu J, Wu S, Niu H. Identification and characterization of an actin filament-associated *Anaplasma phagocytophilum* protein. Microb Pathog. 2020;147:104439. https://doi.org/10.1016/j.micpath.2020.104439.
64. Guzman N, Beidas SO. *Anaplasma Phagocytophilum* (Anaplasmosis). StatPearls, Treasure Island (FL): StatPearls Publishing; 2018.
65. Brouqui P, Bacellar F, Baranton G, Birtles RJ, Bjo BjoPrff A, Blanco JR, et al. Guidelines for the diagnosis of tick-borne bacterial diseases in Europe. Clin Microbiol Infect Off Publ Eur Soc Clin Microbiol Infect Dis. 2004;10:1108–32. https://doi.org/10.1111/j.1469-0691.2004.01019.x.
66. Sigurjonsdottir VK, Feder HM, Wormser GP. Anaplasmosis in pediatric patients: case report and review. Diagn Microbiol Infect Dis. 2017;89:230–4. https://doi.org/10.1016/j.diagmicrobio.2017.08.003.
67. Hansmann Y, Jaulhac B, Kieffer P, Martinot M, Wurtz E, Dukic R, et al. Value of PCR, serology, and blood smears for human granulocytic anaplasmosis diagnosis, France. Emerg Infect Dis. 2019;25:996–8. https://doi.org/10.3201/eid2505.171751.
68. Koebel C, Kern A, Edouard S, Hoang AT, Celestin N, Hansmann Y, et al. Human granulocytic anaplasmosis in eastern France: clinical presentation and laboratory diagnosis. Diagn Microbiol Infect Dis. 2012;72:214–8. https://doi.org/10.1016/j.diagmicrobio.2011.12.005.
69. Kawahara M, Rikihisa Y, Isogai E, Takahashi M, Misumi H, Suto C, et al. Ultrastructure and phylogenetic analysis of "Candidatus Neoehrlichia mikurensis" in the family Anaplasmataceae, isolated from wild rats and found in Ixodes ovatus ticks. Int J Syst Evol Microbiol. 2004;54:1837–43. https://doi.org/10.1099/ijs.0.63260-0.
70. Brouqui P, Sanogo YO, Caruso G, Merola F, Raoult D. *Candidatus* Ehrlichia walkerii: a new *Ehrlichia* detected in *Ixodes ricinus* tick collected from asymptomatic humans in Northern Italy. Ann N Y Acad Sci. 2003;990:134–40.
71. Alekseev AN, Dubinina HV, Van De Pol I, Schouls LM. Identification of *Ehrlichia* spp. and *Borrelia burgdorferi* in *Ixodes* ticks in the Baltic regions of Russia. J Clin Microbiol. 2001;39:2237–42. https://doi.org/10.1128/JCM.39.6.2237-2242.2001.

72. Schouls LM, Van De Pol I, Rijpkema SG, Schot CS. Detection and identification of *Ehrlichia*, *Borrelia burgdorferi* sensu lato, and *Bartonella* species in Dutch *Ixodes ricinus* ticks. J Clin Microbiol. 1999;37:2215–22.
73. Wass L, Grankvist A, Bell-Sakyi L, Bergström M, Ulfhammer E, Lingblom C, et al. Cultivation of the causative agent of human neoehrlichiosis from clinical isolates identifies vascular endothelium as a target of infection. Emerg. Microbes Infect. 2019;8:413–25. https://doi.org/10.1080/22221751.2019.1584017.
74. von Loewenich FD, Geissdörfer W, Disqué C, Matten J, Schett G, Sakka SG, et al. Detection of "*Candidatus* Neoehrlichia mikurensis" in two patients with severe febrile illnesses: evidence for a European sequence variant. J Clin Microbiol. 2010;48:2630–5. https://doi.org/10.1128/JCM.00588-10.
75. Li H, Jiang J, Tang F, Sun Y, Li Z, Zhang W, et al. Wide distribution and genetic diversity of "*Candidatus* Neoehrlichia mikurensis" in rodents from China. Appl Environ Microbiol. 2013;79:1024–7. https://doi.org/10.1128/AEM.02917-12.
76. Wennerås C. Infections with the tick-borne bacterium *Candidatus* Neoehrlichia mikurensis. Clin Microbiol Infect. 2015;21:621–30. https://doi.org/10.1016/j.cmi.2015.02.030.
77. Coipan EC, Jahfari S, Fonville M, Maassen CB, van der Giessen J, Takken W, et al. Spatiotemporal dynamics of emerging pathogens in questing *Ixodes ricinus*. Front Cell Infect Microbiol. 2013;3:36. https://doi.org/10.3389/fcimb.2013.00036.
78. Movila A, Toderas I, Uspenskaia I, Conovalov J. Molecular detection of tick-borne pathogens in *Ixodes ricinus* from Moldova collected in 1960. Ticks Tick-Borne Dis. 2013;4:359–61. https://doi.org/10.1016/j.ttbdis.2012.12.004.
79. Derdáková M, Václav R, Pangrácova-Blaňárová L, Selyemová D, Koči J, Walder G, et al. *Candidatus* Neoehrlichia mikurensis and its co-circulation with *Anaplasma phagocytophilum* in *Ixodes ricinus* ticks across ecologically different habitats of Central Europe. Parasit Vectors. 2014;(7):160. https://doi.org/10.1186/1756-3305-7-160.
80. Jahfari S, Hofhuis A, Fonville M, van der Giessen J, van Pelt W, Sprong H. Molecular detection of tick-borne pathogens in humans with tick bites and erythema migrans, in the Netherlands. PLoS Negl Trop Dis. 2016;10:e0005042. https://doi.org/10.1371/journal.pntd.0005042.
81. Welc-Falęciak R, Siński E, Kowalec M, Zajkowska J, Pancewicz SA. Asymptomatic "*Candidatus* Neoehrlichia mikurensis" infections in immunocompetent humans. J Clin Microbiol. 2014;52:3072–4. https://doi.org/10.1128/JCM.00741-14.
82. Boyer PH, Baldinger L, Degeilh B, Wirth X, Kamdem CM, Hansmann Y, et al. The emerging tick borne pathogen *Neoehrlichia mikurensis* : first French case series and vector epidemiology. Emerg Microbes Infect. 2021:1–21. https://doi.org/10.1080/22221751.2021.1973347.
83. Welinder-Olsson C, Kjellin E, Vaht K, Jacobsson S, Wennerås C. First case of human "*Candidatus* Neoehrlichia mikurensis" infection in a febrile patient with chronic lymphocytic leukemia. J Clin Microbiol. 2010;48:1956–9. https://doi.org/10.1128/JCM.02423-09.
84. Pekova S, Vydra J, Kabickova H, Frankova S, Haugvicova R, Mazal O, et al. *Candidatus* Neoehrlichia mikurensis infection identified in 2 hematooncologic patients: benefit of molecular techniques for rare pathogen detection. Diagn Microbiol Infect Dis. 2011;69:266–70. https://doi.org/10.1016/j.diagmicrobio.2010.10.004.
85. Grankvist A, Sandelin LL, Andersson J, Fryland L, Wilhelmsson P, Lindgren P-E, et al. Infections with *Candidatus* Neoehrlichia mikurensis and cytokine responses in 2 persons bitten by ticks, Sweden. Emerg Infect Dis. 2015;21:1462–5. https://doi.org/10.3201/eid2108.150060.
86. Dadgar A, Grankvist A, Wernbro L, Wennerås C. Fever of unknown origin in a multiple sclerosis patient on immunomodulatory therapy was due to neoehrlichiosis. Lakartidningen. 2017:114.
87. Quarsten H, Salte T, Lorentzen ÅR, Hansen IJW, Hamre R, Forselv KJN, et al. Tick-Borne pathogens detected in the blood of immunosuppressed Norwegian patients living in a tick-endemic area. Clin Infect Dis Off Publ Infect Dis Soc Am 2020. https://doi.org/10.1093/cid/ciaa971.

88. Fehr JS, Bloemberg GV, Ritter C, Hombach M, Lüscher TF, Weber R, et al. Septicemia caused by tick-borne bacterial pathogen *Candidatus* Neoehrlichia mikurensis. Emerg Infect Dis 2010;16:1127–9. https://doi.org/10.3201/eid1607.091907.
89. Li H, Jiang J-F, Liu W, Zheng Y-C, Huo Q-B, Tang K, et al. Human infection with *Candidatus* Neoehrlichia mikurensis, China. Emerg Infect Dis. 2012;18:1636–9. https://doi.org/10.3201/eid1810.120594.
90. Lenart M, Simoniti M, Strašek-Smrdel K, Špik VC, Selič-Kurinčič T, Avšič-Županc T. Case report: first symptomatic *Candidatus* Neoehrlichia mikurensis infection in Slovenia. BMC Infect Dis. 2021;21:579. https://doi.org/10.1186/s12879-021-06297-z.
91. Portillo A, Santibáñez P, Palomar AM, Santibáñez S, Oteo JA. '*Candidatus* Neoehrlichia mikurensis' in Europe. New Microbes New Infect. 2018;22:30–6. https://doi.org/10.1016/j.nmni.2017.12.011.
92. Grankvist A, Andersson P-O, Mattsson M, Sender M, Vaht K, Höper L, et al. Infections with the tick-borne bacterium "*Candidatus Neoehrlichia mikurensis*" mimic noninfectious conditions in patients with B cell malignancies or autoimmune diseases. Clin Infect Dis. 2014;58:1716–22. https://doi.org/10.1093/cid/ciu189.
93. Höper L, Skoog E, Stenson M, Grankvist A, Wass L, Olsen B, et al. Vasculitis due to *Candidatus* Neoehrlichia mikurensis: a cohort study of 40 Swedish patients. Clin Infect Dis Off Publ Infect Dis Soc Am. 2020:ciaa1217. https://doi.org/10.1093/cid/ciaa1217.
94. Moniuszko A, Dunaj J, Czupryna P, Zajkowska J, Pancewicz S. Neoehrlichiosis—a new tick-borne disease—is there a threat in Poland? Przegl Epidemiol. 2015;69(23–6):131–3.
95. Wass L, Grankvist A, Mattsson M, Gustafsson H, Krogfelt K, Olsen B, et al. Serological reactivity to *Anaplasma phagocytophilum* in neoehrlichiosis patients. Eur J Clin Microbiol Infect Dis Off Publ Eur Soc Clin Microbiol. 2018;37:1673–8. https://doi.org/10.1007/s10096-018-3298-3.
96. Yu X, Walker DH. Rickettsiaceae. In: Whitman WB, Rainey F, Kämpfer P, Trujillo M, Chun J, DeVos P, et al. editors. Bergeys Man. Syst. Archaea Bact., Chichester, UK: John Wiley & Sons, Ltd; 2015 pp. 1–2. doi: https://doi.org/10.1002/9781118960608.fbm00178.
97. Merhej V, Raoult D. Rickettsial evolution in the light of comparative genomics. Biol Rev. 2011;86:379–405. https://doi.org/10.1111/j.1469-185X.2010.00151.x.
98. Beati L, Péter O, Burgdorfer W, Aeschlimann A, Raoult D. Confirmation that *Rickettsia helvetica* sp. nov. is a distinct species of the spotted fever group of Rickettsiae. Int J Syst Evol Microbiol 1993;43:521–6. https://doi.org/10.1099/00207713-43-3-521.
99. Fournier PE, Grunnenberger F, Jaulhac B, Gastinger G, Raoult D. Evidence of *Rickettsia helvetica* infection in humans, eastern France. Emerg Infect Dis. 2000;6:389–92. https://doi.org/10.3201/eid0604.000412.
100. Fournier P-E, Allombert C, Supputamongkol Y, Caruso G, Brouqui P, Raoult D. Aneruptive fever associated with antibodies to *Rickettsia helvetica* in Europe and Thailand. J Clin Microbiol. 2004;42:816–8.
101. Nilsson K, Lukinius A, Pahlson C, Moron C, Hajem N, Olsson B, et al. Evidence of *Rickettsia* spp. infection in Sweden: a clinical, ultrastructural and serological study. APMIS Acta Pathol Microbiol Immunol Scand. 2005;113:126–34. https://doi.org/10.1111/j.1600-0463.2005.apm1130206.x.
102. Nilsson K. Septicaemia with *Rickettsia helvetica* in a patient with acute febrile illness, rash and myasthenia. J Infect. 2009;58:79–82. https://doi.org/10.1016/j.jinf.2008.06.005.
103. Parola P, Miller RS, McDaniel P, Telford SR, Rolain J-M, Wongsrichanalai C, et al. Emerging rickettsioses of the Thai-Myanmar border. Emerg Infect Dis. 2003;9:592–5.
104. Nilsson K, Wallmenius K, Pahlson C. Coinfection with *Rickettsia helvetica* and Herpes Simplex Virus 2 in a young woman with meningoencephalitis. Case Rep Infect Dis. 2011;2011:469194. https://doi.org/10.1155/2011/469194.
105. Nilsson K, Elfving K, Pahlson C. *Rickettsia helvetica* in patient with meningitis, Sweden, 2006. Emerg Infect Dis. 2010;16:490–2. https://doi.org/10.3201/eid1603.090184.
106. Koetsveld J, Tijsse-Klasen E, Herremans T, Hovius JWR, Sprong H. Serological and molecular evidence for spotted fever group *Rickettsia* and *Borrelia burgdorferi* sensu lato co-

infections in The Netherlands. Ticks Tick-Borne Dis. 2016;7:371–7. https://doi.org/10.1016/j.ttbdis.2015.12.010.
107. Nilsson K, Lindquist O, Pahlson C. Association of *Rickettsia helvetica* with chronic perimyocarditis in sudden cardiac death. Lancet Lond Engl. 1999;354:1169–73. https://doi.org/10.1016/S0140-6736(99)04093-3.
108. Speck S, Kern T, Aistleitner K, Dilcher M, Dobler G, Essbauer S. In vitro studies of *Rickettsia*-host cell interactions: confocal laser scanning microscopy of *Rickettsia helvetica*-infected eukaryotic cell lines. PLoS Negl Trop Dis. 2018;12:e0006151. https://doi.org/10.1371/journal.pntd.0006151.
109. Karbowiak G, Biernat B, Stańczak J, Szewczyk T, Werszko J. The role of particular tick developmental stages in the circulation of tick-borne pathogens affecting humans in Central Europe. 3. Rickettsiae. Ann Parasitol. 2016;62:89–100. https://doi.org/10.17420/ap6202.38.
110. Elfving K, Olsen B, Bergström S, Waldenström J, Lundkvist A, Sjöstedt A, et al. Dissemination of spotted fever rickettsia agents in Europe by migrating birds. PLoS One. 2010;5:e8572. https://doi.org/10.1371/journal.pone.0008572.
111. Severinsson K, Jaenson TG, Pettersson J, Falk K, Nilsson K. Detection and prevalence of *Anaplasma phagocytophilum* and *Rickettsia helvetica* in *Ixodes ricinus* ticks in seven study areas in Sweden. Parasit Vectors. 2010;3:66. https://doi.org/10.1186/1756-3305-3-66.
112. Overzier E, Pfister K, Herb I, Mahling M, Böck G, Silaghi C. Detection of tick-borne pathogens in roe deer (*Capreolus capreolus*), in questing ticks (*Ixodes ricinus*), and in ticks infesting roe deer in southern Germany. Ticks Tick-Borne Dis 2013;4:320–8. https://doi.org/10.1016/j.ttbdis.2013.01.004.
113. Stefanidesova K, Kocianova E, Boldis V, Kostanova Z, Kanka P, Nemethova D, et al. Evidence of *Anaplasma phagocytophilum* and *Rickettsia helvetica* infection in free-ranging ungulates in central Slovakia. Eur J Wildl Res. 2008;54:519–24. https://doi.org/10.1007/s10344-007-0161-8.
114. Nielsen H, Fournier P-E, Pedersen IS, Krarup H, Ejlertsen T, Raoult D. Serological and molecular evidence of *Rickettsia helvetica* in Denmark. Scand J Infect Dis. 2004;36:559–63. https://doi.org/10.1080/00365540410020776.
115. Boretti FS, Perreten A, Meli ML, Cattori V, Willi B, Wengi N, et al. Molecular investigations of *Rickettsia helvetica* infection in dogs, foxes, humans, and *Ixodes* ticks. Appl Environ Microbiol. 2009;75:3230–7. https://doi.org/10.1128/AEM.00220-09.
116. Schex S, Dobler G, Riehm J, Müller J, Essbauer S. *Rickettsia* spp. in wild small mammals in Lower Bavaria, South-Eastern Germany. Vector Borne Zoonotic Dis Larchmt N. 2011;11:493–502. https://doi.org/10.1089/vbz.2010.0060.
117. Fischer S, Spierling NG, Heuser E, Kling C, Schmidt S, Rosenfeld UM, et al. High prevalence of *Rickettsia helvetica* in wild small mammal populations in Germany. Ticks Tick-Borne Dis. 2018;9:500. https://doi.org/10.1016/j.ttbdis.2018.01.009.
118. Simser JA, Palmer AT, Fingerle V, Wilske B, Kurtti TJ, Munderloh UG. *Rickettsia monacensis* sp. nov., a spotted fever group *Rickettsia*, from ticks (*Ixodes ricinus*) collected in a European city park. Appl Environ Microbiol. 2002;68:4559–66.
119. Brouqui P, Bacellar F, Baranton G, Birtles RJ, Bjoërsdorff A, Blanco JR, et al. Guidelines for the diagnosis of tick-borne bacterial diseases in Europe. Clin Microbiol Infect. 2004;10:1108–32. https://doi.org/10.1111/j.1469-0691.2004.01019.x.
120. Maurin M, Gyuranecz M. Tularaemia: clinical aspects in Europe. Lancet Infect Dis. 2016;16:113–24. https://doi.org/10.1016/S1473-3099(15)00355-2.
121. Chaudhuri RR, Ren C-P, Desmond L, Vincent GA, Silman NJ, Brehm JK, et al. Genome sequencing shows that European isolates of *Francisella tularensis* subspecies *tularensis* are almost identical to US laboratory strain Schu S4. PLoS One. 2007;2:e352. https://doi.org/10.1371/journal.pone.0000352.
122. Hopla CE. The ecology of tularemia. Adv Vet Sci Comp Med. 1974;18:25–53.
123. Chitadze N, Kuchuloria T, Clark DV, Tsertsvadze E, Chokheli M, Tsertsvadze N, et al. Waterborne outbreak of oropharyngeal and glandular tularemia in Georgia: investigation and follow-up. Infection. 2009;37:514–21. https://doi.org/10.1007/s15010-009-8193-5.

124. Parker RR, Spencer RR, Francis E. Tularæmia: XI. Tularæmia infection in ticks of the species *Dermacentor andersoni* Stiles in the Bitterroot Valley, Mont. Public Health Rep 1896-1970 1924;39:1057–73. https://doi.org/10.2307/4577151.
125. Petersen JM, Mead PS, Schriefer ME. *Francisella tularensis*: an arthropod-borne pathogen. Vet Res. 2009;40 https://doi.org/10.1051/vetres:2008045.
126. Mailles A, Vaillant V. Bilan de 10 années de surveillance de la tularémie chez l'homme en France. [in French]. Saint-Maurice: Institut de veille sanitaire 2013.
127. Boone I, Hassler D, Nguyen T, Splettstoesser WD, Wagner-Wiening C, Pfaff G. Tularaemia in southwest Germany: three cases of tick-borne transmission. Ticks Tick-Borne Dis. 2015;6:611–4. https://doi.org/10.1016/j.ttbdis.2015.05.004.
128. Rigaud E, Jaulhac B, Garcia-Bonnet N, Hunfeld K-P, Femenia F, Huet D, et al. Seroprevalence of seven pathogens transmitted by the *Ixodes ricinus* tick in forestry workers in France. Clin Microbiol Infect. 2016:735.e1–9. https://doi.org/10.1016/j.cmi.2016.05.014.
129. Výrosteková V. Transstadial transmission of *Francisella tularensis* in the tick, *Ixodes ricinus*, infected during the larval stage. Cesk Epidemiol Mikrobiol Imunol. 1993;42:71–5.
130. Výrosteková V. Transstadial transmission of *Francisella tularensis* by *Ixodes ricinus* ticks infected during the nymphal stage. Epidemiol Mikrobiol Imunol Cas Spolecnosti Epidemiol Mikrobiol Ceske Lek Spolecnosti JE Purkyne. 1994;43:166–70.
131. Gehringer H, Schacht E, Maylaender N, Zeman E, Kaysser P, Oehme R, et al. Presence of an emerging subclone of *Francisella tularensis* holarctica in *Ixodes ricinus* ticks from south-western Germany. Ticks Tick-Borne Dis. 2013;4:93–100. https://doi.org/10.1016/j.ttbdis.2012.09.001.
132. Genchi M, Prati P, Vicari N, Manfredini A, Sacchi L, Clementi E, et al. *Francisella tularensis*: no evidence for transovarial transmission in the tularemia tick-vectors *Dermacentor reticulatus* and *Ixodes ricinus*. PloS One. 2015;10:e0133593. https://doi.org/10.1371/journal.pone.0133593.
133. Reif KE, Ujczo JK, Alperin DC, Noh SM. *Francisella tularensis novicida* infection competence differs in cell lines derived from United States populations of *Dermacentor andersoni* and *Ixodes scapularis*. Sci Rep. n.d.;8:12685. https://doi.org/10.1038/s41598-018-30419-4.
134. Byington CL, Bender JM, Ampofo K, Pavia AT, Korgenski K, Daly J, et al. Tularemia with vesicular skin lesions may be mistaken for infection with herpes viruses. Clin Infect Dis Off Publ Infect Dis Soc Am. 2008;47:e4–6. https://doi.org/10.1086/588843.
135. WHO. WHO guidelines on tularaemia. Geneva: World Health Organization Press; 2007.
136. Maurin M, Mersali NF, Raoult D. Bactericidal activities of antibiotics against intracellular *Francisella tularensis*. Antimicrob Agents Chemother. 2000;44:3428–31. https://doi.org/10.1128/aac.44.12.3428-3431.2000.
137. Antunes NT, Frase H, Toth M, Vakulenko SB. The class A β-lactamase FTU-1 is native to *Francisella tularensis*. Antimicrob Agents Chemother. 2012;56:666–71. https://doi.org/10.1128/AAC.05305-11.
138. Hepburn MJ, Simpson AJH. Tularemia: current diagnosis and treatment options. Expert Rev Anti Infect Ther. 2008;6:231–40. https://doi.org/10.1586/14787210.6.2.231.
139. Assadian O, Stanek G. Theobald Smith--the discoverer of ticks as vectors of disease. Wien Klin Wochenschr. 2002;114:479–81.
140. Swei A, O'Connor KE, Couper LI, Thekkiniath J, Conrad PA, Padgett KA, et al. Evidence for transmission of the zoonotic apicomplexan parasite *Babesia duncani* by the tick *Dermacentor* albipictus. Int J Parasitol 2018. https://doi.org/10.1016/j.ijpara.2018.07.002.
141. Krause PJ. Human babesiosis. Int J Parasitol. 2019; https://doi.org/10.1016/j.ijpara.2018.11.007.
142. Schreeg ME, Marr HS, Tarigo JL, Cohn LA, Bird DM, Scholl EH, et al. Mitochondrial genome sequences and structures aid in the resolution of *Piroplasmida* phylogeny. PLoS ONE. 2016;11:e0165702. https://doi.org/10.1371/journal.pone.0165702.
143. Zamoto-Niikura A, Morikawa S, Hanaki K-I, Holman PJ, Ishihara C. *Ixodes persulcatus* ticks as vectors for the *Babesia microti* U.S. lineage in Japan. Appl Env Microbiol. 2016;82:6624–32. https://doi.org/10.1128/AEM.02373-16.

144. Sevilla E, González LM, Luque D, Gray J, Montero E. Kinetics of the invasion and egress processes of *Babesia divergens*, observed by time-lapse video microscopy. Sci Rep. 2018;8:14116. https://doi.org/10.1038/s41598-018-32349-7.
145. Jalovecka M, Hajdusek O, Sojka D, Kopacek P, Malandrin L. The complexity of piroplasms life cycles. Front Cell Infect Microbiol. 2018;8:248. https://doi.org/10.3389/fcimb.2018.00248.
146. Spielman A, Wilson ML, Levine JF, Piesman J. Ecology of *Ixodes dammini*-borne human babesiosis and Lyme disease. Annu Rev Entomol. 1985;30:439–60. https://doi.org/10.1146/annurev.en.30.010185.002255.
147. Zintl A, Mulcahy G, Skerrett HE, Taylor SM, Gray JS. *Babesia divergens*, a bovine blood parasite of veterinary and zoonotic importance. Clin Microbiol Rev. 2003;16:622–36.
148. Piesman J, Spielman A. Human babesiosis on Nantucket Island: prevalence of *Babesia microti* in ticks. Am J Trop Med Hyg. 1980;29:742–6. https://doi.org/10.4269/ajtmh.1980.29.742.
149. Tang TTM, Tran M-H. Transfusion transmitted babesiosis: A systematic review of reported cases. Transfus Apher Sci. 2020:102843. https://doi.org/10.1016/j.transci.2020.102843.
150. Iyer S, Goodman K. Congenital babesiosis from maternal exposure: a case report. J Emerg Med. 2019;56:e39. https://doi.org/10.1016/j.jemermed.2018.12.044.
151. Gray EB, Herwaldt BL. Babesiosis surveillance—United States, 2011–2015. Morb Mortal Wkly Rep Surveill Summ Wash DC. 2002;2019(68):1–11. https://doi.org/10.15585/mmwr.ss6806a1.
152. Klevens RM, Cumming MA, Caten E, Stramer SL, Townsend RL, Tonnetti L, et al. Transfusion-transmitted babesiosis: one state's experience. Transfusion (Paris). 2018;58:2611–6. https://doi.org/10.1111/trf.14943.
153. Hunfeld K-P, Hildebrandt A, Gray JS. Babesiosis: recent insights into an ancient disease. Int J Parasitol. 2008;38:1219–37. https://doi.org/10.1016/j.ijpara.2008.03.001.
154. Foppa IM, Krause PJ, Spielman A, Goethert H, Gern L, Brand B, et al. Entomologic and serologic evidence of zoonotic transmission of *Babesia microti*, eastern Switzerland. Emerg Infect Dis. 2002;8:722–6. https://doi.org/10.3201/eid0807.010459.
155. Obiegala A, Pfeffer M, Pfister K, Karnath C, Silaghi C. Molecular examinations of *Babesia microti* in rodents and rodent-attached ticks from urban and sylvatic habitats in Germany. Ticks Tick-Borne Dis. 2015;6:445–9. https://doi.org/10.1016/j.ttbdis.2015.03.005.
156. Hildebrandt A, Hunfeld K-P, Baier M, Krumbholz A, Sachse S, Lorenzen T, et al. First confirmed autochthonous case of human *Babesia microti* infection in Europe. Eur J Clin Microbiol Infect Dis Off Publ Eur Soc Clin Microbiol. 2007;26:595–601. https://doi.org/10.1007/s10096-007-0333-1.
157. Moniuszko-Malinowska A, Swiecicka I, Dunaj J, Zajkowska J, Czupryna P, Zambrowski G, et al. Infection with *Babesia microti* in humans with non-specific symptoms in North East Poland. Infect Dis Lond Engl. 2016;48:537–43. https://doi.org/10.3109/23744235.2016.1164339.
158. Svensson J, Hunfeld K-P, Persson KEM. High seroprevalence of *Babesia* antibodies among *Borrelia burgdorferi*-infected humans in Sweden. Ticks Tick-Borne Dis. 2019;10:186–90. https://doi.org/10.1016/j.ttbdis.2018.10.007.
159. Martinot M, Zadeh MM, Hansmann Y, Grawey I, Christmann D, Aguillon S, et al. Babesiosis in immunocompetent patients, Europe. Emerg Infect Dis. 2011;17:114–6. https://doi.org/10.3201/eid1701.100737.
160. Moritz ED, Winton CS, Tonnetti L, Townsend RL, Berardi VP, Hewins M-E, et al. Screening for *Babesia microti* in the U.S. Blood Supply. N Engl J Med. 2016;375:2236–45.
161. Villatoro T, Karp JK. Transfusion-transmitted babesiosis. Arch Pathol Lab Med. 2019;143:130–4. https://doi.org/10.5858/arpa.2017-0250-RS.
162. Arsuaga M, González LM, Padial ES, Dinkessa AW, Sevilla E, Trigo E, et al. Misdiagnosis of babesiosis as malaria, Equatorial Guinea, 2014. Emerg Infect Dis 2018;24:1588–9. https://doi.org/10.3201/eid2408.180180.
163. Greig JR, Brownlee A, Wilson DR, Gordon SW. The nature of louping-ill. Vet Res. 1931;
164. Davidson MM, Williams H, Macleod JA. Louping ill in man: a forgotten disease. J Infect. 1991;23:241–9.

165. Lindquist L, Vapalahti O. Tick-borne encephalitis. Lancet. 2008;371:1861. https://doi.org/10.5858/arpa.201.
166. Rampas J, Gallia F. Isolation of an encephalitis virus from *Ixodes ricinus* ticks. Cas Lék Ces. 1949;88(41):1179–80.
167. McLean DM, Donohue WL. Powassan virus: isolation of virus from a fatal case of encephalitis. Can Med Assoc J. 1959;80:708.
168. Jeffries CL, Mansfield KL, Phipps LP, Wakeley PR, Mearns R, Schock A, et al. Louping ill virus: an endemic tick-borne disease of Great Britain. J Gen Virol. 2014;95:1005–14. https://doi.org/10.1099/vir.0.062356-0.
169. Velay A, Paz M, Cesbron M, Gantner P, Solis M, Soulier E, et al. Tick-borne encephalitis virus: molecular determinants of neuropathogenesis of an emerging pathogen. Crit Rev Microbiol. 2019;45:472–93. https://doi.org/10.1080/1040841X.2019.1629872.
170. Ruzek D, Županc TA, Borde J, Chrdle A, Eyer L, Karganova G, et al. Tick-borne encephalitis in Europe and Russia: review of pathogenesis, clinical features, therapy, and vaccines. Antiviral Res. 2019;164:23–51. https://doi.org/10.1016/j.antiviral.2019.01.014.
171. Randolph SE. Transmission of tick-borne pathogens between co-feeding ticks: Milan Labuda's enduring paradigm. Ticks Tick Borne Dis. 2011;2(4):179–82. https://doi.org/10.1016/j.ttbdis.2011.07.004.
172. Jones LD, Gaunt M, Hails RS, Laurenson K, Hudson PJ, Reid H, et al. Transmission of louping ill virus between infected and uninfected ticks co-feeding on mountain hares. Med Vet Entomol. 1997;11(1721):1.
173. Karbowiak G, Biernat B. The role of particular tick developmental stages in the circulation of tick-borne pathogens affecting humans in Central Europe. 2. Tick-borne encephalitis virus. Ann Parasitol. 2016;62:3–9. https://doi.org/10.17420/ap6201.25.
174. Hermance ME, Thangamani S. Tick-virus-host interactions at the cutaneous interface: the nidus of flavivirus transmission. Viruses. 2018;10 https://doi.org/10.3390/v10070362.
175. Kemenesi G, Bányai K. Tick-Borne flaviviruses, with a focus on Powassan virus. Clin Microbiol Rev. 2019;32(1):e00106–17. https://doi.org/10.1128/CMR.00106-17.
176. Michelitsch A, Wernike K, Klaus C, Dobler G, Beer M. Exploring the reservoir hosts of tick-borne encephalitis virus. Viruses. 2019;11 https://doi.org/10.3390/v11070669.
177. Gilbert L. Louping ill virus in the UK: a review of the hosts, transmission and ecological consequences of control. Exp Appl Acarol. 2016;68:363–74. https://doi.org/10.1007/s10493-015-9952-x.
178. Lindqvist R, Upadhyay A, Överby AK. Tick-borne flaviviruses and the Type I interferon response. Viruses. 2018;10 https://doi.org/10.3390/v10070340.
179. Ecker M, Allison SL, Meixner T, Heinz FX. Sequence analysis and genetic classification of tick-borne encephalitis viruses from Europe and Asia. J Gen Virol. 1999;80(Pt 1):179–85. https://doi.org/10.1099/0022-1317-80-1-179.
180. Labuda M, Randolph SE. Survival strategy of tick-borne encephalitis virus: Cellular basis and environmental determinants. Zentralblatt Für Bakteriol. 1999;289:513–24. https://doi.org/10.1016/S0934-8840(99)80005-X.
181. Beauté J, Spiteri G, Warns-Petit E, Zeller Hervé. Tick-borne encephalitis in Europe, 2012 to 2016. Euro Surveill. 2018;23(45):pii=1800201. https://doi.org/10.2807/1560-7917.ES.2018.23.45.1800201.
182. Velay A, Solis M, Kack-Kack W, Gantner P, Maquart M, Martinot M, et al. A new hot spot for tick-borne encephalitis (TBE): a marked increase of TBE cases in France in 2016. Ticks Tick-Borne Dis. 2018;9(1):120–5. https://doi.org/10.17420/ap6201.25.115.
183. UE. Commission Implementing Decision of 8 August 2012 amending Decision 2002/253/EC laying down case definitions for reporting communicable diseases to the Community network under Decision No 2119/98/EC of the European Parliament and of the Council (notified under document C(2012) 5538)Text with EEA relevance; 2012:57.
184. Taba P, Schmutzhard E, Forsberg P, Lutsar I, Ljøstad U, Mygland Å, Levchenko I, Strle F, Steiner I. EAN consensus review on prevention, diagnosis and management of tick-borne encephalitis. Eur J Neurol. 2017;24(10):1214-e61. https://doi.org/10.1111/ene.13356.

185. Health Protection Agency. Louping ill; 2011. https://webarchive.nationalarchives.gov.uk/20140714084610/http://www.hpa.org.uk:80/webw/HPAweb&Page&HPAwebAutoListName/Page/1191942172074?p=1191942172074.
186. Charrel RN, Attoui H, Butenko AM, Clegg JC, Deubel V, Frolova TV, et al. Tick-borne virus diseases of human interest in Europe. Clin Microbiol Infect Off Publ Eur Soc Clin Microbiol Infect Dis. 2004;10:1040. https://doi.org/10.1111/ene.13356.t. and of the Council04.01022.x
187. Padfield S, Fogg C. A case of louping ill. Zoonoses Network Newsletter, Number 12. London: Health Protection Agency 2011.
188. Krow-Lucal ER, Lindsey NP, Fischer M, Hills SL. Powassan virus disease in the United States, 2006–2016. Vector Borne Zoonotic Dis. 2018;18:286–90. https://doi.org/10.1089/vbz.2017.2239.
189. Piesman J, Hicks TC, Sinsky RJ, Obiri G. Simultaneous transmission of *Borrelia burgdorferi* and *Babesia microti* by individual nymphal *Ixodes dammini* ticks. J Clin Microbiol. 1987;25:2012ri.
190. Boyer PH, Kieffer P, de Martino SJ, Zilliox L, Vogel JY, Jaulhac B, et al. *Borrelia burgdorferi* sl and tick-borne encephalitis virus coinfection in Eastern France. Med Mal Infect. 2018;48(3):218–20.
191. Bhanot P, Parveen N. Investigating disease severity in an animal model of concurrent babesiosis and Lyme disease. Int J Parasitol. 2019;49:145–51. https://doi.org/10.1016/j.ijpara.2018.06.006.
192. Stanek G, Wormser GP, Gray J, Strle F. Lyme borreliosis. Lancet. 2012;379:461–73.

GPSR Compliance

The European Union's (EU) General Product Safety Regulation (GPSR) is a set of rules that requires consumer products to be safe and our obligations to ensure this.

If you have any concerns about our products, you can contact us on ProductSafety@springernature.com

In case Publisher is established outside the EU, the EU authorized representative is:

Springer Nature Customer Service Center GmbH
Europaplatz 3
69115 Heidelberg, Germany

Batch number: 10732044

Printed by Printforce, the Netherlands